Synthesis, Properties, and Applications of Novel Polymer-Based Gels

Synthesis, Properties, and Applications of Novel Polymer-Based Gels

Guest Editors

Peng Zhang
Yuanxun Zheng
Zhen Gao

MDPI

Basel • Beijing • Wuhan • Barcelona • Belgrade • Novi Sad • Cluj • Manchester

Guest Editors
Peng Zhang
School of Water Conservancy and Transportation
Zhengzhou University
Zhengzhou
China

Yuanxun Zheng
School of Water Conservancy and Transportation
Zhengzhou University
Zhengzhou
China

Zhen Gao
School of Water Conservancy and Transportation
Zhengzhou University
Zhengzhou
China

Editorial Office
MDPI AG
Grosspeteranlage 5
4052 Basel, Switzerland

This is a reprint of the Special Issue, published open access by the journal *Gels* (ISSN 2310-2861), freely accessible at: https://www.mdpi.com/journal/gels/special_issues/68Z1F0X85D.

For citation purposes, cite each article independently as indicated on the article page online and as indicated below:

Lastname, A.A.; Lastname, B.B. Article Title. *Journal Name* **Year**, *Volume Number*, Page Range.

ISBN 978-3-7258-7476-7 (Hbk)
ISBN 978-3-7258-7477-4 (PDF)
https://doi.org/10.3390/books978-3-7258-7477-4

Contents

About the Editors

Peng Zhang

Peng Zhang is a professor at Zhengzhou University and received a PhD in properties of low-carbon and higher-performance concrete materials and structures from Dalian University of Technology in 2008. Afterwards, he completed a post-doctoral fellowship at Zhengzhou University. He is currently a professor and doctoral supervisor at the School of Water Conservancy Engineering at Zhengzhou University. He was the winner of the Fund for Outstanding Young Scholars and was recognized as an Academic Technology Leader and Distinguished Professor of Henan Province, China. He has also been honored with the following awards: Academic and Technical Leader of the Education Department of Henan Province in China, Science & Technology Innovation Talent in Universities of Henan Province in China, and Outstanding Young Backbone Teacher of Henan Province in China. His research interests include geopolymer concretes, green concretes containing solid wastes, fiber- and nanoparticle-reinforced high-performance concretes, and cementitious composites. He has published more than 280 peer-reviewed academic papers and 11 books. As the principal investigator, he has hosted more than 20 research projects sponsored by the National Natural Sciences Foundation of China, Chinese Postdoctoral Science Special Foundation, Chinese Postdoctoral Science Foundation, and others. He has won 4 prizes at the Provincial Science & Technology Awards and 15 other Science & Technology Awards.

Yuanxun Zheng

Yuanxun Zheng is a professor at Zhengzhou University. After receiving his PhD in properties of solid waste resource utilization from Dalian University of Technology in 2009, he completed a post-doctoral fellowship at Zhengzhou University and currently serves as a professor and doctoral supervisor at the School of Water Conservancy Engineering there. He was the winner of the Fund for Outstanding Young Scholars and recognized as an Academic Technology Leader. He has also been honored with the following awards: Academic and Technical Leader of the Education Department of Henan Province in China, Outstanding Young Backbone Teacher of Henan Province in China, the recipient of the list of top 2% global scientists by Stanford (2024, 2025), and an outstanding teacher of Henan Province. His research interests include recycled cement, recycling of waste concrete, high-performance concrete, etc. He has published more than 220 peer-reviewed academic papers and 9 books. As the principal investigator, he has hosted more than 30 research projects sponsored by the National Natural Sciences Foundation of China, the Chinese Postdoctoral Science Foundation, and others. He has won 5 prizes at the Provincial Science & Technology Awards and 15 other Science & Technology Awards.

Zhen Gao

Zhen Gao is an associate researcher and master's supervisor at Zhengzhou University. She received her PhD in low-carbon high-performance concrete materials and structural performance from Zhengzhou University in 2024. Her research interests include geopolymer concrete, high-performance concrete, and cement-based composites. She has published 21 papers in internationally authoritative journals as the first author or corresponding author, including 10 SCI papers in the 1st category of SCI from the Chinese Academy of Sciences. She has been granted six national invention patents and registered two software copyrights. She is currently leading the Youth Project of the Henan Provincial Natural Science Foundation.

Preface

Recent advancements in polymer science have led to the development of novel polymer-based gels with unique properties and diverse applications. These gels are synthesized through various methods, including free-radical polymerization, click chemistry, and supramolecular assembly, allowing precise control over their structure and functionality. Key innovations include stimuli-responsive hydrogels that adapt to environmental changes (e.g., pH, temperature, or light), self-healing gels with dynamic covalent bonds, and nanocomposite gels reinforced with nanoparticles or 2D materials for enhanced mechanical strength.

The aim of this Reprint is to gather contributions that demonstrate how polymer gels can provide functional, economical, and ecologically responsible solutions for improving the freeze–thaw durability of concrete, the valorization of river sediments, dust control in silt soils, flexible sensing, asphalt modification and reinforcement, structural health monitoring, rapid detection of biomarkers, and the protection of cement-based materials. The purpose of assembling these contributions is to highlight the interdisciplinary advances that connect polymer chemistry, civil engineering, materials science, biotechnology, and environmental science, and to stimulate further research in order to establish sustainable technological pathways for green infrastructure construction.

This Reprint is aimed at researchers, practitioners, industry professionals, and policymakers interested in advanced gel materials, green construction technologies, infrastructure durability, and sustainable development strategies. It aims to serve as both a scientific reference and a source of inspiration for those seeking to develop innovative approaches to mitigating engineering and environmental pressures through materials science.

Peng Zhang, Yuanxun Zheng, and Zhen Gao
Guest Editors

gels

Editorial

Synthesis, Properties, and Applications of Novel Polymer-Based Gels

Zhen Gao, Peng Zhang * and Yuanxun Zheng

School of Water Conservancy and Transportation, Zhengzhou University, Zhengzhou 450001, China; gao-zhen@zzu.edu.cn (Z.G.); yxzheng@zzu.edu.cn (Y.Z.)
* Correspondence: zhangpeng@zzu.edu.cn

1. Introduction

Polymer gels, as a class of soft materials with three-dimensional cross-linked networks, have garnered escalating attention in recent decades due to their exceptional capacity to absorb and retain solvents, coupled with tunable mechanical, chemical, and responsive properties [1]. These unique characteristics enable polymer gels to bridge the gap between traditional rigid materials and flexible substrates, finding widespread applications across diverse fields ranging from construction and transportation to biomedicine and environmental engineering [2]. In recent years, advances in synthesis technologies—such as enzyme-induced precipitation, alkali activation, and composite modification—have expanded the functional boundaries of polymer gels, allowing for precise control over their microstructure, reactivity, and performance [3]. Simultaneously, the growing emphasis on sustainability has driven the development of gel systems derived from industrial by-products, waste materials, and bio-based precursors, aligning with global efforts toward carbon neutrality and resource recycling [4].

The versatility of polymer gels is reflected in their diverse functional adaptations. For instance, in construction and geotechnical engineering, gel composites have been developed to enhance the freeze–thaw resistance of cementitious materials, stabilize weak soils, and improve the durability of concrete structures against chloride ion penetration [5]. In transportation infrastructure, gel-modified asphalt mixtures and anti-skid wear layers have emerged as effective solutions to address pavement aging, ice formation, and structural degradation [6]. The biomedical sector has witnessed the development of self-healing hydrogels for strain sensing and molecularly imprinted gel sensors for rapid biomarker detection, leveraging the biocompatibility and responsiveness of gel networks [7]. Additionally, environmental applications of polymer gels include dust suppression in silt soils and the valorization of waste materials (e.g., river sediments and rubber particles) into high-performance gel composites [8].

Cutting-edge research on polymer gels is characterized by interdisciplinary integration, combining insights from materials science, chemistry, engineering, and biology to address complex real-world challenges [9]. Key advancements include the development of multifunctional gels with synergistic properties (e.g., self-healing, high stretchability, and sensitivity), the optimization of synthesis processes for improved sustainability, and the exploration of novel application scenarios in harsh or specialized environments [10]. To capture these latest developments and foster knowledge exchange, the *Gels* journal presents this Special Issue, "Synthesis, Properties, and Applications of Novel Polymer-Based Gels," featuring eleven high-quality contributions that showcase the state of the art in polymer gel research. These studies span synthesis innovations, performance optimization, and

 https://doi.org/10.3390/gels12020143

practical applications, reflecting the dynamic and interdisciplinary nature of the field. In the following section, we provide an overview of each contribution, highlighting the study's aims, key findings, and relevance to the broader context of gel materials and technology.

2. Overview of the Papers Published in This Special Issue

The paper "A State-of-the-Art Review on the Freeze–Thaw Resistance of Sustainable Geopolymer Gel Composites: Mechanisms, Determinants, and Models" conducts a comprehensive and in-depth review on the freeze–thaw (F-T) resistance of geopolymer gel composites (GCs), a topic of great significance for promoting the practical application of geopolymer materials. The authors focus on geopolymers, a sustainable and low-carbon gel binder regarded as a potential alternative to cement, and emphasize that F-T resistance is a crucial indicator for evaluating the durability of GCs, as it exerts a profound impact on the service life of structures. To clarify the intrinsic principles of F-T damage in geopolymers, the authors systematically synthesize several commonly used theories related to F-T damage, while also meticulously elaborating on the key factors that influence the F-T resistance of GCs, including raw materials, curing conditions, and modified materials. The review findings indicate that the F-T resistance of GCs can be significantly enhanced by adopting high-calcium-content precursors, mixed alkali activators, and rubber aggregates; appropriately increasing the curing temperature also improves F-T resistance, especially for GCs made with low-calcium-content precursors. Among modified materials, most fibers and nano-materials remarkably boost the F-T resistance of GCs, whereas air-entraining agents have a negligible effect on this property. Furthermore, the authors summarize evaluation and prediction models for F-T damage of GCs, encompassing empirical models and machine learning models, and note that machine learning-based models exhibit higher predictive accuracy compared to empirical ones. The review's findings are highly relevant for the construction and materials science industries, promoting a deeper understanding of the factors affecting the F-T resistance of GCs and their underlying mechanisms, thus providing a solid foundation for both engineering practice and academic research in this field.

The second article, "Valorization of River Sediments in Sustainable Cementitious Gel Materials: A Review of Characteristics, Activation, and Performance" explores the high-value utilization of river sediments as alternative raw materials for sustainable cementitious gel materials, addressing the dual goals of resource recycling and carbon reduction in the construction industry. The authors highlight that river sediments, abundant in supply and rich in silica-alumina components, have emerged as promising substitutes for traditional raw materials in cementitious systems, aligning with global sustainability initiatives. To conduct a comprehensive review, they performed a systematic literature search on Web of Science and Google Scholar using keywords such as "river sediment," "cementitious materials," "activation," and "pozzolanic activity," covering publications up to July 2025, and employed the Connected Papers citation network tool to ensure the inclusion of emerging studies. The review systematically examines the properties of river sediments from diverse regions, analyzes activation and modification techniques (including alkali/acid activation, thermal calcination, and mechanical milling), and evaluates their applications in various cementitious systems by comparing mix design models to clarify the effects of replacing fine aggregates, coarse aggregates, and cement on workability, strength, and durability. Multi-scale characterization via XRD, FTIR, and TG-DSC reveals the underlying mechanisms, including the formation of C-S-H and C-A-S-H gels, pore refinement, and densification of the interfacial transition zone. Three key findings are emphasized: (1) moderate sediment replacement (20–30%) enhances strength without compromising flowability; (2) alkali–water glass activation and calcination at 600–850 °C effectively im-

https://doi.org/10.3390/gels12020143

prove pozzolanic activity; and (3) combining the minimum paste thickness theory with additives like water reducers, fibers, or biochar enables the design of high-performance, low-carbon concrete. This work demonstrates a critical trend in sustainable construction materials: leveraging industrial and natural waste (river sediments) in cementitious gels can reduce reliance on traditional raw materials, lower carbon emissions, and promote resource recycling. The study's implications extend to greener building practices and the development of low-CO_2 cementitious materials, providing a comprehensive theoretical foundation and technical pathway for the sustainable valorization of river sediments.

The third article, "Performance and Mechanism Analysis of an Anti-Skid Wear Layer of Active Slow-Release Ice–Snow Melting Modified by Gels" delves into the development of sustainable pavement materials for winter maintenance, addressing the long-standing challenge of balancing large-scale upkeep efficiency and driving safety, particularly in the application of active slow-release ice-melting materials. The authors set out to enhance the ice-melting capacity of pavement through controlled salt release, proposing a gel-modified salt-storing ceramsite asphalt mixture as an innovative solution. They conducted systematic experiments by replacing conventional coarse aggregates with salt-storing ceramsite in SMA-10 graded mixtures (with replacement ratios ranging from 0% to 80%), comprehensively evaluating the mixture's mechanical performance and de-icing functionality. The key experimental results reveal that a 40% salt-storing ceramsite content optimizes the mixture's high-temperature stability while maintaining acceptable low-temperature performance and water resistance—critical balances for winter pavement durability. Microstructural analysis further elucidates the underlying mechanisms: the silicone–acrylic emulsion forms a hydrophobic film on the surface of ceramsite, enabling uniform salt distribution and sustained release, while 10% gel modification achieves effective salt retention and controlled release through pore-structure regulation. A practical salt-storing ceramsite content range of 40–60% is established for winter pavement applications, addressing the core need for durable, effective snow-melting asphalt surfaces. This study represents a significant advancement in winter pavement technology, as it integrates gel modification with salt-storing ceramsite to realize active slow-release ice-melting, avoiding the trade-offs between mechanical performance and de-icing efficiency that plague traditional materials. The findings provide valuable insights for the design of long-lasting, safe winter pavement surfaces, offering a reliable technical solution to improve driving safety in cold regions while optimizing maintenance efficiency.

In "Bio-Gel Formation Through Enzyme-Induced Carbonate Precipitation for Dust Control in Yellow River Silt", address an environmental challenge in silt management using gel-enhanced bio-cementation technology. Yellow River silt is prone to dust emission, which poses ecological and health risks, and traditional dust control methods often lack durability or environmental sustainability. This study explored a novel hydrogel-modified enzyme-induced carbonate precipitation (EICP) approach to form reinforced bio-cemented crusts, aiming to enhance the compressive strength and resistance to wind–rain erosion of silt soils. The authors optimized the cementation solution—adopting equimolar concentrations of urea and $CaCl_2$ at 1.25 mol/L to improve the uniformity of $CaCO_3$ precipitation—and determined a spraying volume of 4 L/m^2 (applying urea-$CaCl_2$ solution first, followed by urease solution) as the optimal parameter. Experimental results showed this setup yielded a 14.9 mm thick hybrid gel-$CaCO_3$ crust with a compressive strength exceeding 752 kPa. Mechanistic analysis via SEM confirmed the synergistic interaction between $CaCO_3$ crystals and the gel matrix: the hydrogel network acted as a nucleation template, enhancing crystal bridging and pore-filling efficiency, while XRD analysis validated the formation of a stable gel-$CaCO_3$ composite structure. The treated silt exhibited superior resistance to wind–rain erosion and mechanical wear compared to untreated samples.

https://doi.org/10.3390/gels12020143

By establishing a positive correlation between gel-modified EICP and enhanced dust suppression performance, this work highlights a novel application of bio-gel composites in environmental engineering—one that enables sustainable dust mitigation in silt soils without relying on harsh chemicals. It underscores cross-disciplinary innovation where insights from bio-cementation and polymer gel technology are integrated to solve practical ecological challenges in silt management.

In "Self-Healing and Tough Polyacrylic Acid-Based Hydrogels for Micro-Strain Sensors", the authors delve into the development of advanced hydrogel materials for smart sensing applications in bioengineering and intelligent systems. Self-healing hydrogels are widely recognized for their potential in these fields, yet they face a critical challenge: balancing excellent self-healing ability with sufficient mechanical strength. To address this bottleneck, the authors set out to develop a self-healing hydrogel with superior stretchability, employing a novel strategy of embedding a combination of hydrogen bonding and dynamic metal coordination interactions into a covalent polyacrylic acid (PAA) matrix. These interactions are introduced by three key components: modified fenugreek galactomannan, ferric ions, and lignin silver nanoparticles. Using this approach, Liu et al. successfully achieved a synergistic effect between covalent bonds and multiple non-covalent interactions, endowing the hydrogel with both high self-healing capacity and enhanced mechanical performance. In particular, the introduction of multiple energy dissipation mechanisms—most notably migrative dynamic metal coordination interactions-enabled the hydrogel to exhibit ultra-high stretchability, reaching up to 2000%. Furthermore, the incorporation of lignin silver nanoparticles and ferric ions endowed the hydrogel with excellent strain sensitivity, boasting a gauge factor of approximately 3.94, along with stable and repeatable resistance signals. When assembled into a flexible strain sensor, the hydrogel effectively detected subtle human motions and organ vibrations; it even demonstrated practical applicability by replacing conductive rubber in gaming controllers for real-time input functions. This development represents a significant innovation, as it overcomes the long-standing trade-off between self-healing ability and mechanical strength in hydrogels. The study provides a versatile strategy for designing multifunctional hydrogels, laying a foundation for their broader application in advanced sensing scenarios within bioengineering and intelligent systems.

"Study on Road Performance and Ice-Breaking Effect of Rubber Polyurethane Gel Mixture" delves into the development of high-efficiency, low-carbon, and environmentally friendly pavement materials for active snow melting and ice breaking, focusing on addressing critical challenges in road engineering. Inspired by the urgent need to solve a series of pressing issues-severe pavement temperature diseases, low efficiency and high loss of traditional ice-breaking methods, high occupancy rate of waste tires, and low utilization rate and insufficient durability of rubber particles, the authors set out to improve road service levels and ensure winter pavement safety. They adopted a systematic three-step research approach: (1) the optimization of rubber particle treatment using three different solutions-NaOH, NaClO, and KH550—along with the study of hydrophilic properties, surface morphology, and phase composition of rubber particles before and after optimization to determine the optimal treatment method; (2) the replacement of natural aggregates in polyurethane gel mixtures with the optimized rubber particles via the volume substitution method, coupled with the determination of optimal polyurethane gel dosage and molding-curing processes; and (3) the comparative analysis of the influence law of rubber particle content on the road performance of Rubber Polyurethane Gel Mixture (RPGM) through indoor tests, as well as the exploration of its ice-breaking effect. Using this approach, Chen et al. successfully obtained significant experimental findings: the contact angles of rubber particles treated with the three solutions were reduced by 22.5%, 30.2%, and

https://doi.org/10.3390/gels12020143

36.7%, respectively, with improved surface energy, reduced surface element types, and effective removal of surface impurities—among which the KH550 solution exhibited the most remarkable improvement effect. As rubber particle content increased from 0% to 15%, the dynamic stability of the mixture gradually increased (with a maximum increase of 23.5%), the maximum bending strain increased correspondingly, the residual stability first increased then decreased (with increased ranges of 1.4%, 3.3%, and 0.5%, respectively), and the anti-scattering performance improved—even with excessive rubber content, the scattering loss rate remained below 5%. Additionally, the fatigue life of polyurethane gel mixtures with 0%, 5%, 10%, and 15% rubber particles was 2.9 times, 3.8 times, 4.3 times, and 4.0 times higher than that of AC-13 asphalt mixture, demonstrating excellent anti-fatigue performance; the friction coefficient could be increased by up to 22.3% compared with ordinary asphalt mixtures. RPGM showed superior de-icing performance to traditional asphalt mixtures, with ice-breaking ability effectively enhanced as rubber particle content increased—though the ability weakened significantly when the ice layer thickness exceeded 9 mm. The ice-breaking mechanism was mainly achieved through the synergistic effect of stress coupling, thermal effect, and interface failure: under cyclic driving loads, the bonding performance of the ice–pavement interface was weakened, leading to loosening, breaking, and peeling of the ice layer to achieve efficient de-icing. This research represents a significant innovation, as it simultaneously resolves the problems of waste tire recycling and winter pavement safety, realizing the dual value of environmental protection and engineering practicality. The study provides a proof-of-concept for designing high-performance active snow-melting and ice-breaking pavement materials, where the integration of optimized rubber particles and polyurethane gel effectively improves both road durability and winter driving safety, offering valuable technical insights for practical engineering applications.

"A Study on the Performance of Gel-Based Polyurethane Prepolymer/Ceramic Fiber Composite-Modified Asphalt" delves into the development of composite-modified asphalt using gel-based materials, aiming to solve various problems in traditional roads and extend their service life—a critical focus as new road materials have become a research hotspot. Inspired by the unique and synergistic properties of polyurethane prepolymers (PUPs) and ceramic fibers (CFs)—where PUPs provide elasticity and gel-like behavior while CFs contribute to structural stability and high-temperature resistance—the authors set out to enhance asphalt performance by integrating these two materials. They adopted a systematic research approach combining optimization and comprehensive characterization: (1) the use of response surface methodology to investigate an optimized preparation scheme for PUP/CF composite-modified asphalt; and (2) the employment of multiple advanced testing techniques, including aging tests, dynamic shear rate (DSR) testing, bending rate (BBR) testing, multiple stress creep recovery (MSCR) testing, scanning electron microscopy (SEM), atomic force microscopy (AFM), and infrared spectroscopy (IR), to explore the aging performance, rheological properties, permanent deformation resistance, microstructure, and modification mechanism of the composite-modified asphalt. Using this approach, Guo et al. successfully determined the optimal preparation scheme: a PUP content of 7.4%, a CF content of 2.1%, and a shear time of 40 min. The experimental results indicate that the addition of PUP and CF significantly enhances the asphalt's aging resistance; compared with single-CF-modified asphalt and base asphalt, the PUP/CF composite-modified asphalt exhibits superior high- and low-temperature rheological properties and stronger strain recovery capability. Microstructural analysis reveals that PUP forms a gel network structure in the material, effectively filling the gaps between CF and asphalt, enhancing interfacial bonding strength, and stabilizing overall performance. AFM microscopic morphology further shows that the PUP/CF composite-modified asphalt has more "honeycomb struc-

https://doi.org/10.3390/gels12020143

tures" than matrix asphalt and CF-modified asphalt, forming more structural asphalt and improving overall structural stability. This research represents a significant innovation, as it leverages the synergistic effect of PUP gel and CF to significantly improve both the macro and micro properties of asphalt-with the PUP forming a three-dimensional elastic gel network to enhance adhesion and deformation resistance. The study provides a proof-of-concept for designing high-performance modified asphalt materials, where the optimized formulation (7.4% PUP, 2.1% CF) effectively improves key asphalt properties (penetration ↓ 41.5%, softening point ↑ 6.7 °C, ductility ↑ 9%), demonstrating the great relevance of gel-based composites for asphalt modification in practical road engineering.

The paper "Study on the Adaptability of FBG Sensors Encapsulated in CNT-Modified Gel Material for Asphalt Pavement" explores an innovative application of modified gel materials in asphalt pavement strain monitoring. The authors develop a fiber Bragg grating (FBG) sensor encapsulated in carboxylated carbon nanotube (CNT-COOH)-modified gel material, which is designed to address the needs of prolonging asphalt pavement service life and reducing maintenance costs. While traditional FBG sensors may lack sufficient compatibility and durability when applied directly to asphalt pavement, the CNT-modified gel encapsulation is intended to enhance the sensor's mechanical performance and adaptability to the pavement's working environment. To optimize this encapsulation material, Guo et al. conduct tensile and bending tests to evaluate the effect of different CNT-COOH dosages on the mechanical properties of the gel material, ultimately determining the optimal dosage. They also use infrared spectroscopy and scanning electron microscopy to compare and analyze the infrared spectra and microstructure of carbon nanotubes before and after carboxyl functionalization, as well as the microstructure of the modified gel material. Laboratory test results show that the incorporation of CNT-COOH significantly improves the mechanical properties of the gel material: tensile strength, elongation at break, and tensile modulus increase by 36.2%, 47%, and 17.2%, respectively, while flexural strength, flexural modulus, and flexural strain increase by 89.7%, 7.5%, and 63.8%, respectively. Infrared spectrum analysis confirms the successful introduction of carboxyl (COOH) and hydroxyl (OH) groups on the surface of carbon nanotubes, and microstructure analysis reveals that carboxyl functionalization reduces CNT agglomeration, making the tensile section of the modified gel material rougher with obvious plastic deformation and improved toughness. Calibration experiments indicate that the strain and temperature sensitivity coefficients of the encapsulated sensor are 1.9864 pm/μm and 0.0383 nm/°C, which are 1.63 times and 3.61 times higher than those of bare FBG sensors. Applicability studies and ANSYS finite element analysis verify that the internal strain of asphalt rutting specimens changes linearly with external static load (with a fitting sensitivity of 0.0286 με/N), and simulation results are consistent with measured data, confirming the sensor's effectiveness and monitoring accuracy. Dynamic load tests further reflect the internal strain change trend of asphalt mixture under external rutting load. The study's findings are highly relevant for the road engineering industry, demonstrating how CNT-modified gel encapsulation can enhance FBG sensor performance, thereby providing a reliable technical solution for long-term strain monitoring of asphalt pavement.

"Quantum-Dot-Based Molecularly Imprinted Hydrogel for Rapid Detection of Homocysteine" delves into the development of advanced hydrogel-based detection materials, focusing on addressing the need for rapid and selective detection of homocysteine (Hcy)—a biomolecule whose elevated levels are associated with various pathological conditions including atherosclerosis, hypertension, and cardiovascular diseases. Inspired by the potential of quantum dots (QDs) for fluorescence-based detection and molecular imprinting technology for high selectivity, the authors set out to develop quantum-dot-based molecularly imprinted hydrogels (QD@MIHs) as a novel tool for rapid Hcy detection. They combined

https://doi.org/10.3390/gels12020143

two key technologies: (1) the integration of L-cysteine-modified ZnS quantum dots (QDs) with highly selective molecular imprinting technology; and (2) the fabrication of QD@MIHs using a dual-functional monomer system (acrylamide and methacrylic acid) via surface coating of the Hcy molecularly imprinted polymer gel onto the QDs. Using this approach, Zhang et al. successfully developed the QD@MIHs and characterized their detection performance under optimal conditions. The experimental results showed that the response time of the QD@MIHs for Hcy detection was only 5 min, enabling rapid analysis. When the Hcy concentration ranged from 0.1 to 10.0 μM, the fluorescence quenching of the QD@MIHs exhibited a good linear relationship with Hcy concentration (R^2 = 0.9972), with a corresponding detection limit as low as 0.027 μM, demonstrating high sensitivity. Additionally, the constructed QD@MIHs showed no significant response to other interfering substances, confirming the high selectivity of the prepared material. Practical sample analysis further validated the reliability of the method: the recovery rates of Hcy ranged from 94.34% to 104.1%, with relative standard deviations (RSD, n = 3) between 3.56% and 7.17%. This QD@MIH-based detection method represents a significant innovation, as it achieves rapid, selective, and sensitive Hcy detection with simple operation, overcoming the limitations of traditional detection methods that may be time-consuming or lack selectivity. The study provides a proof-of-concept for designing next-generation biomolecular detection tools—particularly for biomedical diagnostics and preventive-healthcare applications—where the integration of quantum dots and molecularly imprinted hydrogels enables efficient and reliable detection of key pathological markers.

"Polymer–Silicate Composite Gel Systems for Enhanced Chloride Resistance of Cement-Based Materials" delves into the development of advanced gel-based protective materials, focusing on addressing the critical issues of insufficient protection and poor durability of concrete during service. Inspired by the potential of silane and fluorocarbon resin emulsion to improve material protection performance, the authors set out to develop a novel polymer–silicate composite gel system and apply it to mortar specimens to enhance their chloride ion resistance. They combined two key components and testing approaches: (1) the development of the composite gel system by integrating silane with fluorocarbon resin emulsion; and (2) the evaluation of its chloride ion resistance enhancement effect using the RCM method and natural chloride ion penetration tests, coupled with SEM images to analyze the anti-permeation mechanism. Using this approach, Zhang et al. successfully developed the novel polymer–silicate composite gel system and systematically characterized its performance on mortar specimens. The experimental results indicate that the chloride ion migration coefficient of the composite gel system is 4.91×10^{-12} m^2/s, representing a 63.97% reduction compared to the single fluorocarbon gel system, demonstrating a significant improvement in anti-chloride penetration ability. Within the 0–5 mm depth range, the free chloride ion contents at 14, 28, and 56 days decreased by 55.35%, 50.10%, and 43.64%, respectively, further confirming its excellent resistance to chloride penetration. Acid and alkali resistance tests showed that the system retained the inherent corrosion resistance of the fluorocarbon component, ensuring its stability in harsh environments. While carbonation tests demonstrated a slight decrease in carbonation resistance compared with the pure fluorocarbon gel system, the composite gel system still maintained a satisfactory performance level. This polymer–silicate composite gel system represents a significant innovation, as it effectively enhances the mortar's resistance to chloride ion penetration while retaining key protective properties, overcoming the limitations of single-component gel systems that may lack comprehensive performance. The study provides a proof-of-concept for designing next-generation protective materials for cement-based materials—particularly for concrete structures in chloride-rich environments—where the

https://doi.org/10.3390/gels12020143

integration of silane and fluorocarbon resin emulsion enables improved durability and service life, offering valuable technical insights for practical engineering applications.

The paper "Investigation of Toughening Mechanism of Virgin Asphalt by Blending with Waste Battery Powder" explores an innovative application of waste battery powder (WBP) in enhancing the fatigue resistance of sol–gel structured virgin asphalt. The authors develop a WBP-modified asphalt by incorporating a 12% content of WBP, which is designed to address the need for improving pavement service life and achieving resource utilization of waste batteries. While virgin asphalt itself may lack sufficient durability under repeated loading, the WBP modification is intended to enhance its cracking resistance and toughening performance. To clarify this toughening mechanism, the authors conduct linear amplitude, non-damage, and damage time sweep tests to evaluate the fatigue performance of the modified asphalt. They also establish a cracking area model using energy–mechanics balance equations, taking the asphalt cracking area as an index to quantify induced damage and determine the representative rate for the cracking damage process (k_{cd}). Furthermore, they employ the activation energy for cracking damage (E_{acd}) to quantify the difficulty of the cracking process. Laboratory test results show that WBP-modified asphalt exhibits three nonlinear cracking stages and has a lower cracking rate compared to virgin asphalt. Its cracking damage shows an overall increasing trend over time, and the damage evolution parameter β can serve as the representative k_{cd}. Microstructural analysis via scanning electron microscopy reveals that the micro-grooves and wrinkles on the WBP surface enhance its bonding with the asphalt matrix, which significantly increases the E_{acd} of sol–gel 70# virgin asphalt from 10.6 to 23.88 kJ·mol^{-1}, thereby achieving effective toughening. The study's findings demonstrate that the unique micromorphology of WBP is the core factor in improving the toughening performance, and the fatigue damage process can be accurately characterized by the kinetic parameters β and E_{acd}. This provides a novel mechanical characterization method for modified asphalt and offers theoretical and technical support for the high-value utilization of waste battery resources in road engineering.

3. Conclusions and Outlook

The contributions to this Special Issue highlight the remarkable diversity and innovation in modern polymer gel research, spanning synthesis, characterization, and application across construction, transportation, environment, and biomedicine. Key themes emerging from these studies include the pursuit of sustainability through waste valorization and low-carbon formulations, the development of multifunctional gels with synergistic properties (e.g., self-healing, responsiveness, and durability), and the expansion of application boundaries to address complex engineering and societal challenges.

A critical trend observed is the interdisciplinary integration of polymer gel science with other fields, such as microbiology (EICP technology), nanotechnology (quantum dots, carbon nanotubes), and data science (machine learning models for performance prediction). This cross-disciplinary approach enables the design of advanced gel systems that meet stringent performance requirements while adhering to environmental and economic constraints. Additionally, the emphasis on practical applicability—evidenced by numerous laboratory tests and engineering validation—ensures that these innovations can be translated from the lab to real-world scenarios.

Looking ahead, future research in polymer gels will likely focus on several directions: (1) further optimizing sustainable synthesis routes using bio-based precursors and industrial by-products; (2) developing smart gel systems with real-time responsiveness to multiple stimuli (temperature, pH, stress); (3) enhancing the long-term durability and scalability of gel composites for large-scale engineering applications; and (4) expanding biomedical and sensing applications through improved biocompatibility and sensitivity.

https://doi.org/10.3390/gels12020143

Collaboration across academia, industry, and research institutions will be essential to address remaining challenges, such as standardization of performance evaluation, cost reduction, and long-term environmental impact assessment.

In conclusion, this Special Issue showcases the vibrant and evolving nature of polymer gel research, demonstrating its potential to provide innovative solutions to global challenges in sustainability, infrastructure, healthcare, and environmental protection. We anticipate that the findings and insights presented herein will inspire further advancements, foster new collaborations, and drive the development of next-generation polymer gel technologies that are smarter, greener, and more impactful.

Funding: This research received no external funding.

Acknowledgments: As Guest Editor, I would like to express my sincere appreciation to all the authors who contributed their high-quality work to this Special Issue. I am also grateful to the editorial team of *Gels* for their invaluable support and careful handling of the publication process, and special thanks to the reviewers for their constructive comments and suggestions, which significantly improved the quality of the included papers. Given the success and strong engagement this Special Issue has received, I am pleased to announce that we have initiated the second edition of "Synthesis, Properties, and Applications of Novel Polymer-Based Gels" to continue highlighting cutting-edge research in this dynamic field. I warmly invite colleagues across academia and industry to contribute to this ongoing effort.

Conflicts of Interest: The authors declare no conflicts of interest.

List of Contributions:

1. Zhang, P.; Shi, B.; Dai, X.; Chen, C.; Lai, C. A State-of-the-Art Review on the Freeze–Thaw Resistance of Sustainable Geopolymer Gel Composites: Mechanisms, Determinants, and Models. *Gels* **2025**, *11*, 537. https://doi.org/10.3390/gels11070537.
2. Zheng, Y.; Xie, Y.; Zhang, Y.; Wan, C.; Miao, L.; Zhang, P. Valorization of River Sediments in Sustainable Cementitious Gel Materials: A Review of Characteristics, Activation, and Performance. *Gels* **2025**, *11*, 755. https://doi.org/10.3390/gels11090755.
3. Chen, Y.; Li, Z.; Guo, T.; Fang, C.; Guo, P.; Wang, C.; Bai, B.; Zhang, W.; Yan, H.; Chen, Q. Performance and Mechanism Analysis of an Anti-Skid Wear Layer of Active Slow-Release Ice–Snow Melting Modified by Gels. *Gels* **2025**, *11*, 449. https://doi.org/10.3390/gels11060449.
4. Zhang, J.; Jia, H.; Li, J.; Chen, X.; Wang, L.; Wang, S.; Liu, L. Bio-Gel Formation Through Enzyme-Induced Carbonate Precipitation for Dust Control in Yellow River Silt. *Gels* **2025**, *11*, 452. https://doi.org/10.3390/gels11060452.
5. Liu, C.; Lu, B. Self-Healing and Tough Polyacrylic Acid-Based Hydrogels for Micro-Strain Sensors. *Gels* **2025**, *11*, 475. https://doi.org/10.3390/gels11070475.
6. Chen, Y.; Li, Z.; Guo, T.; Fang, C.; Yang, J.; Guo, P.; Wang, C.; Bai, B.; Zhang, W.; Tang, D.; et al. Study on Road Performance and Ice-Breaking Effect of Rubber Polyurethane Gel Mixture. *Gels* **2025**, *11*, 505. https://doi.org/10.3390/gels11070505.
7. Guo, T.; Guo, X.; Chen, Y.; Fang, C.; Yang, J.; Li, Z.; Feng, J.; Huang, H.; Li, Z.; Chen, H.; et al. A Study on the Performance of Gel-Based Polyurethane Prepolymer/Ceramic Fiber Composite-Modified Asphalt. *Gels* **2025**, *11*, 558. https://doi.org/10.3390/gels11070558.
8. Guo, T.; Guo, X.; Chen, Y.; Fang, C.; Yang, J.; Li, Z.; Feng, J.; Kong, J.; Chen, H.; Wang, C.; et al. Study on the Adaptability of FBG Sensors Encapsulated in CNT-Modified Gel Material for Asphalt Pavement. *Gels* **2025**, *11*, 590. https://doi.org/10.3390/gels11080590.
9. Zhang, X.; Liang, J.; Zheng, B.; Jia, P.; Xu, Q. Quantum-Dot-Based Molecularly Imprinted Hydrogel for Rapid Detection of Homocysteine. *Gels* **2025**, *11*, 632. https://doi.org/10.3390/gels11080632.
10. Zhang, T.; Dai, Y.; Ren, S.; Huang, Z.; Han, C.; Ding, W. Polymer–Silicate Composite Gel Systems for Enhanced Chloride Resistance of Cement-Based Materials. *Gels* **2025**, *11*, 936. https://doi.org/10.3390/gels11120936.

https://doi.org/10.3390/gels12020143

11. Fang, C.; Guo, X.; Chen, Y.; Li, H.; Guo, N.; Li, Z.; Wu, Z.; Yang, J.; Guo, T. Investigation of Toughening Mechanism of Virgin Asphalt by Blending with Waste Battery Powder. *Gels* **2026**, *12*, 117. https://doi.org/10.3390/gels12020117.

References

1. Osada, Y.; Gong, J.P. Soft and Wet Materials: Polymer Gels. *Adv. Mater.* **1998**, *10*, 827–837. [CrossRef]
2. Zhang, T.; Wang, K.; Wang, H.; Wei, M.; Chen, Z.; Zhong, D.; Chen, Y.; Pei, P. Polymer Gels for Aqueous Metal Batteries. *Prog. Mater. Sci.* **2025**, *151*, 101426. [CrossRef]
3. Parvin, N.; Kumar, V.; Joo, S.W.; Mandal, T.K. Cutting-Edge Hydrogel Technologies in Tissue Engineering and Biosensing: An Updated Review. *Materials* **2024**, *17*, 4792. [CrossRef] [PubMed]
4. Babaei-Ghazvini, A.; Vafakish, B.; Patel, R.; Falua, K.J.; Dunlop, M.J.; Acharya, B. Cellulose Nanocrystals in the Development of Biodegradable Materials: A Review on CNC Resources, Modification, and Their Hybridization. *Int. J. Biol. Macromol.* **2024**, *258*, 128834. [CrossRef] [PubMed]
5. Zhang, P.; Shi, B.; Dai, X.; Chen, C.; Lai, C. A State-of-the-Art Review on the Freeze–Thaw Resistance of Sustainable Geopolymer Gel Composites: Mechanisms, Determinants, and Models. *Gels* **2025**, *11*, 537. [CrossRef] [PubMed]
6. Chen, Y.; Li, Z.; Guo, T.; Fang, C.; Guo, P.; Wang, C.; Bai, B.; Zhang, W.; Yan, H.; Chen, Q. Performance and Mechanism Analysis of an Anti-Skid Wear Layer of Active Slow-Release Ice–Snow Melting Modified by Gels. *Gels* **2025**, *11*, 449. [CrossRef] [PubMed]
7. Liu, C.; Lu, B. Self-Healing and Tough Polyacrylic Acid-Based Hydrogels for Micro-Strain Sensors. *Gels* **2025**, *11*, 475. [CrossRef] [PubMed]
8. Zhang, J.; Jia, H.; Li, J.; Chen, X.; Wang, L.; Wang, S.; Liu, L. Bio-Gel Formation Through Enzyme-Induced Carbonate Precipitation for Dust Control in Yellow River Silt. *Gels* **2025**, *11*, 452. [CrossRef] [PubMed]
9. Correa, S.; Grosskopf, A.K.; Lopez Hernandez, H.; Chan, D.; Yu, A.C.; Stapleton, L.M.; Appel, E.A. Translational Applications of Hydrogels. *Chem. Rev.* **2021**, *121*, 11385. [CrossRef] [PubMed]
10. Nandi, A.K.; Chatterjee, D.P. Hybrid Polymer Gels for Energy Applications. *J. Mater. Chem. A* **2023**, *11*, 12593–12642. [CrossRef]

https://doi.org/10.3390/gels12020143

gels

MDPI

Article

Performance and Mechanism Analysis of an Anti-Skid Wear Layer of Active Slow-Release Ice–Snow Melting Modified by Gels

Yuanzhao Chen [1,2,3,4,*], Zhenxia Li [1,2,3,4], Tengteng Guo [1,2,3,4], Chenze Fang [1,2,3,4], Peng Guo [5], Chaohui Wang [6], Bing Bai [1], Weiguang Zhang [7], Haobo Yan [1] and Qi Chen [1]

1 School of Civil Engineering and Transportation, North China University of Water Resources and Electric Power, Zhengzhou 450045, China; zhenxiali2009@ncwu.edu.cn (Z.L.); guotth@ncwu.edu.cn (T.G.); fangchenze@126.com (C.F.); baibing7777@ncwu.edu.cn (B.B.); 15737993622@163.com (H.Y.); chq319666@163.com (Q.C.)

2 Henan Province Engineering Technology Research Center of Environment Friendly and High-Performance Pavement Materials, Zhengzhou 450045, China

3 Technology Innovation Center of Henan Transport Industry of Utilization of Solid Waste Resources in Traffic Engineering, North China University of Water Resources and Electric Power, Zhengzhou 450045, China

4 Henan Province University-Enterprise Research and Development Center for Green, Low-Carbon and High-Performance Road Materials, Zhengzhou 450045, China

5 National and Local Joint Engineering Laboratory of Traffic Civil Engineering Materials, Chongqing Jiaotong University, Chongqing 400074, China; guopeng@cqjtu.edu.cn

6 School of Highway, Chang'an University, Xi'an 710064, China; wchh0205@chd.edu.cn

7 School of Transportation, Southeast University, Nanjing 210096, China; wgzhang@seu.edu.cn

* Correspondence: cyz740513@ncwu.edu.cn; Tel.: +86-13673359605; Fax: +86-0371-69127209

Abstract: Winter pavement maintenance faces challenges in balancing large-scale upkeep and driving safety, particularly regarding the application of active slow-release materials. This study proposes a gel-modified salt-storing ceramsite asphalt mixture to enhance ice-melting capabilities through controlled salt release. By replacing a conventional coarse aggregate with salt-storing ceramsite in SMA-10 graded mixtures (0–80% content), we systematically evaluate its mechanical performance and de-icing functionality. The experimental results demonstrate that 40% salt-storing ceramsite content optimizes high-temperature stability while maintaining acceptable low-temperature performance and water resistance. Microstructural analysis reveals that silicone–acrylic emulsion forms a hydrophobic film on ceramsite surfaces, enabling uniform salt distribution and sustained release. The optimal 10% gel modification achieves effective salt retention and controlled release through pore-structure regulation. These findings establish a 40–60% salt-storing ceramsite content range as the practical range for winter pavement applications, offering insights into the design of durable snow-melting asphalt surfaces.

Keywords: pavement materials; slow-release de-icing material; microscopic; characterization; cold-climate pavement; ceramsite; road performance; slow-release mechanism; gel material

1. Introduction

With an increasing amount of road traffic, road surfacees will exhibit the phenomenon of tectonic depth attenuation and flatness reduction [1]. At present, the treatment methods of China's highway maintenance include washing and planing the original road surface to lay a new asphalt surface layer, micro-surface or thin slurry sealing layer, and paving anti-skid wear layer [2]. When an anti-skid wear layer is applied to a road surface, damage to the structural layer of the road surface is reduced, improving the performance of the surface and extending its service life [3]. When the paving thickness is small, usually in the range of 15~25 mm, it can reduce the consumption of materials and energy, reduce initial costs and maintenance costs, and is an environmentally friendly road paving technology, in-line with the concept of global environmental protection.

At present, in most of the northern regions of China in winter, snow and ice phenomena appear on road surfaces in rainy and snowy weather, resulting in a reduced friction coefficient of automobile tires, resulting in vehicle slippage and braking difficulties, which can easily lead to loss of control of vehicles and, therefore, traffic accidents. An active slow-release type of snow- and ice-melting material combined with asphalt pavement pre-conservation technology, salt-storing pavement de-icing, and snow-removal technology are needed, based on an innovative anti-slip wear layer with excellent anti-skid and wear-resistant performance [4], in order to prepare asphalt pavement for active pre-maintenance and achieve the effect of actively melting ice and snow on road surfaces. This can not only serve a winter pavement snow-melting and de-icing function, but also can effectively reduce the adverse effects of salt-storing snowmelt on asphalt pavements. Therefore, it is of great significance to develop pavement materials with snow-melting and ice-melting effects and maintenance functions.

Ice- and snow-melting salt material is coated on the salt-storing carrier using a modification process based on slow-release gel technology, prepared as a powder or granular composite materials [5], that can replace the aggregate and mineral powder in the asphalt mixture [6]. In recent years, experts have introduced wear layer technology into ice- and snow-melting pavements, and the results have proved that the developed materials have certain ice- and snow-melting effects. Therefore, in this paper, through the development of a slow-release composite snow-melting agent, attached to the pores of a porous aggregate, combined with anti-skid wear layer maintenance technology and salt-storing aggregate-replacing parts of aggregates of the same particle size, we study the ice- and snow-melting performance of a road treated with an active slow-release snow-melting anti-skid wear layer so as to achieve an active and lasting snow- and ice-melting function from the pavement. This is of positive significance for the coordinated and sustainable development of our society, economy, and environment, as well as for the promotion of the high-quality development of transportation engineering. Anti-skid wearing layer technology research first began in France, and scholars worldwide have proposed a thin asphalt concrete surface layer, ultra-thin asphalt concrete (UTAC), a Novachip anti-skid wearing layer based on synchronized paving technology, a Novachip ultra-thin wearing layer, and an open-graded anti-skid wearing layer (OGFC). On the basis of previous research, American scholars successively launched SUP-5 and SMA-5, two more advanced fine-grained ultra-thin wearing layer technologies. In recent years, domestic and foreign ultra-thin wearing course technology has developed rapidly, with different types and functions of thin-layer technology emerging frequently, such as high-toughness ultra-thin asphalt wearing course [7–9], SMC warm-mixed thin layer [10], ECA easy-to-consolidate ultra-thin wearing course [11], temperature-controlled ultra-thin wearing course [12], as well as active-melting snow and ice ultra-thin wearing course, etc. At present, active-melting snow and ice anti-skid layer is the most advanced thin-layer technology. At present, the active ice- and snow-melting anti-skid wear layer is divided into salt-storing ice- and snow-melting anti-skid wear layer and energy-conversion anti-skid wear layer according to the principle of melting ice and snow. Energy-transforming anti-skid wear layer melting ice and snow consumes a lot of energy, and the energy and heat inevitably affect the pavement structure [13,14], which can be avoided using a salt-storage melting ice and snow anti-skid wear layer. Ice- and snow-melting materials are combined in some form (filler or aggregate) with ultra-thin wear layer materials, thus introducing three new influencing factors, i.e., changes in the oil/gravel ratio due to differences in filler properties [15,16], changes in the mix structure due to particle interferences [17,18], and changes in the voids caused by the salt that is removed [19,20]. Based on the above problems, researchers have carried out related research work. For example, Sun Dahang [21] proposed a new evaluation index and design method for an ice-suppressing anti-skid wear layer; Liu Yang [22] investigated the impact of slow-release ice-melting and snow-melting material doping on the road performance of ultra-thin wear layer by using single-factor analysis and constructed an optimal custom model to optimize the composition of the material based on the Response Surface Analysis method; Chen Shuanfa [23] obtained the basic composition and key design parameters of the material from three aspects, namely, the composition of the mineral grades, asphalt paste characteristics, and road performance of TSSAM, and verified the basic material composition and long-lasting snow-melting performance and road performance of TSSAM under different conditions. Chen Shuanfa [23], regarding the TSSAM mineral gradation composition, asphalt slurry characteristics, and road performance, researched the basic composition of the material and the key design parameters, and verified snow-melting performance and snow-melting long-lasting performance under different conditions; Chen Xiao [24] used SMA-5 gradation as an ultra-thin snow melting cover, and, through the study of road performance and snow-melting and ice suppression function, concluded that, when the mixing amount of the snow-melting agent is 33%, the ultra-thin snow-melting covers with various road performance and snow-melting performance all meet the requirements. The road performance and snow- and ice-melting performance of the ultra-thin snow-melting cover meet the requirements.

Comprehensive research has shown that an active slow-release ice-melting snow anti-skid wear layer, compared to other salt-storing pavement de-icing and snow-removal technology [25], can improve asphalt pavement skid resistance and abrasion resistance, can be considered to extend the service life of the pavement, and represents a new technology for snow-melting and de-icing, offering better road performance. However, due to the lack of actual engineering experience, design specifications, and evaluation standards, active slow-release ice-melting and snow-melting anti-skid wear layer pre-maintenance technology is still in its infancy. How to prepare slow-release composite snow-melting agents, combined with anti-skid wear layer maintenance technology, salt-storing aggregates [26–29] as a partial replacement for aggregates of the same particle size, the study of active slow-release ice-melting and snow-melting [30–33], and the performance of the snow-melting wear layer, as well as snow- and ice-melting performance, in order to achieve active and durable road melting and snow-melting functions, is an important issue to be solved at present [34–36]. Function is an important problem to be solved at present. Many scholars have performed research on the anti-slip performance of the anti-skid wear layer, surface functional layer performance, and snow-melting on pavements, mainly including the anti-skid performance of wear layers, surface functional layer performance, and a series of research and development work on snow-melting technology on pavements; however, in the current literature, few studies have addressed snow-melting performance and the mechanisms of active slow-release anti-ice wear layers. This paper, therefore, investigates the performance and underlying mechanisms of gel-modified salt-storing ceramsite in anti-skid wearing layers, addressing this identified gap in knowledge. Compared to traditional de-icing methods (e.g., bulk salt application or heated pavements), our gel-modified salt-storing ceramsite approach has comparable initial costs, but significantly lower long-term maintenance requirements, and its slow-release functionality extends the economic service life of pavements. This paper explores the advantages of anti-skid wear layers with environmentally friendly slow-release snow- and ice-melting functions.

2. Results and Discussion

2.1. Road Performance Test Results

Referring to JTG E20-2011 [37], the road performance test was carried out on the salt-storing ceramic granule wear layer mixes with volume dosages of salt-storing ceramic granules of 0%, 20%, 40%, 60% and 80%, respectively, and the effect of different slow-release salt-storing ceramic granule dosages on the road performance of the active ice-melting and anti-skid wear layer was analyzed by combining the results of the tests in each group. The experimental research plan is shown in Figure 1.

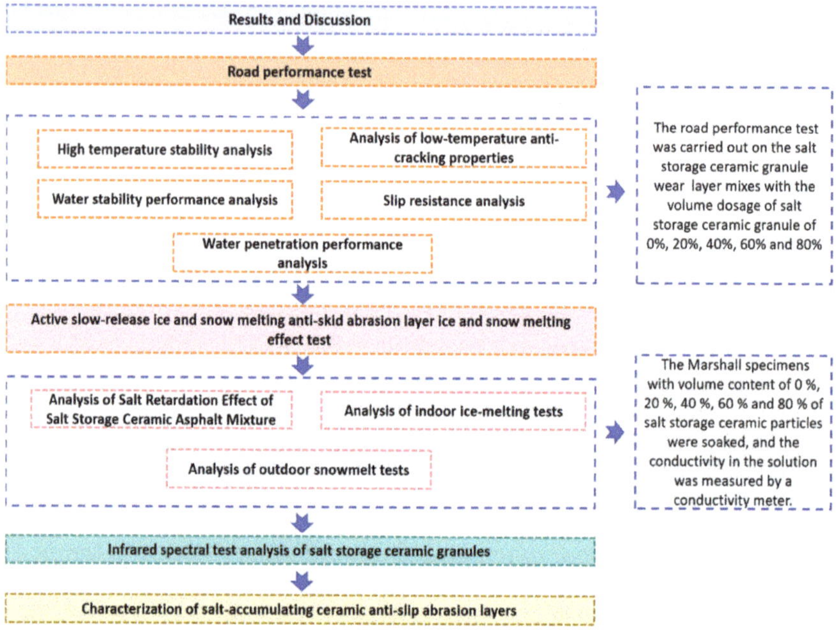

Figure 1. Technology roadmap.

2.1.1. High-Temperature Stability Analysis

The rutting test was used to evaluate the high-temperature stability. Five rutted plate specimens doped with salt-accumulated ceramic grains were molded, and the rutting test was carried out by holding the heat for 4 h at 60 °C; the rutting results of different salt-accumulated ceramic grain-doped specimens are shown in Figure 2.

As can be seen in Figure 2, the dynamic stability of the anti-slip wear layer mix under different salt-storing ceramic granule dosages meets the specification requirements. The dynamic stability of the wear layer mix with the increase in salt-storing ceramic particles showed a trend of increasing and then decreasing; when the dosage of salt-storing ceramic particles was 40%, the dynamic stability of the wear layer mix reached the maximum, and its dynamic stability increased by 40.4% compared to the mix without salt-storing ceramic particles. It can be concluded from the test results that more salt-storage ceramic particles does not necessarily mean the better the high-temperature stability of the mixture; as far as high-temperature stability is concerned, the optimal proportion of salt-storage ceramic particles is 40%. These results align with the findings of Chen Xiao et al. [24], who reported an optimal snow-melting agent content (~33%) for an ultra-thin asphalt layer, indicating consistency across studies. Salt-storing ceramic particles improve the high-temperature stability of the wear layer mixture: (1) Slow-release salt-storing ceramic particles and polymer-modified cement mortar coat the salt-storing ceramic particles due to the alkaline cement, so that modified cement mortar parcel salt-storing ceramic particles and asphalt have good adhesion; adding salt-storing ceramic particles after polymer-modified cement mortar parcel means that its strength improves and that it shows better wear resistance, and so the mixture is good. The strength of salt-accumulating ceramic granules is improved after the polymer-modified cement mortar is wrapped, and the abrasion resistance is better, so the high-temperature stability of the mix is good. (2) Shale grains are mainly shale materials, as raw materials calcined at high temperatures have certain activity on their surfaces, so that, as the contact surface strength of the grains and asphalt increases, the friction of the wear layer mixture increases; the salt-storing grains of the ceramic anti-skid wear layer with high-temperature stability have a certain effect of enhancement. (3) Due to the structural characteristics of ceramic grains, the surface is rough and there are a large number of pore structures, and the salt storage ceramic grains are larger than the ordinary crushed stone. The effective surface area of the aggregate is large, so that, as the bonding area between the asphalt and the salt grains increases, its adsorbs effective asphalt and also adsorbs excess asphalt, improving the internal cohesion of the mixture, which in turn increases the shear resistance of the salt-grain anti-skid wear layer.

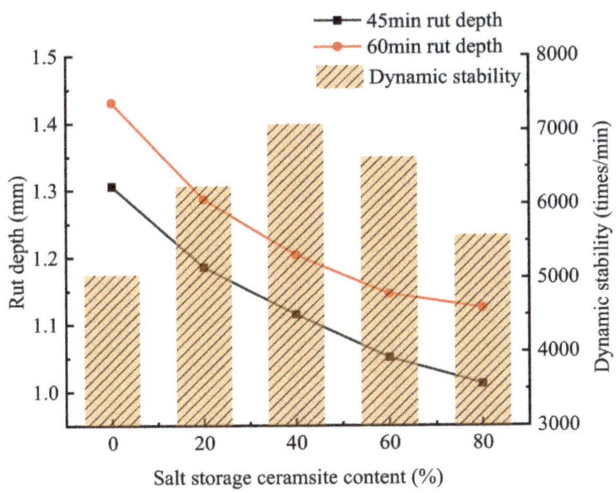

Figure 2. Wheel-tracking test results.

2.1.2. Analysis of Low-Temperature Anti-Cracking Properties

The low-temperature trabecular bending test was used to evaluate the low-temperature performance of salt-storing ceramic grain wear layer mixtures which were placed in a constant temperature box at -10 ± 0.5 °C for 5 h and loaded with a universal testing machine at a constant rate until the destruction of the specimen; the results of the low-temperature trabecular bending test with different salt-storing ceramic grain admixtures are shown in Figure 3.

As can be seen in Figure 3, the maximum bending strain and flexural tensile strength of the salt-storing ceramic grain abraded layer mixtures showed different degrees of reduction with increases in salt-storing ceramic grain dosage, which indicates that the salt-accumulated ceramic grain dosage has a greater impact on their low-temperature performance. At 20%, 40%, 60%, and 80% of the volume of salt-storing grains, the flexural tensile strength of the wear layer mix was reduced by 14.3%, 27.3%, 35.0%, and 41.9%, respectively, and the maximum flexural strain was reduced by 5.5%, 15.4%, 21.0%, and 25.7%, respectively, compared to that of the control mix without salt-storing grains. The main reasons are as follows: (1) Due to the crushed-stone shale grains after the addition of the polymer-modified cement mortar package and after the angularity becomes poor, the salt-storing grains in the anti-skid wear layer mixture cannot form a strong embedded structure, resulting in insufficient internal friction, which causes the wear layer mixture with salt-storing grains to deform easily under external force. (2) Due to the low strength of the salt-accumulated ceramic particles, the ceramic particles become brittle after freezing at −10 °C, the overall resistance of the specimen becomes insufficient, and the ceramic particles fracture earlier than common gravel; therefore, the low-temperature performance will deteriorate.

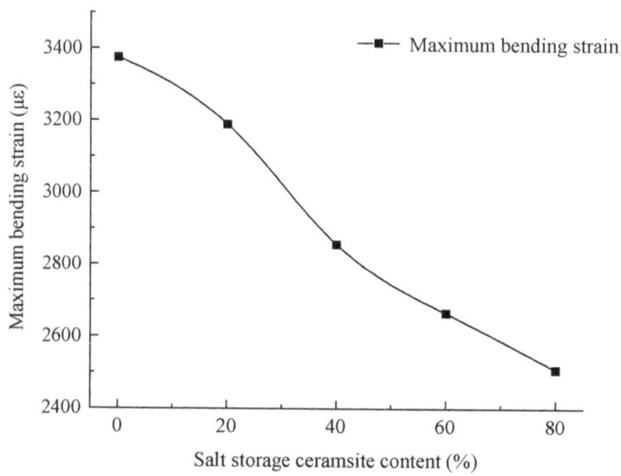

Figure 3. Test results of the maximum bending strain of trabecular.

2.1.3. Water Stability Performance Analysis

Water stability was evaluated using the immersion Marshall Test and the freeze–thaw splitting test. The results are as follows.

Immersion Marshall Test

Five different dosages of salt-storing ceramic asphalt mixtures were used to mold two groups of Marshall specimens, each containing four specimens: Group 1 was immersed in a constant-temperature water tank at 60 °C for 30 min to test stability; and Group 2 was immersed at 60 °C for 48 h to test stability by calculating the residual stability of the specimens to evaluate the water stability of different dosages of salt-storing ceramic asphalt mixes. The results of the immersion Marshall test with different salt-storing ceramic grain dosages are shown in Figure 4.

As can be seen from Figure 4, 20%, 40%, and 60% dosages of salt-storing ceramic grain wear layer mixture residual stability meet the MSR $\geq$ 80% specification requirements. Compared to the 0% dosage of salt-storing ceramic grains asphalt mixture, the addition of salt-storing ceramic grains reduces the residual stability of the wear layer mix. The higher the dosage of salt-storing ceramic grains, the lower the residual stability of the Marshall specimens. This is mainly due to the structural characteristics of the ceramic grains; salt-storing ceramic grains, compared to ordinary aggregate strength, are relatively insufficient and have a high water absorption rate. Therefore, with more ceramic particles mixed, water in the asphalt mixture damage is more significant, and the worse the water stability is. Doping with amounts of 20%, 40%, and 60% of salt-storing ceramic grains meants that residual stability, compared to the ordinary asphalt mixture, decreased by 2.3%, 4.5%, and 8.4%; when the salt-storing ceramic grain dosage increased to 80%, the residual stability of the wear layer mixture no longer met the specification requirements. This means that a certain amount of slow-release salt-storing ceramic particles reduces the water stability of the wear layer asphalt mixture; the dosage is too high, meaning that the residual stability does not meet specification requirements.

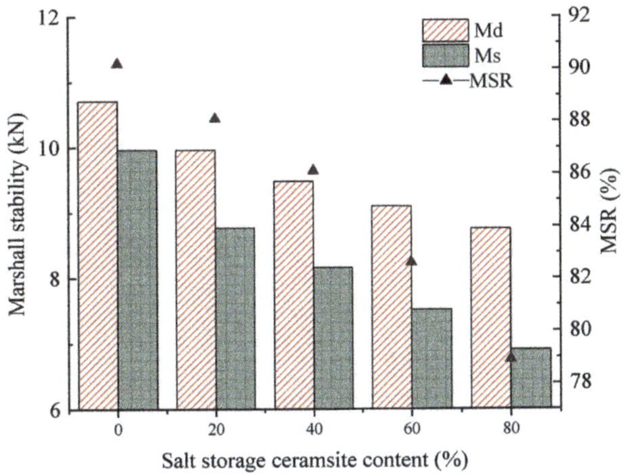

Figure 4. Immersion Marshall test results.

Freeze–Thaw Splitting Test

We referred to T 0729 in JTG E20-2011 [37] to perform the execute the freeze–thaw splitting test. The results of the freeze–thaw splitting test with different salt-storing ceramic granule dosages are shown in Figure 5.

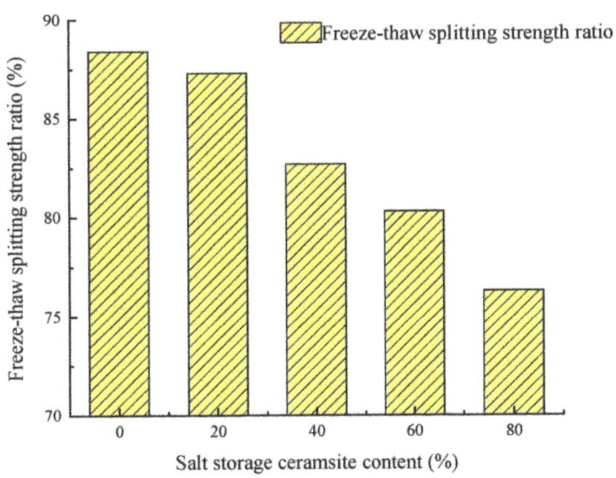

Figure 5. Freeze–thaw splitting strength ratio test results.

The larger the value of the split strength ratio, the stronger the mix's resistance to water damage. In Figure 5, it can be seen that the split strength ratio decreases gradually with the increase in salt-storing ceramic granule doping, and the split strength of 20%, 40%, and 60% salt-storing ceramic granule-doped wear layer mixes was reduced by 1.2%, 6.4%, and 9.2% compared with that of the ordinary wear layer mix. In the test process, it was found that, after the freezing and thawing of the Marshall specimen, a particle spalling phenomenon could be seen, and, as the salt-storing ceramic granule dosage increased from

20% to 80%, the spalling phenomenon became more severe; when the dosage reaches 80%, the splitting strength of the mixture no longer meets the specification requirements.

In the test results, it can be seen that the salt-storing ceramic particles mixed into the wear layer mixture have a significant impact on water stability. There are two main reasons for this: First of all, asphalt and ceramic particles on the surface of the combination are weak, resulting in low cohesion within the mixture; in the role of the dynamic hydraulic force, large-scale peeling of the asphalt overlay layer may occur, which affects the water stability of the salt-storing ceramic particle wear layer. Secondly, the structures of the salt-storing ceramic particles and of the specific salt grains themselves are also an important factor due to the high water absorption rate and the strong water retention, meaning that water can enter the mixture easily and is difficult to dissipate; therefore, water absorption and retention are significant characteristics, and, under vehicle loading, the mix becomes loose, which causes the salt grain wear layer mixture to become easily damaged under the action of external forces or the freeze–thaw cycle.

According to the salt grains wear layer mixture of the immersion Marshall test and freeze–thaw ratio test, it can be seen that, at 80% salt grain dosage, the Marshall stability of the mixture and split ratio do not meet the requirements; at 60% dosage, the split strength ratio is 80.2%, which just meets the specification requirements. In order to ensure that the salt-storing ceramic wear layer mixture has good water stability, the salt-storing ceramic mix dosage should be less than 60%.

2.1.4. Slip-Resistance Analysis

Anti-sliding performance was evaluated using the sanding method and pendulum instrument. The results are as follows.

Sand-Laying Method

We used the sand-laying method to determine the construction depth of different salt-storing ceramic granule dosages of ice- and snow-melting anti-skid wear layer mixture; the test results are shown in Table 1 below.

Table 1. Structural depth test results.

Salt-Storing Ceramsite Content (%)	Paving Diameter (mm)	Structure Depth TD (mm)	Technical Requirement (mm)
0	176.8	1.018	
20	179.7	0.986	
40	181.4	0.967	≥0.55
60	185.0	0.930	
80	186.1	0.919	

As can be seen in Table 1, the construction depth of asphalt mixtures with five different ceramic granule dosages satisfies the technical requirements of the specification (TD ≥ 0.55 mm). With the increase in salt-storing ceramic particles, the pavement diameter gradually becomes larger, the construction depth gradually decreases, and the rutting depth of the rutting plate with 20%, 40%, 60%, and 80% salt-storing ceramic particle dosages decreases by 3.1%, 5.0%, 8.6%, and 9.7%, respectively, compared to that of the rutting plate with 0% salt-storing ceramic particles. This is due to the poor angularity of the salt-accumulated ceramic particles after wrapping with silica–propylene emulsion-modified cement mortar, but the effect of salt-accumulated ceramic particles on the depth of the structure is not significant, and the reduction in the depth of the structure is less than 10%. This is due to the use of grading type SMA-10, which is an intermittent grading and skeleton-dense structure, which compacts the surface of the structural depth with a large and good anti-skid performance, so the ceramic particles do not affect the anti-skid performance of the pavement.

Pendulum Instrument

The anti-skid performance of a slow-release salt-storing ceramic asphalt mixture rutting plate was studied using a BM-III type pendulum friction coefficient tester, and the test results are shown in Figure 6.

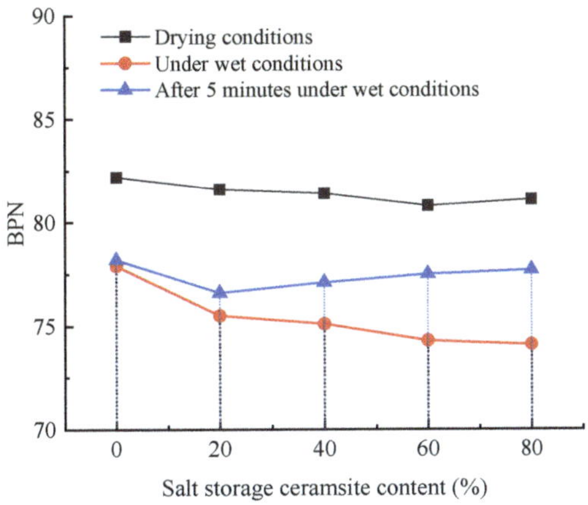

Figure 6. Anti-sliding performance test results.

As can be seen in Figure 6, under dry conditions, the addition of ceramic granules results in a slight decrease in the BPN value of rutted slabs, which is almost negligible and does not affect the pavement's skid resistance. Under wet conditions, the BPN values of all test groups decreased to a certain extent, and the BPN values of rutted slabs with 0%, 20%, 40%, 60%, and 80% salt-storing ceramic granule dosages decreased by 5.2%, 7.4%, 7.7%, 8.0%, and 8.6%, respectively, under wet conditions, and the BPN value of rutted slabs under wet conditions decreased by a larger and larger rate with the increase in the dosage of ceramic granules. This is due to the fact that the ceramic granules become less angular after being wrapped in cement mortar, and the anti-slip performance is weakened under wet conditions with the increase in ceramic granule doping. After 5 min, the wetted rutted plate was tested, and the BPN value of the rutted plate recovered to some extent, and, compared to the BPN under the wetting condition, the BPN values of rutted slabs tiwht 0%, 20%, 40%, 60%, and 80% salt-storing ceramic granule dosages increased by 0.4%, 1.5%, 2.7%, 4.3%, and 4.9%, respectively, which was due to the fact that the ceramic granules have a porous structure and high water absorption and, after wrapping the cement net mortar, the cement will also absorb part of the water so that the water dissipation of the rutted slab doped with salt-storing ceramic granules is faster than that of the rutted slab not doped with salt-storing ceramic granules, so that the BPN value increases more rapidly and the anti-skid performance is partially restored. According to this comprehensive analysis, the addition of salt-storing ceramic granules will not affect the anti-skid performance of the pavement.

2.1.5. Water-Penetration Performance Analysis

Water seepage performance was evaluated using a water seepage test.

The results of percolation tests with different salt-storing ceramic granule dosages are shown in Table 2.

Table 2. Water seepage test results.

Salt Storage Ceramsite Content (%)	3 Minutes of Water Seepage (mL)	C_W Water Permeability Coefficient (mL/min)	Specification Requirement
0	180	40	≤80 mL/min
20	189	43	
40	195	45	
60	204	48	
80	213	51	

The results in Table 2 show that, with the increase in salt-storing ceramic granule doping, the water permeability coefficient gradually became larger; this is because the ceramic granule itself is highly absorbent and, after the cement mortar package, the cement also absorbs part of the water. The water permeability coefficient of the SMA-10 anti-slip wear layer is below the specification value of 80 mL/min, which indicates that the salt-storing ceramic granule will not have an effect on the salt-storing ceramic granule wear layer of the mixing material's seepage performance.

2.2. *Active Slow-Release Ice and Snow-Melting Anti-Skid Wear Layer Ice in the Snow-Melting Effect Test*

The salt-storing ceramic asphalt mixture conductivity test, indoor ice-melting test, and outdoor snow-melting test were performed to analyze the different dosages of salt-storing ceramic asphalt mixtures' snow- and ice-melting performance, combined with the road performance, to determine the optimal dosage of salt-storing ceramic.

2.2.1. Analysis of the Salt-Retardation Effect of Salt-Storing Ceramic Asphalt Mixture

In this section, Marshall specimens are soaked, and the conductivity of the solutions are measured using a conductivity meter to test the salt-release pattern of asphalt mixtures with different volumetric dosages of salt-storing ceramic grains and the long-term effectiveness of the salt release of the slow-release storage melting ice and snow anti-skid wear layer. The results of short-term conductivity for different salt-storing ceramic granule dosages are shown in Figure 7a, and the long-term conductivity is shown in Figure 7b.

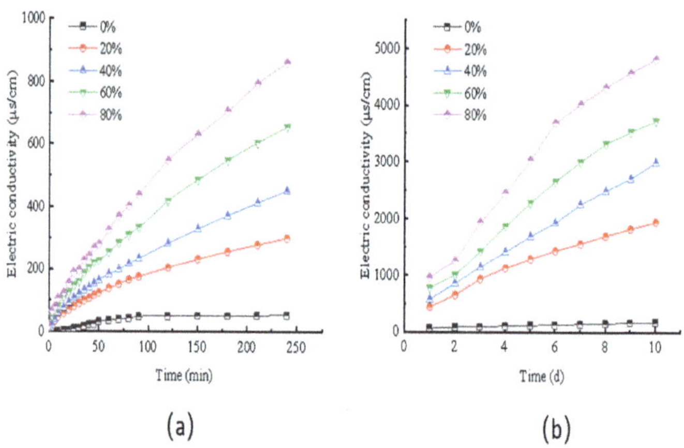

Figure 7. Short-term (**a**) and long-term (**b**) conductivity of salt-storing ceramide asphalt mixture.

As can be seen from Figure 7, the salt-storing ceramic particles mixed with 20%, 40%, 60%, and 80% of the mixture, compared to the ordinary asphalt mixture of snow-melting salt, shows significant synthesis, indicating that the presence of salt-storing ceramic particles in the asphalt mixture does not hinder salt precipitation, which also proves that the salt-storing ceramic particles in the asphalt mixture can melt ice and snow. From the short-term conductivity graph of the mixture in Figure 7a, it can be seen that, with an increase in salt-storing granules, the conductivity in the solution gradually increases—that is, the concentration of the snow-melting salt solution increases. The larger the dosage of salt-storing ceramic granules, the more snow-melting salt is precipitated per unit of time and the more significant the melting effect on snow and ice is. In Figure 7b, a long-term conductivity graph of the mixture can be seen; even when using different amounts of salt-storing ceramic asphalt mixture after 7 days, the conductivity can still ensure that there is a faster rate of growth. This shows that the salt in the mixture is more sufficient and can ensure the long-lasting effect of snow-melting in the actual snow-melting process.

2.2.2. Analysis of Indoor Ice-Melting Tests

Referring to the 'Ice and Snow Melting Material for Highway Asphalt Mixture' (JT/T 1210.2-2018) [38] for the ice-melting rate test, the results of the indoor ice-melting test with different salt-storing ceramic granule dosages are shown in Figure 8.

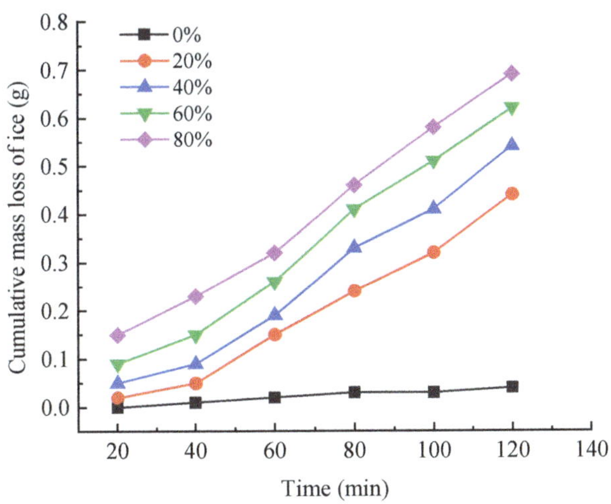

Figure 8. Melting mass loss trend of ice cubes.

As can be seen from Figure 8, under the condition of equal ice contact, with the increase in salt-storing ceramic granules, the mass loss in the ice cubes in the same period of time shows a gradual increasing trend. The amount of ice-melting in the ordinary asphalt mixture (0% salt-storing ceramic granules) is much smaller than the amount of ice-melting in the asphalt mixture with salt-storing ceramic granules. In salt-storing ceramic particles mixed at 20%, 40%, 60%, and 80%, the amount of ice-melting after 120 min, compared to the ordinary asphalt mixture's ice-melting, increased by 10, 12.5, 14.5, 16.25 times; therefore, it can be concluded that salt-storing ceramic particles mixed with asphalt mixture have a better ability to melt ice. Relative to the replacement of the mineral-powder-type snow-melting salt asphalt mixture, the salt-storing ceramic granule replacement of ordinary ice-melting aggregates is not very obvious; in all five groups, the ice-melting amounts were within 1 g, thus appearing to show a relatively low de-icing effect. Taking into account the environment of the box temperature of −5 °C, the loss in mass of ice is relatively small, considering the effect of vehicle load on the road surface, and more salt will seep into the water, further enhancing the melting of ice and snow. Considering that more salt will seep out with water under the effect of vehicle load on the road surface to further enhance the effect of ice- and snow-melting, the results of road use will differ.

2.2.3. Analysis of Outdoor Snow-Melting Tests

Marshall specimens, from left to right, were doped with salt-storing ceramic granules in the order of 0, 20%, 40%, 60%, and 80%; the outdoor snow-melting test snowfall process affecting the specimens' snow accumulation are shown in Figure 9.

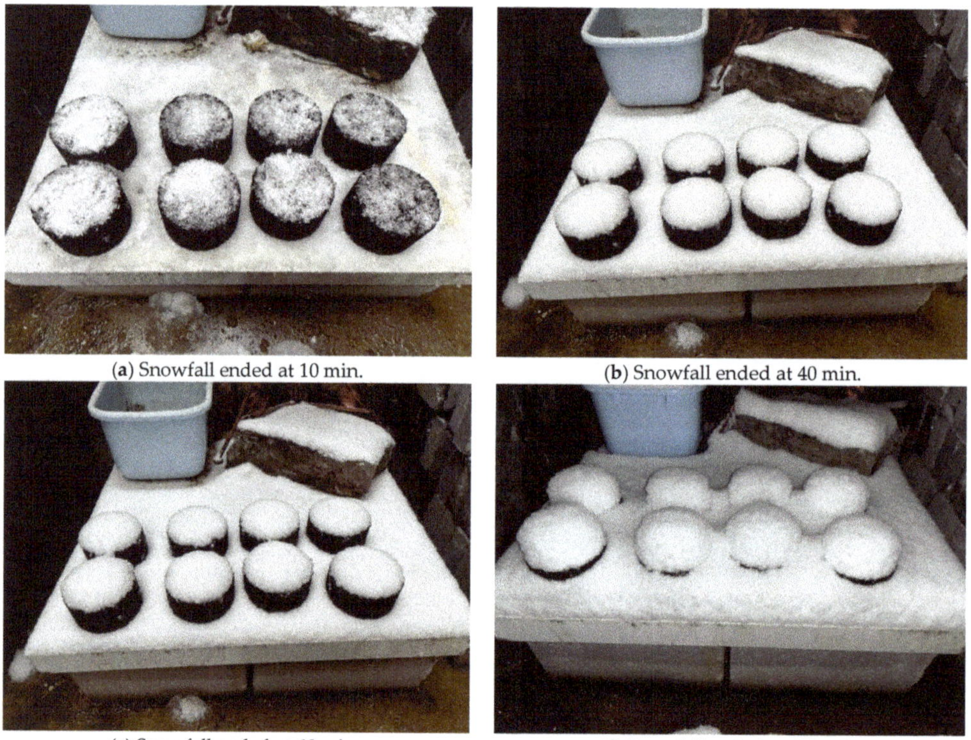

(**a**) Snowfall ended at 10 min. (**b**) Snowfall ended at 40 min.

(**c**) Snowfall ended at 60 min. (**d**) Snowfall ended at 120 min.

Figure 9. Changes in test pieces during snowfall.

From Figure 9a–d, it can be seen, during snowfall, that snow accumulation increased on all five specimens with different dosages. At the same time, different salt-storage dosages of specimens in the snow comparison test found that different specimens of the different snowmelt showed subtle differences in the effect of snow-melting; this is because, if the snowfall amount on that day was too high, the rate of snowfall was greater than the rate of snow melting. In this paper, the salt-storing ceramic granules were used to replace aggregates in the asphalt mixture; this type of aggregate-substituted salt-storing asphalt mixture, compared to mineral-powder-substituted snow-melting asphalt mixture, had a slower snow-melting rate in the first period. Therefore, in this paper, regarding snowfall, different salt-storing ceramic grain dosages of snow retention on the test specimen were observed, compared, and analyzed to examine the snow-melting effects of asphalt mixtures with different dosages of salt-storing ceramic granules.

The snow melting on top of the Marshall specimens at various times after snowfall is shown in Figure 10.

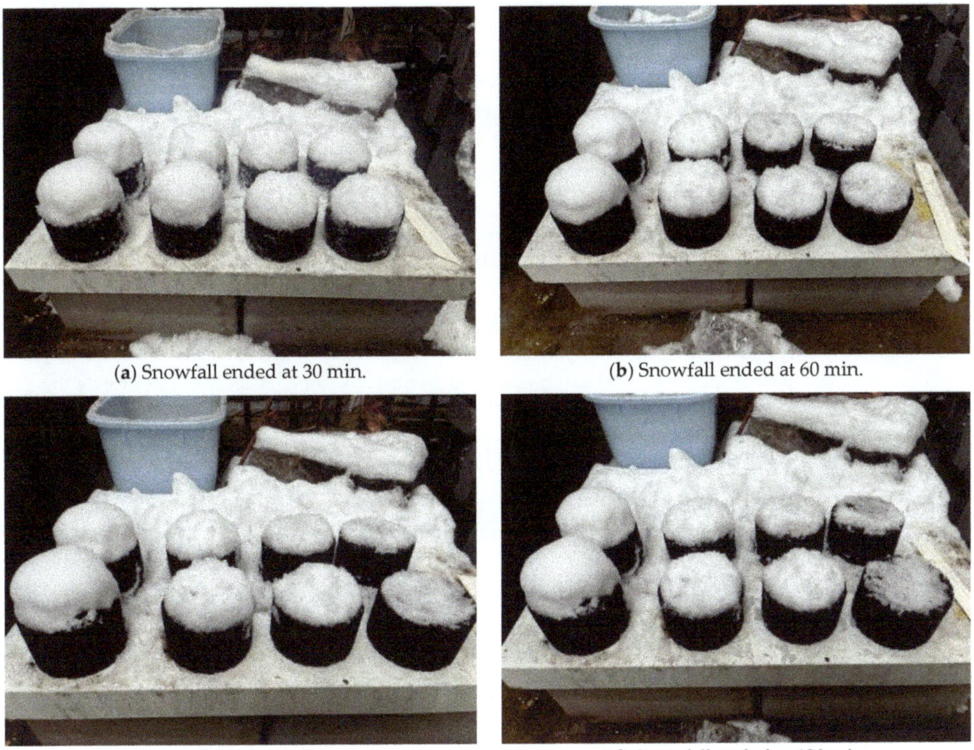

(a) Snowfall ended at 30 min. (b) Snowfall ended at 60 min.

(c) Snowfall ended at 90 min. (d) Snowfall ended at 120 min.

Figure 10. Snow-melting test.

From Figure 10a–d, it can be seen, from left to right, that, with the increase in salt-storing ceramic granule mixing, the amount of snow on the specimen gradually decreases in the 20% dosage of the specimen, with a subtle effect of melting snow; the 60% and 80% dosage specimens' melting snow effect is more significant. As shown in Figure 10, image analysis at t = 120 min demonstrates that the sample with 80% salt-storing ceramsite content exhibits approximately 5% residual snow cover (indicating nearly complete melting), whereas the sample with 20% content retains approximately 80% snow cover. This contrast highlights that higher salt-storing ceramsite content is correlated with enhanced snow-melting capacity. Consequently, the snow-melting rate demonstrates a clear positive correlation with increasing salt-storing ceramsite content, reflecting a significant acceleration in melting efficiency as content rises. In the salt-storing ceramic wear layer mix in the process of snowfall, the initial effect of snow melting is not very apparent, but taking into account the actual road process, under the action of vehicle load, salt will be dissolved into water and the snow-melting effect will improve. In the comprehensive snowfall snow-melting test, it can be concluded that, when mixed, the salt-storing ceramics wear layer mix has a certain snow-melting effect, and at dosages of 40% or higher, the salt-storing ceramic wear layer mix has a more significant ice- and snow-melting effect.

2.3. Infrared Spectral Test Analysis of Salt-Storing Ceramic Granules

Analyzing Figure 11, it can be seen that the infrared spectra of salt-storing ceramic granules before and after being wrapped with polymer-modified cement mortar (slow-release salt-storing ceramic granules) showed an insignificant change in the positions of the wave peaks, but there was a significant change in the areas of the absorption peaks associated with different functional groups [39,40]. The strong and wide absorption peak at wave number 3454 cm^{-1} indicates the presence of an -OH absorption peak in the conjugated state; the absorption peak at 750~700 cm^{-1} indicates that there is a C-Cl group, and the absorption peak at 468 cm^{-1} is determined to be the absorption peak of sodium chloride, indicating that sodium chloride and calcium chloride, the primary snowmelt salts, have adhered to the shale terracotta grains; and the presence of a carboxylate group can be determined by the presence of a C=O bond at 1750~1680, which shows that sodium acetate and calcium acetate have adhered to the shale grains. At the microscopic level, this demonstrates the successful ceramic salt adsorption of snowmelt salts. Located at 2935 cm^{-1}, 2869 cm^{-1}, and 1741 cm^{-1} are three absorption peaks with significantly increased vibration intensities, reflecting the methyl (-CH3-) and methylene (-CH2-) groups, and -C=O increased the number of -CH3- and -CH2- groups, which are often found in a variety of organic compounds and can be introduced into the auxiliary alcohol ester twelve, as well as gel-based silica-propylene emulsion doping caused by the increase in the number of functional groups. The number of functional groups increases. The wave number 1625.31 cm^{-1} is the absorption peak of H_2O, indicating the presence of crystallization water in the material. A clear absorption peak at 799 cm^{-1} is the characteristic absorption peak of the -Si (R) 2O- chain link in organosiloxane, which is the characteristic peak of silicone propylene emulsion. The strong absorption peak at 1043 cm^{-1} corresponds to Si–O–alkyl and Si–O–Si vibrations, which indicates that copolymerization has occurred and suggests that a hydrophobic film has formed due to the action of the silicone–propylene emulsion and the additive alcohol ester XII. This shows that gel-based silicone propylene emulsion completes the hydrophobic modification of cement slurry.

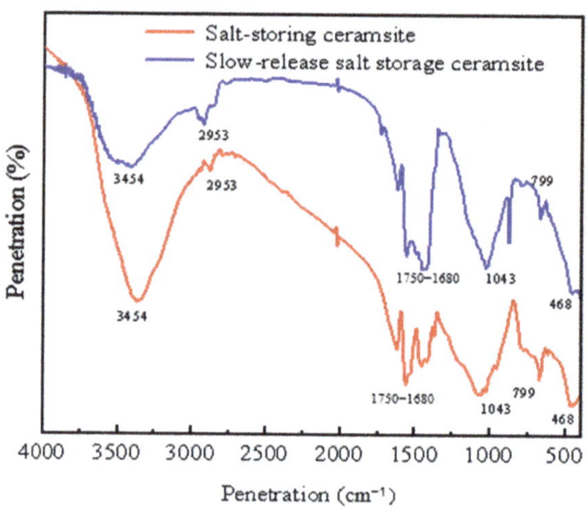

Figure 11. Infrared spectrum of salt-storing ceramsite.

2.4. Characterization of Salt-Storing Ceramic Anti-Slip Wear Layers

The micro-morphology of salt-storing ceramic grains is shown in Figure 12.

The observations obtained from the electron microscope image of the salt-storing ceramic grains in Figure 12a (magnified 1000×) show that the snow-melting salt is attached to the pores of the shale ceramic grains in a relatively uniform distribution, and, in Figure 12b, it can be observed that the snow-melting salt is present in the internal pores of the ceramic grains, and the ceramic grains exhibit better adsorption than the snow-melting salt.

The microscopic morphology of salt-storing ceramic granules wrapped in ordinary cement mortar (0% gel-based silica–propylene emulsion doping) is shown in Figure 13, and that of salt-storing ceramic granules in 6% and 10% gel-based silica–propylene emulsion-modified cement mortar is shown in Figures 14 and 15.

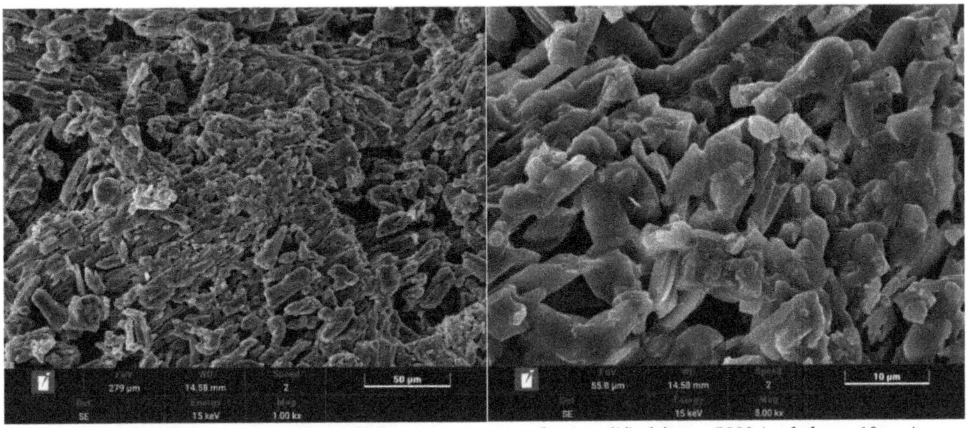

(**a**) Amplified factor 1000 (scale bar = 50 μm) (**b**) Amplified factor 5000 (scale bar = 10 μm)

Figure 12. Two-times zoomed salt-storing ceramsite electron microscope diagram.

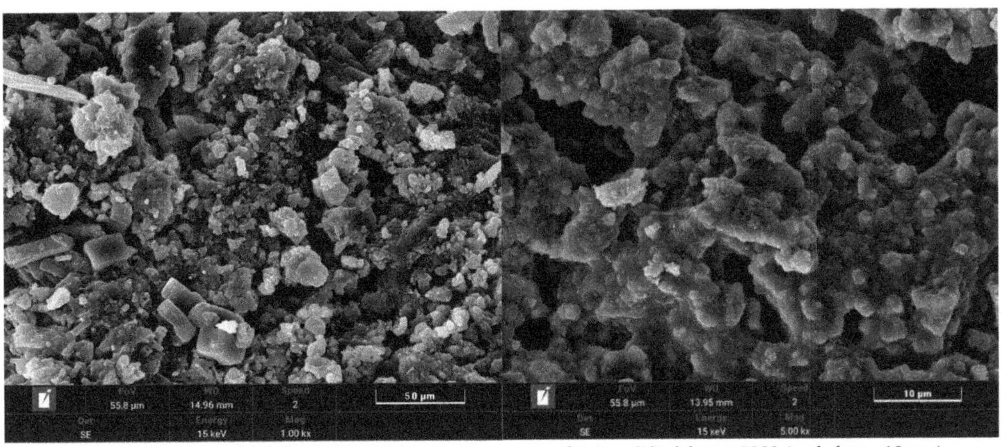

(**a**) Amplified factor 1000 (scale bar = 50 μm) (**b**) Amplified factor 5000 (scale bar = 10 μm)

Figure 13. Silicone acrylic emulsion content is 0%.

From the SEM image of ordinary cement mortar on salt-storing ceramic granules in Figure 13, it can be seen that the structure of the cement mortar wrapping layer without gel-based silica–propylene emulsion doping is relatively rough, and there are a large number of pores on the surface of the wrapping layer; combined with the change in conductivity in the slow-release salt storage ceramic granules in the immersion test (Figure 7) of this paper, the salt release of the slow-release salt-storing ceramic granules with 0% of doping silica–propylene emulsion is faster than that of slow-release salt-storing ceramic granule sdoped with silica–propylene emulsion. The surface roughness of the structural form can be judged using SEM morphology, and the existence of many pores reduces the long-term slow-release performance in water-immersion environments, although the ordinary cement-coating layer can serve a slow-release function in the salt release of the salt-storing grains, and the structural layer on the surface of the slow-release salt-storing grains gradually fails after a long period of immersion, resulting in the rapid release of snow-melting salt and an insufficient slow-release performance.

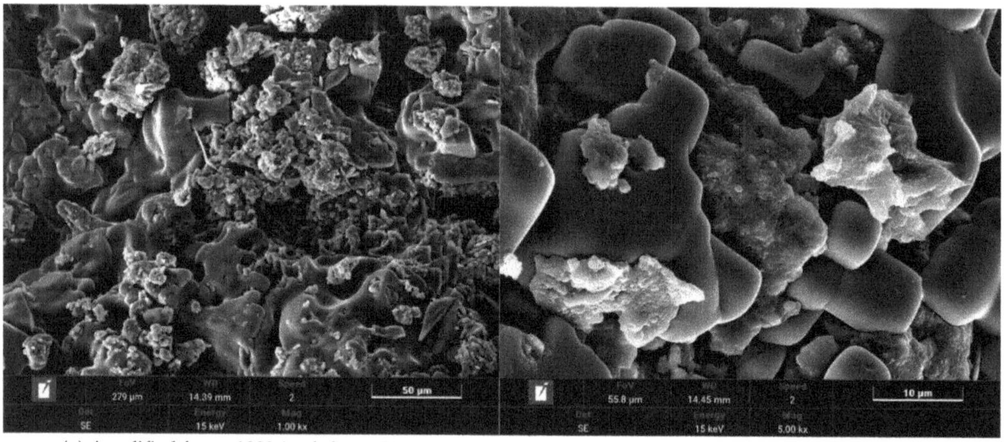

(**a**) Amplified factor 1000 (scale bar = 50 μm) (**b**) Amplified factor 5000 (scale bar = 10 μm)

Figure 14. Silicone acrylic emulsion content is 6%.

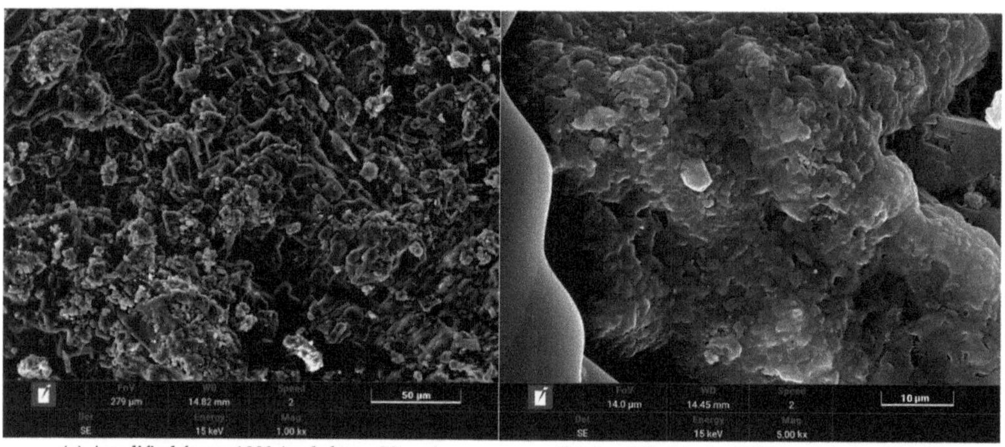

(**a**) Amplified factor 1000 (scale bar = 50 μm) (**b**) Amplified factor 5000 (scale bar = 10 μm)

Figure 15. Silicone acrylic emulsion content is 10%.

A comparative observation of Figure 14, showing 6% gel-based silica–propylene emulsion doping, shows that, with the doping of gel-based silica–propylene emulsion in the cement mortar, the cement mortar layer begins to form a membrane structure, but, as can be seen from Figure 14a, the membrane system is relatively dispersed, and only part of the area is wrapped by the membrane system. In Figure 14b, magnified 5000×, it can be observed that a small number of pores still exist in the slow-release salt-storing ceramic wrapping layer. This is due to the low dosage of silica–propylene emulsion; the amount of membrane formed by the modified cement mortar is too low, resulting in incomplete encapsulation and residual pores, which results in the slow-release salt-storing ceramic particles not reaching optimal performance.

A comparative observation of Figures 15a and 14a shows that, when the dosage of gel-based silica–propylene emulsion is 10%, it can be found that, after more silica–propylene emulsion is added to the cementitious net mortar, the cement mortar structural layer forms a complete membrane, which essentially encapsulates the salt-storing terracotta grains. Observing Figure 15b, it can be seen that the membrane system's structure formed on its surface is more dense and uniform. When the dosage of gel-based silica–propylene emulsion reaches 10%, it is able to form a complete membrane structure on the surface of salt-storing grains. Combined with the conductivity test of different dosages of gel-based silica–propylene emulsion-modified salt-storing ceramic granules in Section 2.2 of this paper, it can be concluded that the membrane structure formed by gel-based silica–propylene emulsion-modified cement mortar effectively improves the impermeability and hydrophobicity of cement mortar layer materials, thus realizing the slow release of snow-melting salt components in salt-storing ceramic granules.

The micro-morphology of the salt-storing ceramic-wear layer mix is shown in Figure 16.

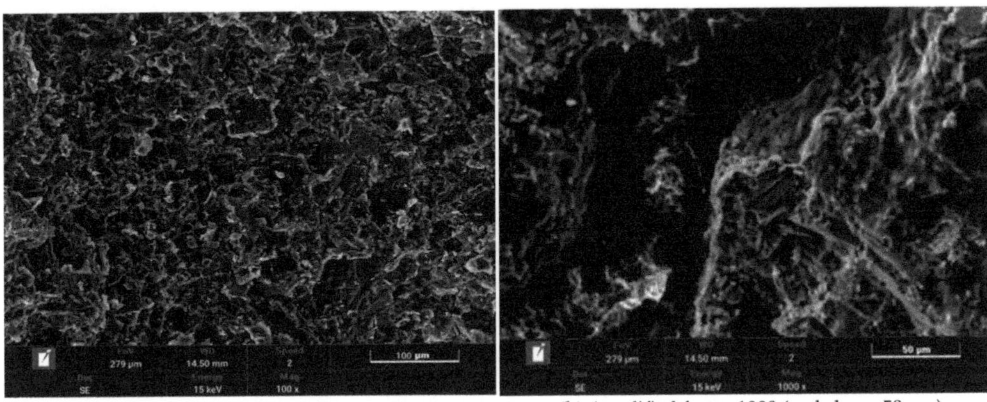

(**a**) Amplified factor 100 (scale bar = 100 μm) (**b**) Amplified factor 1000 (scale bar = 50 μm)

Figure 16. Microscopic topography of salt-storing ceramic-grain-wear layer mixture.

The SMA-10 wear layer mix is formed by the coarse aggregate skeleton, with fine aggregate and asphalt mastic filling the voids, forming a high-density skeleton structure. From the scanning electron microscope image of the salt-storing ceramic grain wear layer mixture in Figure 16a, it can be seen that salt-storing ceramic grains are more uniformly distributed in the mixture, ensuring that the wear layer performs well in melting ice and snow. Voids are present at the mineral–asphalt interface, especially if the bond between ceramic particles and asphalt is not tight and if there is a loose phenomenon. In the 1000× magnified electron microscope image (Figure 16b), it can be clearly seen, in the interface between the mineral material and asphalt transition zone, tha the mineral material surface is bare, and the asphalt shedding phenomenon, visible mineral material, and asphalt mortar bonding force are not enough, and the skeleton still exists in the voids. This indicates that the addition of salt-storing ceramic particles reduces the adhesion between asphalt and mineral material, corresponding to the reduction in road performance of ceramic asphalt mixtures in Section 4.

3. Conclusions

(1) In wear layer type selection SMA-10, with salt-storing ceramic particles of the same size and volume blended into the asphalt mixture, salt-storing ceramic particle dosages of 0%, 20%, 40%, 60%, and 80% corresponded to asphalt mixture oil–stone ratios of 6.2%, 6.4%, 6.8%, 7.2%, and 7.5%, corresponding to the asphalt dosage of the segregation loss rate and the rate of loss of fugitive emissions to meet the specification requirements.

(2) Salt-storing grains have different degrees of increase in dynamic stability, showing a trend of initial increase followed by a decrease; when the salt-storing grains dosage is 40%, the dynamic stability reaches the maximum. With increasing salt-storing ceramic grain content, low-temperature performance, water stability, and anti-skid performance weakened to different degrees; when the salt-storing ceramic grain doping is 80%, the water stability of the wear layer no longer meets the specification requirements. In order to ensure that the active slow-release ice- and snow-melting anti-skid wear layer has good road performance, the dosage of salt-storing ceramic grains should be kept below 60%.

(3) The conductivity results of the wear layer mixture show that the abrasive layer does not affect salt precipitation in the salt-storing granules. With increasing salt-storing granule content, conductivity also increases; the value of the conductivity is still guaranteed to have a fast rate of growth, which can ensure the long-lasting effect of the snow-melting effect. Indoor ice-melting and outdoor snow-melting tests show that, with increasing salt-storing ceramic granule content, the snow-melting effect improves, especially at 60% and 80% dosages. Comprehensive road performance and ice-melting performance analysis determined the recommended range of salt-storing ceramic granule mixing to be from 40% to 60%.

(4) The infrared spectra of salt-storing ceramic grains show that the snow-melting salts, sodium chloride and calcium chloride, are attached to the shale ceramic grains, and the ceramic grains are more successful in the adsorption of snow-melting salts. The incorporation of auxiliary alcohol ester XII and gel-based silica–propylene emulsion caused an increase in the number of functional groups, and gel-based silica–propylene emulsion and auxiliary alcohol ester XII formed a hydrophobic film, indicating that the gel-based silica–propylene emulsion completed the hydrophobic modification of the cement mortar.

(5) Through the analysis of the micro-morphological map of the salt-storing ceramic particles and the coating layer, the distribution of snow-melting salts in the pores of the ceramic particles is relatively uniform, and when the dosage of gel-based silica–propylene emulsion reaches 10%, it forms a complete membrane structure on the surface of the salt-storing ceramic particles to realize the slow-release effect of the snow-melting salt components in the salt-storing ceramic particles. Through the analysis of the micromorphological image of the salt-storing ceramic asphalt mixture, it was found that voids exist at the interface between mineral and asphalt; in particular, the ceramic and asphalt bonding is not closed, and there is a loose phenomenon. The incorporation of ceramic particles reduces the bonding force between asphalt minerals, leading to a decrease in the road performance of ceramic asphalt mixtures.

(6) Compared to commercial de-icing methods (e.g., salt-spreading or electrically heated pavements), the gel-modified salt-storing pavement layer delivers persistent snow-melting without external energy, thus reducing salt usage, maintenance costs, and temperature-induced structural stress.

4. Materials and Methods

4.1. Asphalt and Natural Aggregate

The SBS I-D modified asphalt, provided by Shandong High-speed Construction Materials Co., Ltd. (Jinan, Shandong Province, China), was used in the test, and the basic performance of the modified asphalt was determined according to the 'Highway Engineering Asphalt and Asphalt Mixture Test Procedures' (JTG E20-2011) [37]. The technical indicators are listed in Table 3.

The coarse aggregate used in the experimental study was basalt and self-made salt-storing ceramsite (a porous shale aggregate impregnated with de-icing salts) provided by Zhengzhou Zhengfa Municipal Construction Co., Ltd. (Zhengzhou, Henan Province,

China), and the filler used was ground limestone powder. According to the specification requirements, the indexes were tested in strict accordance with the 'Highway Engineering Aggregate Test Procedure' (JTG E42-2005) [41]. The technical indexes of natural aggregate used in the experimental study are shown in Table 4.

Table 3. Basic performance specifications of SBS I-D modified asphalt.

Pilot Project	Unit	Test Result
Penetration (25 °C, 100 g, 5 s)	0.1 mm	56
Ductility (5 cm/min, 5 °C)	cm	32
Softening point (TR&B)/°C	°C	78

Table 4. Test results of aggregate physical properties.

Performance Index	5~10 mm Crushed Stone	3~5 mm Crushed Stone	3~5 mm Silicone-Acrylic Emulsion Modified Cement Salt Storage Ceramsite	Fine Aggregate
Losangeles wore value (%)	15.1	-	-	-
Apparent specific gravity (g/cm^3)	2.945	2.932	1.503	2.724
Relative density of bulk volume (g/cm^3)	2.829	2.818	-	-
Water absorption (%)	0.52	0.55	8.3	-
Compressive strength of concrete cylinder (MPa)	-	-	7.3	-

According to the test procedure [42], the basic properties of ore powder were tested, and the results are shown in Table 5.

Table 5. Main technical index of mineral powder.

Pilot Project	Unit	Test Result	Standard Requires
Apparent density	t/m^3	2.726	≥2.50
Moisture content	%	0.2	≤1
Particle size range < 0.6 mm	%	100	100
<0.15 mm	%	96.8	90–100
<0.075 mm	%	86.5	75–100
Hydrophilic coefficient	—	0.56	<1.0

Fiber plays the role of adsorption, dispersion, stiffening, and toughening in SMA mixtures. In this paper, lignin fiber was selected, and the content was set at 0.4%. The technical properties are shown in Table 6.

Table 6. Technical index of lignin fiber.

Test Items	Unit	Specification Requirement	Test Result	Test Method
Fiber length	mm	≤6	<6	Observation of aqueous solution by microscope
Ash content	%	18 ± 5	18.5	After burning at a high temperature of 590~600 °C, the residue was determined
PH value	—	7.5 ± 1.0	7.7	PH meter measurement
Moisture content	%	≤5	0.3	It was heated in a 105 °C oven for 2 h and then cooled and weighed

4.2. Preparation of the Slow-Release Salt-Storing Ceramsite

In this experiment, salt-storing ceramsite was prepared using salt-soaking adsorption. Shale ceramsite with a particle size of 3–5 mm was selected and immersed in a saturated composite snow-melting salt solution at a temperature of 60 °C for 12 h. The optimum content of surfactant PEG-400 was 3%; the present study selected a silicon-acrylic emulsion-based gel material with the best modification effect and determined the silicon–acrylic emulsion dosage in the cement paste to be 10%. The following unified expression is silicone–acrylic emulsion-modified cement paste. The composition and technical properties of the raw materials are shown in Table 7.

Table 7. Technical index of raw materials.

Number	Type	Material	Technology Index
1	Gel material	Silicone-acrylic emulsion	Orchid milky liquid, 45% mass fraction of total solid content, PH value: 8.36, glass transition temperature 25 °C, silicone content 11.2%
2	Additives	Alcohol ester twelve	Colorless transparent liquid, no insoluble matter
3	Surfactant	PEG-400	Colorless transparent liquid, PH value: 6.23, viscosity: 83.5 MPa·s
4	Sustained-release materials	Cement	The strength grade is 42.5, the standard consistency water consumption is 25.7, the specific surface area is 343 m^2/kg, the initial setting time is 177 min, and the final setting time is 239 min

First of all, 3–5 mm shale grains were pre-washed and pre-treated to remove the dust and impurities in the pores of the shale grains, which were put into the oven with the temperature adjusted to 100 °C for drying and sparing. Take 500 mL of de-distilled water in a beaker and place it on a magnetic stirrer. The temperature was set to 60 °C; sodium acetate, calcium acetate, sodium chloride, and calcium chloride were added in a 31%:20%:24%:25% ratio and stirred until the solution became saturated; 3% (equivalent to the quality of the ceramic grains) surfactant (PEG-400) was slowly added to the saturated composite snow-melting salt solution, and 500 g of shale grains were then added, soaked for 12 h, removed, and dried for later use.

The specific steps for the slow-release modification of salt-storing ceramic granules are as follows: (1) weigh 400 g of dry salt-storing ceramic granules in a clean tray; (2) mix the polymer emulsions, cement, water, and additives according to specified proportions, and add them to the cement mortar mixing pot and mix, and then mix for 2–3 min to form a cement slurry; (3) add salt-storing ceramic granules to the mixing pot, and then mix for 2 min to perform the slow-release coating of salt-storing ceramic granules; (4) spread the coated granules evenly in a tray and keep for 24 h at room temperature, and then place them in a standard curing environment to complete hardening; and (5) spread the coated salt-storing ceramic granules evenly in a tray and allow them to cure at room temperature for 24 h, and then cure them in a standard environment for 28 days.

In order to determine the optimal dosage of the slow-release treatment agent (silica–propylene emulsion), the test was conducted using modified cement slurry with silica–propylene emulsion dosages of 0%, 6%, 8%, 10%, 12%, and 14% to coat the salt-storing ceramic granules. In total, 400 g of ceramic granules were used, and the cement mass was set to half the mass of the ceramic granules of each group of samples, and the additive used in the silica–propylene emulsion was alcohol ester twelve with a dosage of 6% relative to the emulsion's solid content; the material dosages used in the test are listed in Table 8.

Table 8. Different polymer content per modified cement paste ratio.

Polymer Emulsion Content (%)	Quality of Polymer Emulsion (g)	Additive Dosage (g)	Cement (g)	Water (g)
0	0	0	200	80
6	12	0.72	200	80
8	16	0.96	200	80
10	20	1.2	200	80
12	24	1.44	200	80
14	28	1.68	200	80

Different dosages of silica–propylene emulsion-modified cement mortar significantly wrapped slow-release salt-storing ceramic granules were placed in a standard curing environment for 7 days and 28 days, in reference to the relevant requirements of 'Lightweight Aggregates and Their Test Methods' (GB/T 17431.2-2010) [43]. Samples were tested for cylindrical compressive strength after 7 and 28 days of curing; the relationship between silica–propylene emulsion dosage and cylindrical compressive strength of the slow-release salt-storing ceramic granules is shown in Figure 17.

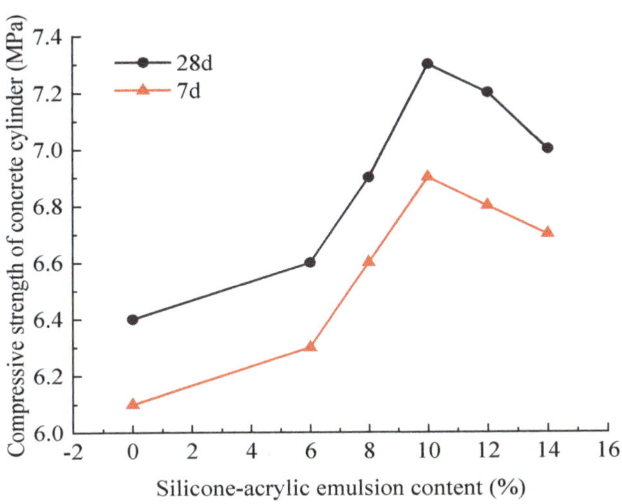

Figure 17. The cylinder compressive strength of salt-storing ceramsite after coating.

From the curves in Figure 17, it can be seen that the cylindrical compressive strength of slow-release salt-storing ceramic granules cured for 7 and 28 days shows a trend of an initial increase followed by a decrease with increasing silica–propylene emulsion dosage. The 7-day and 28-day compressive strengths of the test group with silica–propylene emulsion-modified cement mortar are higher than those of the test group without the emulsion, indicating that the silica–propylene emulsion-modified cement coating effectively improves the compressive strength of the ceramic granules with slow-release salt storage. Comparing the 7-day and 28-day results, compressive strength increases with curing time, especially in groups with higher silica–propylene emulsion content. When the silica–propylene emulsion dosage is 10%, the 7-day and 28-day compressive strengths of the salt-storing granules reach their maximum values. The 7-day and 28-day compressive strengths of the salt-storing ceramic granules with a dosage of 10% increased by 13.1% and 14.1%, respectively, compared to the granules wrapped in the 0% (control) group. Therefore, regarding the effect of silica–propylene emulsion-modified cement slurry on the mechanical properties of salt-storing ceramic granules, the optimal dosage of silica–propylene emulsion is 10%.

The test was conducted using an immersion dissolution method on granule samples coated with different dosages of silica–propylene emulsion-modified cement mortar; 100 g of slow-release salt-storing granule samples with different dosages of silica–propylene emulsion was taken and immersed in the same mass of water. A DDSA-308A digital conductivity meter was used to record the numerical conversion of the conductivity to measure the short-term conductivity of the salt-storing ceramic granules, and, after 4 h of testing, the conductivity was measured every 24 h to monitor long-term changes in the salt-storing ceramic granules; the results of the short-term conductivity test of the salt-storing ceramic granules are shown in Figure 18a, and the results of the long-term conductivity test are shown in Figure 18b.

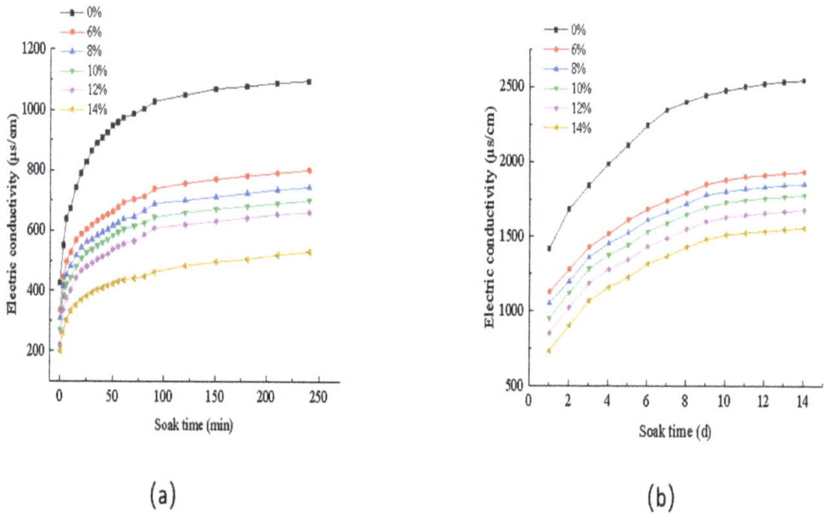

Figure 18. Short-term (**a**) and long-term (**b**) conductivity change in slow-release salt storage ceramsite.

Comparing Figures 18a and 18b, by analyzing the short- and long-term conductivity curves of the salt-storing grains, the salt-release rates across test groups with different silica–propylene emulsion dosages are generally consistent, and, after comparing the conductivity trends at different emulsion dosages, it is found that conductivity decreases as silica–propylene emulsion dosage increases, indicating that the silica–propylene emulsion-modified cement mortar acts as a slow-release coating for salt-storing grains, but the dosage of 14% silica-propylene emulsion is slower than that of other dosages of silica-propylene emulsion, indicating that excessive silica–propylene emulsion dosage may hinder salt release from the salt-storing grains.

By observing the conductivity curves for 6%, 8%, 10%, and 12% dosages, it was concluded that the slow-release performance of the salt-storing ceramic granules increased with the increase in the dosage of silica–propylene emulsion in the cement slurry, and the slopes of the long-term and short-term conductivity curves of each group did not show any significant changes in the soaking cycle. In terms of the salt release rate, the higher the dosage of silica–propylene emulsion, the slower the change in the conductivity of the solution, indicating that salt-storing silica–propylene emulsion-modified cement slurry effectively controls salt release from the ceramic granules. Combined with the test of compression strength of salt-storing grains after being coated with silica–propylene emulsion-modified cement slurry, the optimal dosage of silica–propylene emulsion in the cement slurry was determined to be 10%.

4.3. Preparation of the Active Slow-Release Melting Ice and Snow Anti-Skid Wear Layer

The test adopts SMA-10 as the wear layer gradation, and a Marshall test was conducted to evaluate the effect of salt-storing ceramic granule dosage on the asphalt aggregate ratio of the wear layer mixture; the results of the oil–rock ratio of each dosing are shown in Table 9.

Table 9. Optimum mixture ratio of different ceramide content.

Ceramsite Content (%)	0	20	40	60	80
Optimal asphalt content (%)	6.2	6.4	6.8	7.2	7.5

The optimum asphalt content was verified using the Schellenberg drainage test and the Fort Kentucky fly-away loss test, the results of which are shown in Tables 10 and 11.

Table 10. Leakage test results.

Salt Storage Ceramsite Content (%)	Technology Index	Test Result	Test Method
0	≤0.1	0.045	T 0732
20		0.050	
40		0.053	
60		0.059	
80		0.068	

Table 11. Flying test results.

Salt Storage Ceramsite Content (%)	Technology Index	Test Result	Test Method
0	≤15	4.3	T 0733
20		6.8	
40		7.5	
60		9.3	
80		11.5	

The test results in Tables 10 and 11 show that the results of the segregation leakage test and fly-away test of salt-accumulating ceramic granules in mixes with different volume dosages meet the requirements of the specification [38].

4.4. Road Performance Test

In this test, evaluations of high-temperature stability, low-temperature crack resistance, water stability, anti-slip performance, and permeability were conducted on active slow-release ice- and snow-melting anti-slip wear layers containing different dosages of salt-storing ceramic granules.

(1) Five rutted plate specimens with different salt-storing ceramic granule dosages were molded and held at 60 °C for 4 h during rutting tests to evaluate their high-temperature stability.

(2) Wear layer trabecular specimens were placed in a constant-temperature chamber at -10 ± 0.5 °C for 5 h, and a low-temperature trabecular bending test was conducted using a universal testing machine to evaluate their low-temperature stability performance.

(3) Five types of salt-storing ceramsite asphalt mixtures were formed into two groups of Marshall specimens, with each group consisting of four samples. The first group was immersed in a constant-temperature water tank at 60 °C for 30 min, and the second group was immersed in a constant-temperature water tank at 60 °C for 48 h. The immersion Marshall test was carried out. The test group was vacuum-saturated using a maximum theoretical density device and then placed in a 25 °C water bath for 20 min. The Marshall specimen was loaded into a plastic bag and added to 10 mL of water after sealing. It was placed in a −18 °C low-temperature test chamber for freezing for 17 h. After freezing, it was placed in a 25 °C constant-temperature water bath for 3 h after the stability test. In the control group, a splitting test was performed after soaking at 25 °C for 3 h, and the water stability was comprehensively evaluated.

(4) The sand-paving method was used to determine the construction depth of different salt-storing ceramic granule mixes with different dosages of ice-melting and snow-melting anti-skid wear layer mixes, and the BM-III pendulum friction coefficient tester was used to study the anti-skidding performance of rutted slabs of slow-release salt-storing ceramic granule asphalt mixtures.

(5) Permeability tests were conducted on the rutted asphalt mixture slabs with different dosages of salt-storing ceramic granules to evaluate their permeability performance.

4.5. Active Slow-Release Melting Ice and Snow Anti-Skid Wear Layer Melting Ice in the Snow Effect Test

In order to investigate the ice- and snow-melting performance of the slow-release salt-storing ceramic anti-skid wear layer, specimens with different volume fractions (0%, 20%, 40%, 60%, and 80%) of slow-release salt-storing ceramic particles were tested using a wear layer mixture conductivity test, indoor ice-melting test, and outdoor snow-melting test. The test results were used to analyze the effect of different doping levels of slow-release salt-storing ceramic particles on the ice- and snow-melting capacities of the wear layer and road performance to determine the optimal doping of salt-storing ceramic particles on the active melting of ice and snow on the anti-skid wear layer.

4.5.1. Conductivity Test

In this section, Marshall specimens were immersed, and solution conductivity was measured using a conductivity meter; the more snowmelt salt that was dissolved and released per unit time, the higher the conductivity. The salt concentration was estimated by measuring the change in conductivity of the immersed solution, the numerical change in the conductivity meter was continuously recorded during the test, and, after 4 h of testing, the conductivity of the solution supernatant was measured every other day, with theshort-term and long-term conductivity being measured, respectively.

4.5.2. Indoor Ice-Melting Test Trials

Referring to the ice-melting rate test in 'Ice and snow melting materials for highway asphalt mixture' (JT/T 1210.2-2018) [38], the ability of salts to melt ice and snow was evaluated. First, Marshall specimens were prepared based on the asphalt mix design. A glass dish with a diameter of 100 mm and a height of 20 mm was filled with water and frozen at a temperature of −18 °C for 24 h to ensure complete freezing of the water. Meanwhile, the Marshall specimens were conditioned in an oven at −5 °C for 4 h. The ice in the glass dish was removed, immediately placed on the surface of the specimen, and then both placed at a constant temperature of −5 °C for 2 h, and the remaining mass of the ice and dish was measured at 10 min intervals. The remaining masses of the specimen types in the test were salt-storing ceramic wearing course asphalt mixtures (SMA-10) with dosages of 0%, 20%, 40%, 60%, and 80%, and two specimens were selected for each group of samples to perform the parallel test.

4.5.3. Outdoor Snow-Melting Tests

Marshall specimens with different dosages of salt-storing ceramic granules were used to simulate road conditions and were placed outdoors during rain and snow conditions to observe their snow-melting effects. Marshall specimens with varying dosages were tested simultaneously for comparison; each group used two specimens, arranged from left to right in the order of 0%, 20%, 40%, 60%, and 80% salt-storing ceramic granule content, to observe the different melting times of the Marshall specimens on top of the snow melting, as well as to analyze the ice- and snow-melting performance.

4.6. Infrared Spectroscopy Test

A VERTEX70 Fourier Transform Infrared (FTIR) spectrometer (provided by Shanghai Erdi Instrument Technology Co., Ltd. in Shanghai, China) was used in this experiment. Samples consisted of slow-release salt-storing ceramic granules wrapped with silica–propylene emulsion-modified cement mortar prepared by grinding both types of salt-storing ceramic granules into powder and mixing them with potassium bromide (KBr) in a ratio of 1:100, and then using infrared spectroscopic test presses to prepare presses with good transparency; the infrared spectra were subsequently scanned.

4.7. Scanning Electron Microscope Test

In this experiment, a field emission scanning electron microscope (FESEM), model JSM-7500F, was used to observe the microscopic morphology of salt-storing ceramic particles, salt-accumulated ceramic particles wrapped with modified cement mortar with 0%, 6%, and 10% silicone-propylene (SP) emulsion, and abrasive-layer mixtures containing salt-storing ceramic particles. The distribution of snowmelt salt in the ceramic granules, the morphology of the modified cement mortar coating layer with silicone–propylene emulsion, and the microstructure of the salt-storing ceramic asphalt mixtures were analyzed using the obtained micrographs.

Author Contributions: Y.C.: Conceptualization, Investigation, Project administration, Supervision, Writing—Review and Editing. Z.L.: Conceptualization, Formal analysis, Methodology, Visualization. T.G.: Supervision, Project administration, Data curation, Formal analysis. C.F.: Conceptualization, Writing—Original Draft, Supervision, Investigation. P.G.: Conceptualization, Supervision, Writing—Original Draft. C.W.: Conceptualization, Project administration, Supervision, Investigation. B.B.: Funding acquisition, Investigation. W.Z.: Funding acquisition, Investigation. H.Y.: Project administration, Resources. Q.C.: Project administration, Resources. All authors have read and agreed to the published version of the manuscript.

Funding: This work was supported by a planned project supported by the science and technology innovation team of the universities and colleges in Henan province (24IRTSTHN011); the Central Plains Science and Technology Innovation Leader Project (244200510031); Key scientific and technological projects in Henan province (252102240031); and the special plan for service industry development of key scientific research projects in colleges and universities in Henan Province (25CY022).

Institutional Review Board Statement: Not applicable.

Informed Consent Statement: Not applicable.

Data Availability Statement: The authors confirm that the data supporting the findings of this study are available within the article.

Conflicts of Interest: The authors declare no conflicts of interest.

References

1. Tan, Y.Q.; Li, J.L.; Xu, H.N. Review on Friction Characteristics and Operation Risk Intelligent Management of Ice and Snow Pavement. *China J. Highw. Transp.* **2022**, *35*, 1–17.
2. Wang, Q.S. The optimization design of ultra-thin anti-skid wear layer structure composition. *J. China Foreign Highw.* **2017**, *37*, 254–257.
3. Guan, B.W.; Xue, X.J.; Meng, J.D. Evaluation of road performance and skid resistance of ultra-thin wear layer using calcined bauxite aggregate. *J. Chang. Univ. (Nat. Sci. Ed.)* **2022**, *42*, 10–19.
4. Liu, H.; Wang, Z.; Yang, C.; Chen, S.; Yu, H.; Huang, T.; Li, X.; You, Z. Effect of coarse aggregate characteristics on skid resistance deterioration of the ultrathin wearing course. *J. Mater. Civil. Eng.* **2021**, *33*, 04021051. [CrossRef]
5. Lv, H.; Ma, R.; Guo, R.; Wang, Z.; Xia, Z. Study on effectiveness evaluation of ice melting and snow melting of high elastic salt storage asphalt pavement. In Proceedings of the Fourth International Conference on Optoelectronic Science and Materials (ICOSM 2022), SPIE, Hefei, China, 16–18 September 2022; Volume 12553, pp. 78–85.
6. Gao, Y. Material Composition Design and Performance Study of Slow-Release Anti-icing Fog Seal. Master's Thesis, Chongqing Jiaotong University, Chongqing, China, 2020.
7. Jiangmiao, Y.U.; Fuda, C.H.E.N.; Xinyan, P.E.N.G.; Guohua, L.I.U.; Ke, D.E.N.G.; Xianshu, Y.U.; Junhua, L.I. High-toughness, ultra-thin friction course for the channel on the Zhuhai artificial island of the Hong Kong-Zhuhai-Macao Bridge. *J. Tsinghua Univ. Sci. Technol.* **2020**, *60*, 48–56.
8. Yu, J.; Chen, F.; Deng, W.; Ma, Y.; Yu, H. Design and performance of high-toughness ultra-thin friction course in south China. *Constr. Build. Mater.* **2020**, *246*, 118508. [CrossRef]
9. Yu, J.; Yang, N.; Chen, F.; Chen, Y.; Lin, Z.; Yu, H. Design of cold-mixed high-toughness ultra-thin asphalt layer towards sustainable pavement construction. *Buildings* **2021**, *11*, 619. [CrossRef]
10. He, S.; Gao, L.; Guo, C.; Wu, X. Fatigue performance of steel slag smc ultrathin abrasive layer under strain controlling mode. *Math. Probl. Eng.* **2022**, *2022*, 1017425. [CrossRef]
11. Ding, L.; Wang, X.; Zhang, K.; Zhang, M.; Yang, J.; Chen, Z. Durability evaluation of easy compaction and high-durability ultra-thin overlay. *Constr. Build. Mater.* **2021**, *302*, 124407. [CrossRef]
12. Xie, J.; Chen, J.; Hu, L.; Wu, S.; Wang, Z.; Li, M.; Yang, C. Preparation, thermochromic properties and temperature controlling ability of novel pellets in ultra-thin wearing course. *Constr. Build. Mater.* **2023**, *389*, 131797. [CrossRef]
13. Gao, J.; Zhang, Z.; Han, Z.; Sha, A.; Wang, Z.; Wei, J. A Review of Electromagnetic Wave Absorbing Materials Used in Microwave Deicing Pavement. *Mater. Rev.* **2016**, *30*, 87–95.
14. Liu, Z.S.; Wu, S.B.; Liu, P.F.; Hu, G. Review on Functional Features of Conductive Asphalt Concrete. *Mater. Rev.* **2017**, *31* (Suppl. S1), 374–378+387.
15. Liu, Z.M.; Chen, H.X.; Dou, H.B.; Wang, Y.; Niu, D. Snowmelt Performance of Ultra Thin Saline and Self-Melted Asphalt Mixture. *Bull. Chin. Ceram. Soc.* **2017**, *36*, 262–268.
16. Zhang, L.; Zhao, F.Q. Review of research on the effeet of salt storage deicing material on the preformance of asphalt mixture. *Chem. Ind. Eng. Prog.* **2018**, *37*, 2282–2294.
17. Yu, J.; Yang, N.; Yu, H. Research and application status of high-performance asphalt ultra-thin wearing layer technology. *J. Cent. South Univ. (Sci. Technol.)* **2021**, *52*, 2287–2298.
18. Ma, T.; Geng, L.; Ding, X.; Zhang, D.; Huang, X. Experimental study of deicing asphalt mixture with anti-icing additives. *Constr. Build. Mater.* **2016**, *127*, 653–662. [CrossRef]
19. Cao, L.T.; Guo, S.B.; Lv, X.S.; Chen, S.J. Analysis on Influence of Salt on Antifreezing Asphalt Mixture. *Maint. Constr. Mach.* **2013**, *30*, 72–74.
20. Wu, S.; Yang, J.; Yang, R.; Zhu, J.; Liu, S.; Wang, C. Investigation of microscopic air void structure of anti-freezing asphalt pavement with X-ray CT and MIP. *Constr. Build. Mater.* **2018**, *178*, 473–483. [CrossRef]
21. Sun, D.H. Study on Typical Gradation and Residual Life Prediction Low Freezing Point Ultra-Thin Wear Layers with Considering Anti-Freezing Ice Ability. Master's Thesis, Harbin Institute of Technology, Harbin, China, 2021.
22. Liu, Y. Study on the Application of Slow-release Anticoagulant Ice Material in Ultra-thin Wear Layer. Master's Thesis, Chongqing Jiaotong University, Chongqing, China, 2021.
23. Liu, Z.; Chen, S.; He, R.; Xing, M.; Bai, Y.; Dou, H. Investigation on the properties of asphalt mixtures containing antifreeze fillers. *J. Mater. Civil. Eng.* **2015**, *27*, 04014180. [CrossRef]
24. Chen, X. Pavement performance of asphalt emulsion and asphalt mixture with ultra-thin cover snow melting agent. *J. Chang. Univ. Sci. Technol. (Nat. Sci.)* **2018**, *15*, 8–13.
25. Wu, C.; Gao, D.; Shangguan, H.; Chen, R.; Hou, C. Phase-Change/Salt-Based Slow-Release Composite Material for Anti-Icing and Snow-Melting. *Buildings* **2024**, *14*, 2177. [CrossRef]

26. Liu, Z.; Li, B.; Yao, T.; Sun, M.; Wang, Y.; Niu, L.; Du, Y. Optimization of slow-release salt storage snowmelt aggregate preparation process and its slow-release performance based on response surface methodology-orthogonal test. *Constr. Build. Mater.* **2024**, *449*, 138356. [CrossRef]
27. Yang, Y.; Chen, G.; Yang, Y.; Yue, L.; Xu, J. Advances in salt-storage materials, road and anti-freezing performances of salt-storage asphalt mixture: A review. *Coatings* **2022**, *12*, 1323. [CrossRef]
28. Han, H.; Cui, S.; Lu, Y.; Zhao, P.; Zou, X. Preparation of Salt-Storage Aggregate using Magnesium Oxychloride Cement and Investigation on Salt-Release Performance. *J. Eng. Sci. Technol. Rev.* **2024**, *17*, 71–77. [CrossRef]
29. Roig-Flores, M.; Lucio-Martin, T.; Alonso, M.C.; Guerreiro, L. Evolution of thermo-mechanical properties of concrete with calcium aluminate cement and special aggregates for energy storage. *Cem. Concr. Res.* **2021**, *141*, 106323. [CrossRef]
30. Xu, K.; Chen, Z.; Xiao, H.; Zhu, M.; Wang, Z. Heat Transfer Characteristics of Electrical Heating Deicing and Snow-Melting Asphalt Pavement Under Different Operating Conditions. *Coatings* **2025**, *15*, 367. [CrossRef]
31. Zhang, W.; Dong, S.; Song, Z.; Ding, S.; Yi, J.; Han, B. Snow-melting performance and application method of stainless steel wires-modified conductive asphalt concrete based on electrothermal conversion. *Appl. Therm. Eng.* **2025**, *269*, 126066. [CrossRef]
32. Wang, Y.; Li, Y.; Hu, W.; Xiao, R.; Zhou, H.; Huang, B. Electrically conductive hot mix asphalt mixtures for salt-free snow/ice-melting pavements heated with direct electric energy: A comparison between utilizing carbon-based aggregate and fiber. *J. Clean. Prod.* **2025**, *489*, 144738. [CrossRef]
33. Xu, K.; Chen, Z.; Xiao, H.; Zheng, L.; Wang, J. Analysis of entransy dissipation thermal resistance and heat transfer efficiency of electrical heating snow-melting pavement. *Therm. Sci. Eng. Progress* **2025**, *61*, 103551. [CrossRef]
34. Du, W.; Wang, Q.; Li, Y.; Wang, X.-N.; Liu, X.-C.; Wang, Y.-M.; Li, J. Performances of asphalt mastic incorporating with a home-made sustained-releasing salt storage additive. *Case Stud. Constr. Mater.* **2025**, *22*, e04114. [CrossRef]
35. Meng, Y.; Meng, F.; Chen, J.; Wang, Z.; Li, Y.; Deng, S.; Wei, X.; Gou, C. Preparation of slow-release biologically active anti-icing filler and study on the anti-icing long-lasting performance. *Constr. Build. Mater.* **2024**, *416*, 135150. [CrossRef]
36. He, Z.; Xie, H.; Jamil, M.I.; Li, T.; Zhang, Q. Electro-/Photo-Thermal Promoted Anti-Icing Materials: A New Strategy Combined with Passive Anti-Icing and Active De-Icing. *Adv. Mater. Interfaces* **2022**, *9*, 2200275. [CrossRef]
37. *JTG E20-2011*; Standard Test Methods of Bitumen and Bituminous Mixtures for Highway Engineering. China Communication Press: Beijing, China, 2011.
38. *JT/T 1210.2-2018*; Deicing and Thawy Material Used in Asphalt Mixture-Part 2: Sainization-Based Material. China Communication Press: Beijing, China, 2018.
39. Pretsch, E.; Clerc, T.; Seibl, J.; Simon, W. *Tables of Spectral Data for Structure Determination of Organic Compounds*; Springer Science & Business Media: Berlin/Heidelberg, Germany, 2013.
40. Badertscher, M.; Bühlmann, P.; Pretsch, E. *Structure Determination of Organic Compounds: Tables of Spectral Data*; Springer: Berlin/Heidelberg, Germany, 2009.
41. *JTG E42-2005*; Test Methods of Aggregate for Highway Engineering. China Communication Press: Beijing, China, 2005.
42. *JTG F40-2004*; Tehnical Specifications for Construction of Highway Asphalt Pavements. China Communication Press: Beijing, China, 2004.
43. *GB/T 17431.1-2010*; Lightweight Aggregates and Its Test Methods Part 2: Test Methods for Lightweight Aggregates. Standards Press of China: Beijing, China, 2010.

gels

MDPI

Article

Bio-Gel Formation Through Enzyme-Induced Carbonate Precipitation for Dust Control in Yellow River Silt

Jingwei Zhang [1], Hualing Jia [1], Jia Li [2,*], Xuanyu Chen [3], Lei Wang [1], Shilong Wang [4] and Lin Liu [4]

1 School of Civil Engineering, Zhengzhou University, Zhengzhou 450001, China; zhangjingwei@zzu.edu.cn (J.Z.); jhl969517830@163.com (H.J.); lwang029@zzu.edu.cn (L.W.)
2 School of Water Conservancy and Transportation, Zhengzhou University, Zhengzhou 450001, China
3 School of Transportation, Southeast University, Nanjing 211189, China; cxyyes@163.com
4 Zhengzhou City Construction Group Investment Co., Ltd., Zhengzhou 450007, China; 24384002@163.com (S.W.); 524175404@163.com (L.L.)
* Correspondence: lijia@zzu.edu.cn

Abstract: This study explored the enzymatic formation of gel-like polymeric matrices through carbonate precipitation for dust suppression in Yellow River silt. The hydrogel-modified EICP method effectively enhanced the compressive strength and resistance to wind–rain erosion by forming a reinforced bio-cemented crust. The optimal cementation solution, consisting of urea and $CaCl_2$ at equimolar concentrations of 1.25 mol/L, was applied to improve $CaCO_3$ precipitation uniformity. A spraying volume of 4 L/m^2 (first urea-$CaCl_2$ solution, followed by urease solution) yielded a 14.9 mm thick hybrid gel-$CaCO_3$ crust with compressive strength exceeding 752 kPa. SEM analysis confirmed the synergistic interaction between $CaCO_3$ crystals and the gel matrix, where the hydrogel network acted as a nucleation template, enhancing crystal bridging and pore-filling efficiency. XRD analysis further supported the formation of a stable gel-$CaCO_3$ composite structure, which exhibited superior resistance to wind–rain erosion and mechanical wear. These findings suggest that gel-enhanced EICP represents a novel bio-gel composite technology for sustainable dust mitigation in silt soils.

Keywords: EICP; dust control; wind and rain resistance; wear resistance; bio-cemented crust

1. Introduction

The soil composition in the alluvial plains of the Yellow River in China mainly consists of silt, characterized by low water stability and challenging compaction, leading to the easy generation of dust during construction activities, thereby posing a substantial threat to air quality [1]. The main source of dust generation is construction sites (refer to Figure 1), including exposed surfaces, open earth stacking, and delayed road surface hardening. Conventional dust suppression techniques such as water sprinkling, dust inhibitors, and dustproof nets exhibit specific drawbacks, including their temporary effectiveness [2,3], stringent application requirements [4], and the potential for inducing secondary pollution.

Gels 2025, 11, 452

https://doi.org/10.3390/gels11060452

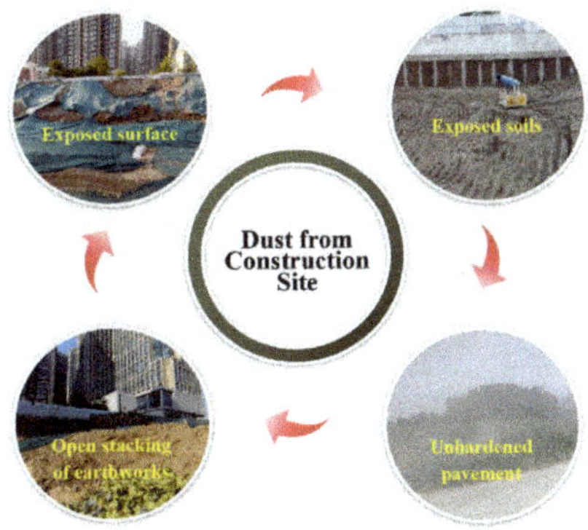

Figure 1. Dust source from construction site.

For the past several years, to address the shortcomings of traditional dust suppression methods, microbially induced carbonate precipitation (MICP) technology has been extensively studied and applied in engineering to enhance the wind erosion resistance of soil [5–7]. However, due to limitations such as the size, aerobic nature, and cost of urease-producing bacteria, the MICP technology has restrictions on the applicable soil types and soil depth [8,9]. Consequently, researchers have proposed enzyme-induced carbonate precipitation (EICP) technology (as shown in Formula (1) and (2)), which offers the following advantages compared to MICP technology: the small size of free urease can penetrate fine-grained soils [10,11], the reaction can be completed without the need for nutrients or air supply [12,13], and the degradability of urease avoids long-term environmental impacts [14]. Researchers have extracted urease from various plant seeds, such as beans [15,16], watermelon seeds [17], and soybeans [18,19], to address the issue of expensive commercial urease prices [20]. Among them, soybeans have become ideal research subjects due to their widespread cultivation in Asia and extensive application in the food industry. Previous studies have confirmed the feasibility of using soybean urease in EICP technology [18,21,22]. The effectiveness of EICP technology in soil solidification is influenced by various factors, including urease activity [23,24], grouting solution concentration [25], environmental conditions [26–28], and construction processes [10,29]. Despite numerous experimental studies on EICP technology, the formulation of EICP dust suppressants for silt soils in the Yellow River alluvial plain region remains undetermined, and the impact of EICP construction processes on the solidification effects of silt soils remains unclear. Understanding of the wind, rain, and wear resistance of the anti-dust solidification layer is still lacking.

$$CO(NH_2)_2 + 2H_2O \overset{urease}{\rightarrow} CO_3^{2-} + 2NH_4^+ \tag{1}$$

$$Ca^{2+} + CO_3^{2-} \rightarrow CaCO_3 \downarrow \tag{2}$$

The objective of this study is to investigate the effectiveness of soybean urease-induced carbonate precipitation in suppressing dust in a typical silt soil environment within the Yellow River alluvial plain region. Through a gradient test and optimization of the EICP dust suppressant formulation, various factors affecting urease activity and curing efficiency were elucidated, along with an investigation into the underlying mechanism for dust suppression. Based on these findings, a construction process for EICP dust suppression was determined, and characteristics such as wear resistance, wind resistance, and rain resistance were evaluated.

2. Results and Discussion

2.1. Optimization of EICP Solution

2.1.1. Particle Size and Solid–Liquid Mass Ratio

According to Figure 2a, when the particle size is 0.50 mm, the urease activity at a solid–liquid ratio of 1:5 is 143.30% higher than that at a ratio of 1:10, and 517.19% higher than that at a ratio of 1:40, indicating a significant increase in urease activity with an increasing solid–liquid ratio. Unit mass urease activity reflects the extraction efficiency of urease. As shown in Figure 2b, the urease extraction efficiency is highest at a solid–liquid ratio of 1:40, remains relatively consistent within the range of 1:30 to 1:10, and significantly decreases at a ratio of 1:5. At a particle size of 0.50 mm, the unit mass urease activity at a solid–liquid ratio of 1:5 is 64.47% of that at a ratio of 1:40 and 71.53% of that at a ratio of 1:10. This urease activity curve can approximately characterize the yield of calcium carbonate precipitation. Higher urease activity accelerates carbonate availability, thereby enhancing precipitation kinetics [9,10].

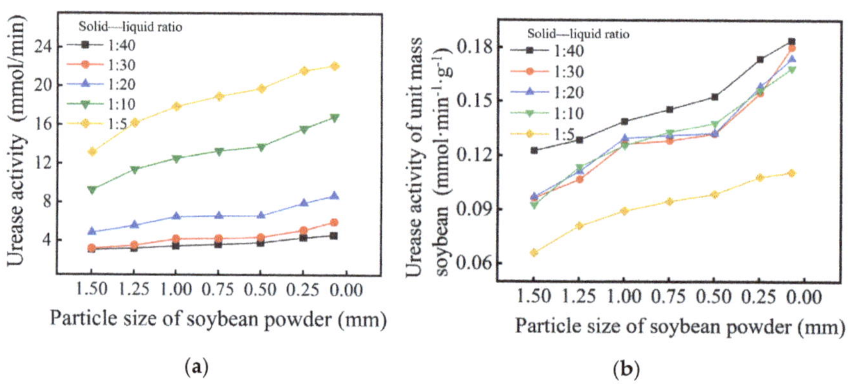

Figure 2. Effect of the nature of soybean powder on urease activity: (**a**) the urease activity; (**b**) the urease activity of unit mass soybean.

In summary, the observed increase in urease activity with smaller soybean powder particle sizes (<0.50 mm) is attributed to the larger specific surface area of finer particles. Reduced particle size enhances the exposure of encapsulated urease enzymes, facilitating more efficient substrate (urea) diffusion and active site accessibility. When the solid–liquid ratio is low (1:40), the total urease content in the soybean urease solution may be insufficient, resulting in lower urease activity and failing to meet experimental requirements. Conversely, when the solid–liquid ratio is high (1:5), the soybean powder solution has a high oil content and viscosity, making infiltration into fine-grained soil difficult and resulting in low urease extraction efficiency. Therefore, considering the requirements for urease activity and cost-effectiveness in engineering applications, this study recommends preparing urease solutions with particle sizes less than 0.50 mm and a solid–liquid ratio of 1:10.

2.1.2. pH Value

The activity of soybean urease demonstrates an initial increase followed by a decrease as the initial pH rises, as depicted in Figure 3. Notably, the urease activity reaches a notable level of 13.40~14.15 mmol/min when the solution's pH ranges between 7 and 9 and reaches peaks at pH 8. Conversely, urease activity diminishes significantly when the solution's pH falls below 2 or exceeds 12. This decline can be attributed to the urease's proteinaceous nature, which renders it susceptible to structural damage under extremely acidic or alkaline conditions, consequently leading to its inactivation. The PH value mainly affects the activity of urease. When the PH is 8, the urease has a relatively high activity, and it can be approximately considered that the yield of calcium carbonate is better at this time. Hence, the optimal activity of the urease solution is discerned at an initial pH of 8.

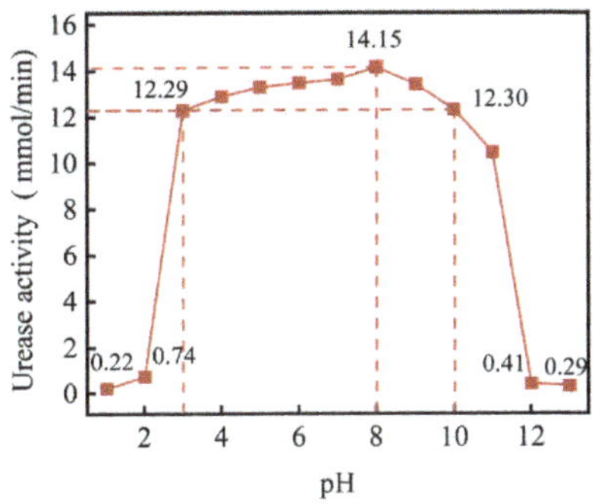

Figure 3. The urease activity at different initial pHs.

2.1.3. Concentration and Volume Ratio of Reaction Solution

Unconfined compressive strength tests were conducted on silty soil samples treated with different concentrations of cementation solutions. Portions of soil samples from the fractured surfaces were taken to measure the calcium carbonate content; the experimental results are shown in Figure 4.

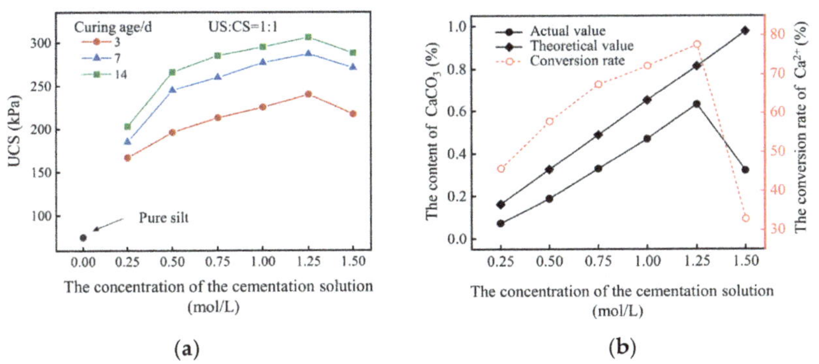

Figure 4. Influence of concentration of CS on solidification effect: (**a**) UCS; (**b**) the content of $CaCO_3$.

From Figure 4a, it can be observed that the unconfined compressive strength of the soil sample increases with the curing age. When the concentration of the cementation solution was 1.25 mol/L, the unconfined compressive strength of the sample cured for 3 days was 240 kPa, which was 83% of the strength at 7 days and 78% of the strength at 14 days. A gradual increase in the unconfined compressive strength of the soil sample was observed when the concentration of the cementation solution increased from 0.25 mol/L to 1.25 mol/L. However, the unconfined compressive strength of the soil sample decreases when the concentration of the cementation solution exceeds 1.25 mol/L. The UCS value approximately indirectly reflects the precipitation content of calcium carbonate. The higher the value, the higher the precipitation yield of calcium carbonate. From Figure 4b, it can be seen that as the concentration of the cementation solution increases from 0.25 mol/L to 1.25 mol/L, the content of $CaCO_3$ in the soil sample gradually increases, reaching a maximum at a cementation solution concentration of 1.25 mol/L, accounting for 0.63% of the total mass of the soil and the conversion rate of Ca^{2+} reaching 77.61%. The presence of excessive plant proteins in the crude soybean urease solution can impede the precipitation of $CaCO_3$. Therefore, a moderate increase in the concentration of the cementation solution will increase the content of $CaCO_3$. However, as the concentration of the cementation solution further rises, the elevated levels of calcium ions therein suppress the activity of soybean urease and diminish the efficacy of urea hydrolysis [30]. This conclusion is consistent with the research results of Carmona et al. [31].

The Impact of the volume ratio of urease to cementation solution on the EICP effect was examined by measuring the unconfined compressive strength (UCS) of soil samples at various curing stages. Subsequently, soil samples taken from the fractured surfaces after UCS testing were analyzed for calcium carbonate content. The experimental findings are presented in Figure 5.

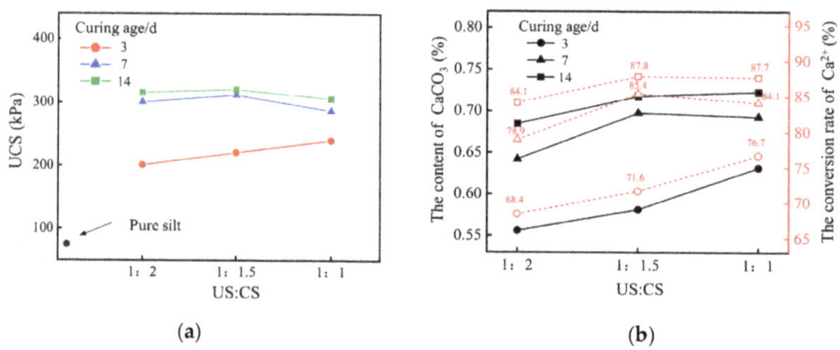

Figure 5. Influence of volume ratio on solidification effect: (**a**) UCS; (**b**) the content of $CaCO_3$.

As shown in Figure 5, at a 3-day curing age, there was a linear increment in UCS as the volume ratio of urease solution to cementation solution increased. Conversely, over the 7- and 14-day curing ages, UCS initially rose with the volume ratio and then decreased. Based on the literature [32], it is evident that as biochemical reactions progress, urease in the soil will gradually lose its activity, reducing the production of $CaCO_3$. Therefore, considering solidification effectiveness and economic factors, the optimal concentration of the cementation solution should be set at 1.25 mol/L, and the volume ratio of urease to cementation solution was 1:1.

2.2. Construction Technology

Spraying solution is the most cost-effective and practical method for mitigating dust issues on sites with silty soil. This approach leverages the solution's penetrating ability in the soil to promote calcium carbonate precipitation among the silty soil particles, leading to the formation of a solidification layer aimed at achieving effective dust control.

2.2.1. Influence of Spraying Scheme on Solidification Effect

Figure 6a illustrates the solidification performance of silt specimens subjected to varying spraying volumes and spraying methods. Initially, with a small spraying volume, the EICP solution failed to penetrate the soil thoroughly, thereby resulting in the formation of a thin solidification layer on the surface and limited curing effect of the silt. As the spraying volume increased, the solution penetrated the silt more effectively, promoting the formation of bio-gel materials through EICP that subsequently enhanced the compressive strength of the specimens. Notably, at a spraying volume of 4 L/m^2, the surface compressive strength of the samples increased to 752.20 kPa, with a solidification layer thickness of 14.97 mm, demonstrating the effective gelation capacity of EICP-generated cementitious materials.

Nevertheless, further increases in spraying volume led to marginal improvements in surface compressive strength and solidification-layer thickness. This phenomenon could be attributed to the formation of calcium carbonate precipitation and subsequent bio-gel network development among soil particles on the surface as the EICP solution volume increased, hindering additional penetration and reaching a critical solidification value. As a result, a spraying volume of 4 L/m^2 was deemed optimal for subsequent experimental spraying procedures.

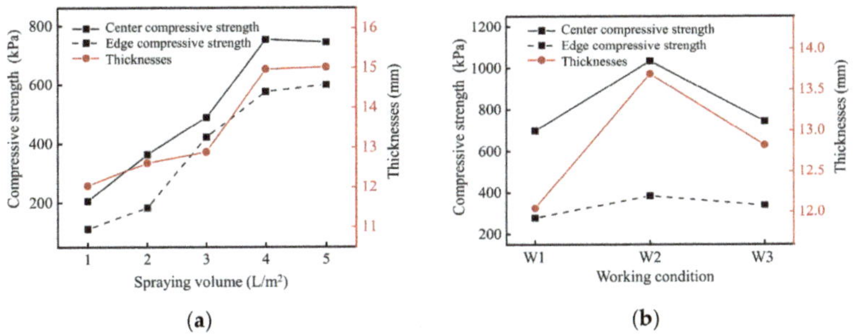

Figure 6. Influence of spraying scheme on solidification effect: (**a**) different spraying volumes on solidification effect; (**b**) different spraying methods on solidification effect.

Working conditions W1, W2, and W3 are shown in Table 1. From Figure 6b, it can be seen that the solidification effects of W1 and W3 were both unsatisfactory. In these conditions, both urease and urea solution were pre-mixed, which means that the hydrolysis reaction of urea had already begun before the EICP solution was sprayed onto the soil surface. This premature formation of $CaCO_3$ created a dense bio-gel layer that binds with soil particles, hindering the penetration of the solution into deeper layers of the silt. In contrast, the EICP solution demonstrates optimal permeation and diffusion into the deep silt in condition W2. After the urease solution was injected, the controlled gelation process allowed the hydrolysis and precipitation reactions to proceed gradually, resulting in a uniform bio-cemented gel matrix with a thicker solidification layer (14.97 mm) and higher soil compressive strength (752.20 kPa) compared to other working conditions. This sequential spraying strategy optimized the in situ gel formation, demonstrating the effectiveness of EICP-generated cementitious materials. Therefore, in subsequent experiments, the practice of initially spraying a mixture of calcium chloride and urea solutions followed by urease solution was maintained.

Table 1. The design of mixing sequences.

Working Conditions	Spray Bottle I			Spray Bottle II		
	Urea Volume/mL	Calcium Chloride Volume/mL	Urease Volume/mL	Urea Volume/mL	Calcium Chloride Volume/mL	Urease Volume/mL
W1	30	0	60	0	30	0
W2	30	30	0	0	0	60
W3	30	30	60	0	0	0

2.2.2. Reaction Time

Figure 7 shows the relationship between time and solidification. The solidification effect increases rapidly in the initial stage of the reaction due to the rapid formation of bio-gel structures through EICP-induced $CaCO_3$ precipitation. The solidification effect can reach 80% at the 15 h mark and further increase to 90% within 24 h, with the surface strength of specimens cured for 72 h serving as the reference benchmark. As the reaction progresses, a bio-cemented gel layer composed of calcium carbonate and silt develops on the specimen surface, whose dense gel-like microstructure halts the further penetration of the EICP solution into the deep silt. The incompletely reacted solution in the deep layers of the silt further precipitated to form $CaCO_3$ until the reaction reached completion, demonstrating the self-limiting nature of EICP gelation. Consequently, the reaction exhibits rapid progress in the initial stage, with a gradual decrease in the reaction rate over time as the bio-gel network matures and stabilizes. In practical engineering applications, the reaction time can be adjusted according to the desired curing effect and time requirements to optimize the balance between gelation efficiency and material penetration depth, thereby achieving optimal benefits.

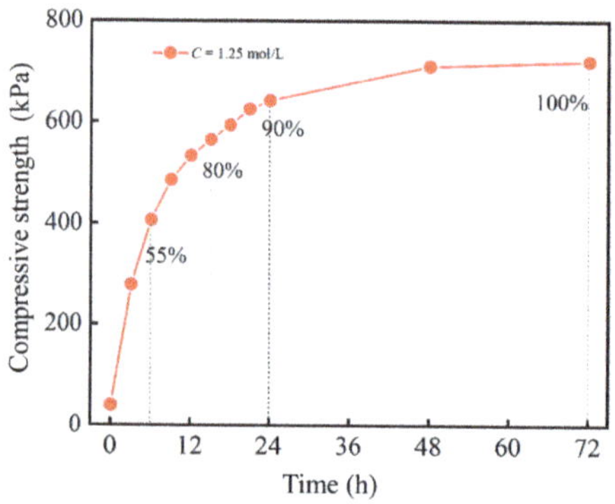

Figure 7. Influence of reaction time on solidification effect.

2.3. *Curing Effect*

2.3.1. Macro Appearance

Spraying EICP solution onto the surface of silt soil can increase the calcium carbonate content and induce the formation of a soil crust through bio-gel bonding, thereby enhancing the cohesion among soil particles and improving surface strength. As depicted in Figure 8, a calcareous layer, namely a bio-cemented gel layer with a dense microstructure, developed, and its thickness serves as one of the evaluation indicators for assessing curing effects. Using a vernier caliper, as illustrated in Figure 8, measurements were taken to determine the thickness of the soil crust, with its maximum value reaching 15.01 mm, demonstrating the structural stability of the EICP-derived gel matrix.

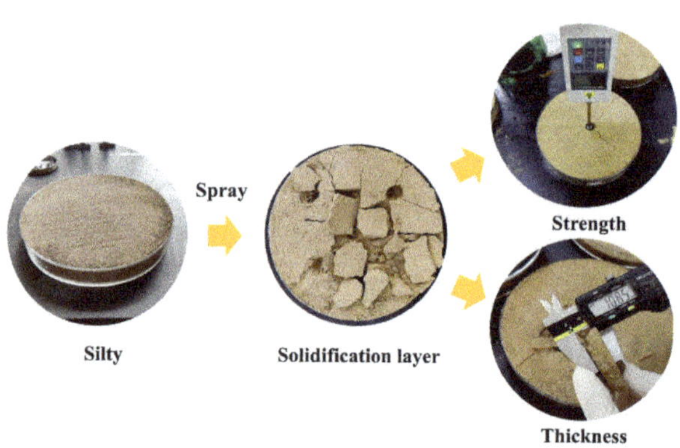

Figure 8. Soil crust induced by EICP.

2.3.2. Micro Analysis

The SEM and XRD results of the soil sample after EICP treatment are shown in Figure 9.

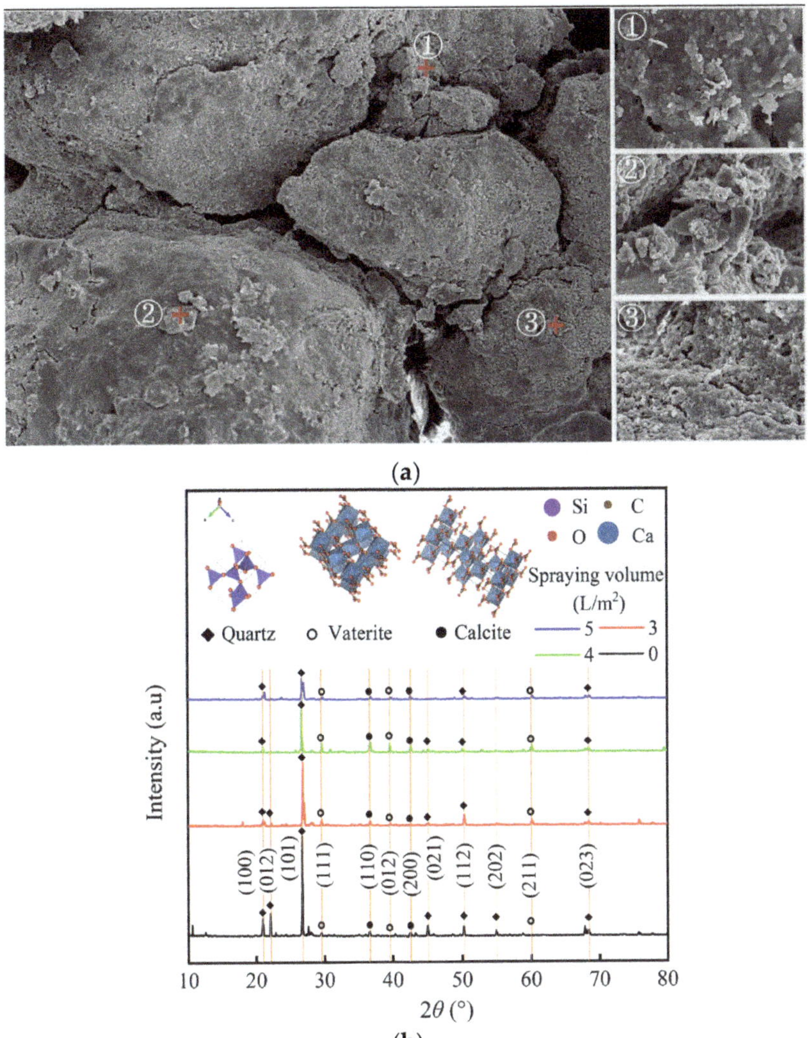

Figure 9. Micro analysis results: (**a**) SEM image of specimen after EICP treatment; (**b**) XRD pattern of silt specimens.

1. SEM

Figure 9a reveals spherical or globular aggregates of irregular size induced by soybean urease. The interaction between soil particles and crystals can be categorized into three types: ① film covering, where crystals cover the surface of soil particles, increasing particle volume and surface area without contact with other soil particles; ② cementation, where crystals primarily precipitate and aggregate near contact points of particles, acting as a bonding agent; ③ bridging, involving the precipitation and aggregation of crystals between neighboring particles to ultimately link them together. These three modes of crystal cementation effectively reduce soil porosity and permeability, while the structural durability and strength rely on crystals that perform cementation and bridging functions. The results confirm the positive effect of EICP on silt solidification.

2. XRD

The distribution of phase composition in silt specimens treated with EICP is depicted in Figure 9b. As the spraying volume increased, there were discernible shifts in the diffraction peak values of crystals, indicative of changes in the relative content of crystal components. Notably, the peak intensities associated with the crystal faces of quartz (SiO_2), such as (100), (012), (101), (021), (112), (202), and (023), have all decreased. Particularly, at a diffraction angle of 26.7°, the peak intensity of the crystal face (101) decreased from 3985 at a spraying volume of 0 L/m^2 to 1434, 339, and 717 at spraying volumes of 3, 4, and 5 L/m^2, respectively. Moreover, in crystal faces representing vaterite (111), (012), (211), and calcite (110), (200), the corresponding diffraction peak intensities increased to varying degrees with the increase in spraying volume. Compared to the untreated silty soil samples, it is evident that the silty soil samples treated with EICP technology exhibit distinct diffraction peaks of calcite and chondraronite. Calcite, being the most thermodynamically stable mineral phase in calcium carbonate polycrystalline form, possesses good mechanical strength capable of cementing silt particles, thereby enhancing the structural stability of silt. Consequently, the compressive strength of silt samples significantly improves after EICP treatment.

2.4. *Dust Control Effect*

2.4.1. Wind–Rain Resistance

As shown in Figure 10, significant morphological changes occurred in the untreated soil sample within 30 min under wind erosion, resulting in substantial soil particle loss and extensive exposure of the mold bottom. The soil sample treated with deionized water exhibited continued soil particle loss, primarily evidenced by the widening of surface cracks. Furthermore, this sample experienced substantial soil particle loss during rain erosion, leading to notable alterations in surface morphology. The specimens treated with EICP showed minimal morphological alterations following wind erosion due to the bio-gel-reinforced crust formed through $CaCO_3$ crystal networking. After 60 min of rain erosion, the gel-like cementation matrix resulted in relatively minor morphological changes. Comparing the morphological alterations among the specimens indicates that the EICP-generated bio-cement gel exerts a discernible inhibitory effect on dust emission in silt.

Figure 11a,b illustrate the results of wind and rain erosion tests on EICP-treated and untreated soil specimens. After 60 min of wind erosion at a wind speed of 15 m/s, the EICP-treated specimen exhibited a wind erosion coefficient of 0.14%, resulting in a mass loss of 8.54 g.

Figure 11c shows the mass loss and erosion coefficients of silt specimens treated with EICP under different working conditions, as listed in Table 1. In the first round of wind erosion tests with wind speeds of 60 min, the bio-gel-reinforced specimens exhibited mass loss less than 8.54 g (accounting for <0.2% of total mass), demonstrating the cohesive strength of the $CaCO_3$-gel composite matrix. After rainfall erosion tests for 60 min, the gel-stabilized samples showed mass loss below 83.50 g (~1.2% of total mass), attributed to the water-resistant nature of the bio-mineral gel network. Following drying, the persistent gel-phase cementation maintained dust suppression ability, with second-round wind erosion mass loss not exceeding 16.66 g per group. These results indicate that the EICP-derived gel-cemented layer can resist Beaufort scale 7 winds (51–61 km/h) and 40 mm/h rainfall rates, where the self-healing gel architecture prevents crack propagation under cyclic wet–dry conditions.

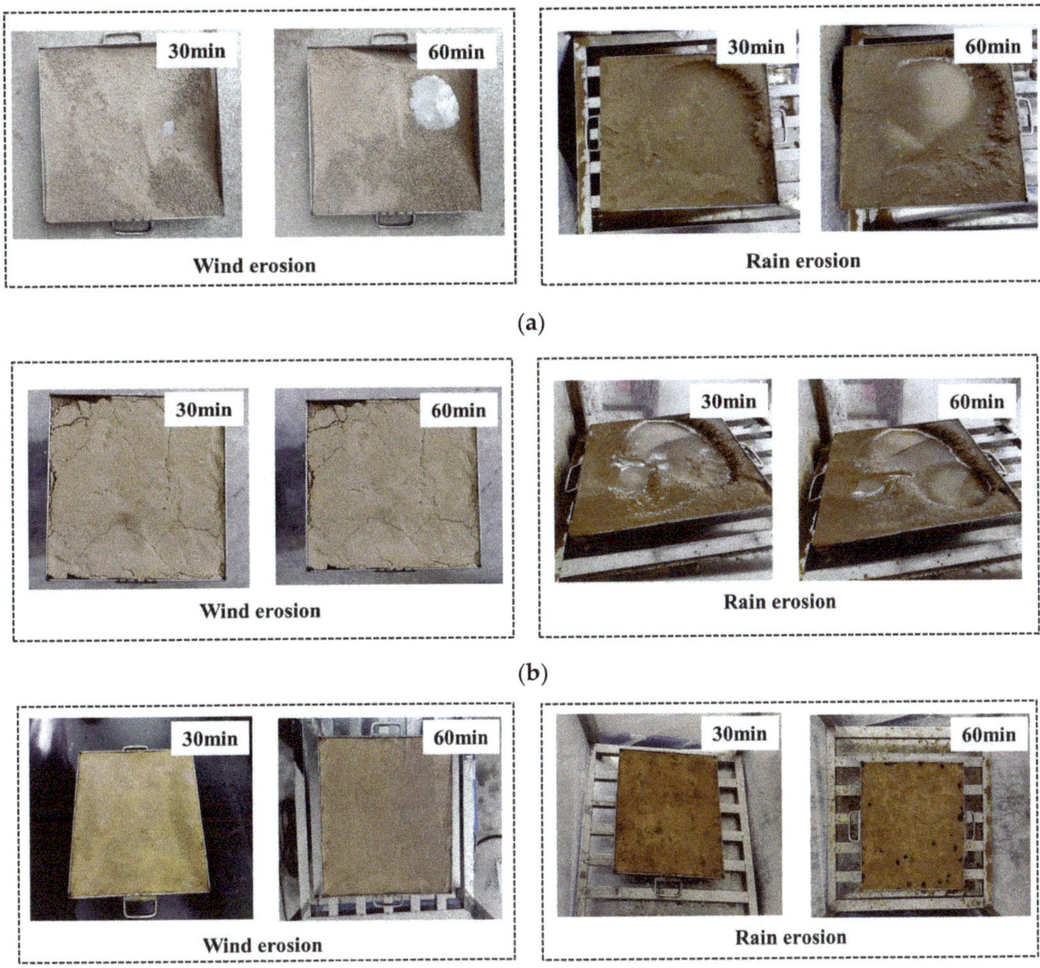

(c)

Figure 10. Morphology analysis of wind and rain erosion: (**a**) untreated specimens; (**b**) deionized water treated specimens; (**c**) EICP treated specimens. In contrast, the untreated specimen experienced a significantly higher mass loss of 2459.38 g under similar conditions. For rainfall erosion, after 60 min at a rate of 40 mm/h, the EICP-treated soil specimen showed a rain erosion coefficient of 1.39%, with a resulting mass loss of 83.50 g. In comparison, the untreated soil specimen lost 1095.63 g in mass under the same rainfall conditions.

These findings align closely with Sun et al. [11], who demonstrated that EICP-PVAc (50 g/L) treatment achieved surface strengths exceeding 500 kPa and near-zero soil loss under extreme rainfall (300 mm/h). Field tests by Sun et al. revealed $CaCO_3$ crystallization within 10–27 mm thick cemented layers, corroborating the cohesive mechanism documented in the present study. While Sun et al. focused on slope-scale stabilization under high-intensity rainfall, the current investigation extends these insights by quantifying the resistance of EICP-gel composites to cyclic wind and rainfall stresses. This advancement builds upon previous methodologies through the systematic evaluation of long-term durability under combined environmental stressors, addressing a critical gap in prior EICP applications focused solely on static hydrological conditions.

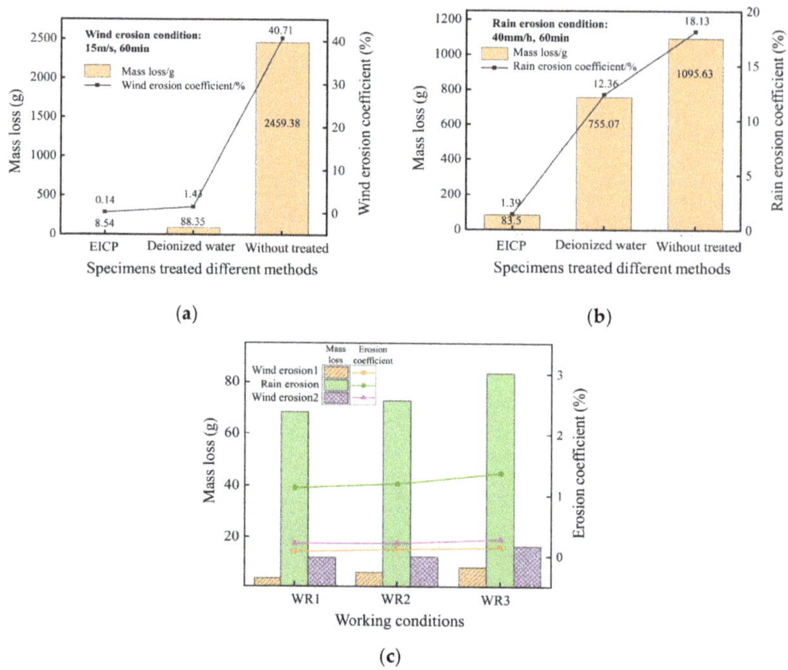

Figure 11. Test results of wind and rain erosion: (**a**) mass loss of wind erosion test; (**b**) mass loss of rain erosion test; (**c**) mass loss of different working conditions.

2.4.2. Wear Resistance

Figure 12 demonstrates that the soil crust remains intact under specific conditions: at 80 kPa pressure with revolution numbers below 30 circles, or at 53.3 kPa pressure with revolution numbers below 50 circles. The maximum values for mass loss and wear depth were 33.67 g and 5.4 mm, respectively, under each condition. The maximum wear rate recorded was 0.670 g/cm^2. Exceeding these critical friction conditions compromises the solidification layer. Here, the insufficient strength of the unconsolidated silt beneath the soil crust fails to resist the abrasion from the rubber friction head, resulting in a rapid increase in wear depth and mass loss. The experimental findings indicate that the soil solidification layer withstands repeated abrasion from fully loaded trucks for 30 cycles and unloaded trucks for 50 cycles.

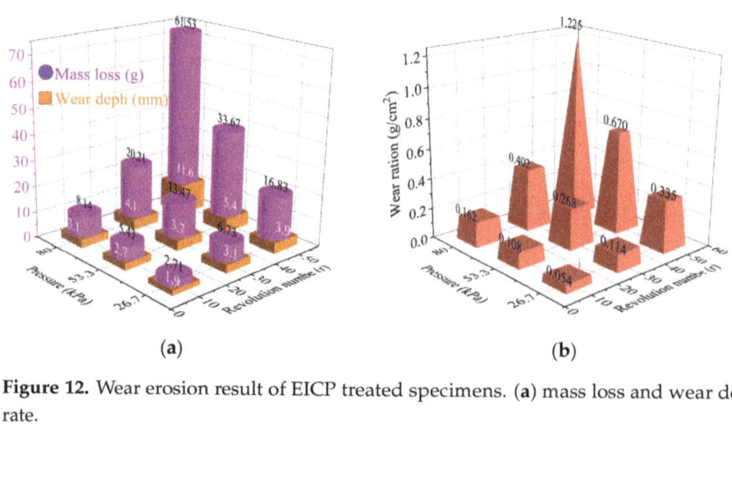

Figure 12. Wear erosion result of EICP treated specimens. (**a**) mass loss and wear depth; (**b**) wear rate.

3. Conclusions

This investigation into the potential of enzyme-induced carbonate precipitation (EICP) to reduce wind erosion of Yellow River silt revealed significant results. The bio-gel formation through EICP was found to enhance the bearing capacity, wind–rain erosion resistance, and wear resistance of the silt through the in situ generation of a mineral gel matrix. The level of improvement was notably affected by the concentration of the cementation solution and the spraying volume.

(1) The optimal cementation solution, consisting of equal concentrations of urea and $CaCl_2$ (1.25 mol/L) applied at 4 L/m^2, enabled controlled gelation through sequential spraying (first urea-$CaCl_2$ solution, then urease).
(2) This protocol produced a 14.9 mm thick bio-cemented gel layer with compressive strength exceeding 752 kPa, where $CaCO_3$ crystallization created a self-reinforcing gel architecture.
(3) The gel-stabilized crust maintained integrity under Beaufort scale 7 winds (51–61 km/h), resisted 40 mm/h rainfall erosion, and endured 30 cycles of fully loaded truck abrasion.

These findings establish EICP as a novel bio-gel technology that strengthens silt via natural gel-phase cementation, providing an effective biological solution for dust mitigation in the Yellow River region.

Limitations and Future Work:

(1) Our tests focused on short-term performance; long-term durability under freeze–thaw cycles and microbial degradation needs validation.
(2) Field-scale cost analysis (USD 0.32/m^2 for lab trials) should be conducted to assess economic viability.
(3) Combining EICP with biopolymers may further improve erosion resistance in high-shear environments.

4. Materials and Methods

4.1. Materials

4.1.1. Yellow River Silt

The silt used in this experiment was collected from Zhengzhou City in the central Yellow River alluvial plains, Province of Henan, China. The D_{10}, D_{50}, and D_{90} values of the silt are 75 μm, 91 μm, and 158 μm, respectively. Figure 13a presents a depiction of the distribution of particles sizes in the soil that was utilized. X-ray diffraction analysis identified quartz as the predominant mineral and SiO_2 as the compound within the silt, as shown in Figure 13b. Detailed physical properties of the soil can be found in Table 2.

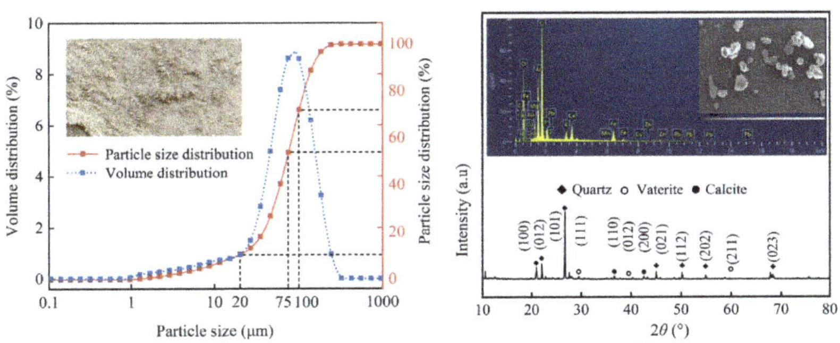

Figure 13. Particle size and microscale identification of the test silt: (**a**) particle size distribution and grain gradation; (**b**) microscopic view of the silt with the XRD and SEM images.

Table 2. Basic properties of test silt.

Density ρ/g·cm^{-3}	Water Content W_{op}/%	Void Ratio e	Maximum Dry Density ρ/g·cm^{-3}	Specific Gravitys G_s/g·cm^{-3}	Permeability Coefficient K_T/cm·s^{-1}
1.39	10.34	1.14	1.26	2.7	2.5×10^{-4}

4.1.2. EICP Solution

The EICP solution consists of soybean urease solution (US) and cementation solution (CS). The bean powder was sifted into various particle sizes: 1.5, 1.0, 0.75, 0.5, 0.25, and 0.075. Subsequently, the powder was mixed with PBS liquid at mass ratios of 1:40, 1:30, 1:20, 1:10, and 1:5. After thorough stirring, the mixture was centrifuged at 3000 rpm for 15 min, and the clear liquid at the top was collected to obtain the soybean urease solution. These solutions were then adjusted to pH levels ranging from 1 to 13 and stored at temperatures of 4 °C and 25 °C for urease activity analysis. The selection of 4 °C and 25 °C reflects standard enzymatic storage (4 °C) and application (25 °C) conditions, where 25 °C represents a practical ambient baseline for activity comparison, while 4 °C minimizes enzymatic degradation without inducing freezing damage, as validated in prior soybean urease studies [9–11]. The cementation solution primarily consists of urea and calcium chloride, with concentrations maintained between 0.25 mol/L and 1.5 mol/L. The soybean urease solution and cementation solution are combined in ratios of 1:2, 1:1.5, and 1:1 to create the EICP solution, as depicted in Figure 14.

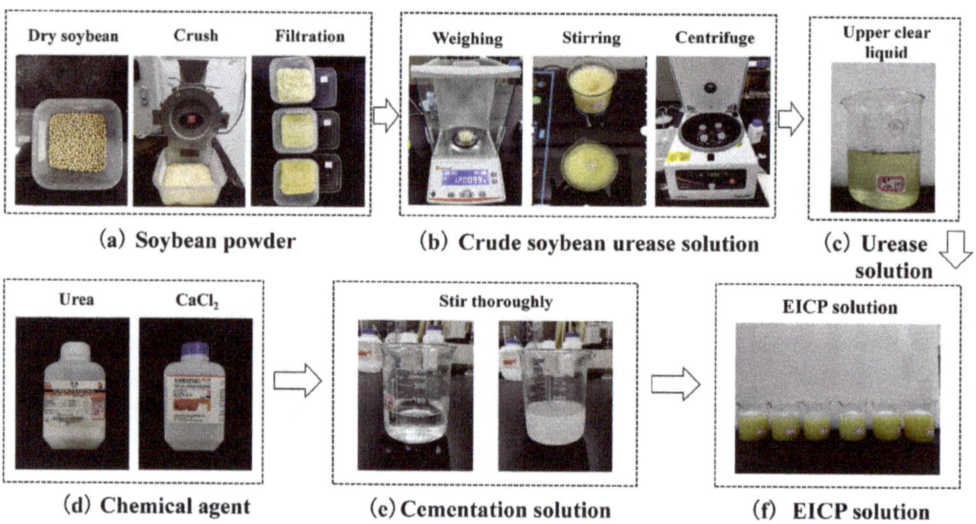

Figure 14. Schematic steps for preparing EICP solution: (**a**) soybean powder; (**b**) initial solution; (**c**) urease solution; (**d**) chemical agent; (**e**) cementation solution; (**f**) EICP solution.

4.1.3. Specimens

This EICP solution comprises urease, urea, and calcium chloride solutions, which were sprayed onto the silt surface in varying volumes and sequences. Subsequently, the disk-shaped specimens, with a diameter of 200 mm and a height of 30 mm, and square disk-shaped specimens, with a side length of 300 mm and a height of 40 mm, were placed in a constant temperature box with curing at 25 °C. In order to meet the requirements of rainwater infiltration, square specimens should be prepared by drilling holes in the bottom of the mold and laying geotextiles.

4.2. Test Methods

4.2.1. Urease Activity Measurement

Since the changes in the amount of conductivity of the urease solution are directly proportional to urea hydrolysis, the urease activity can be determined using the amount of hydrolyzed urea conductivity method. Specifically, 3 mL of urease solution was mixed with 27 mL of urea solution at a concentration of 1.11 mol/L. The changes in conductivity of the solution were then monitored for the initial 30 min at 25 °C. The urease activity can be obtained based on the conductivity change using the following equation proposed by Whiffin [33]:

$$U = k\frac{\Delta\sigma}{\Delta t}F \tag{3}$$

where U is the urease activity (mmol/min); $\Delta\sigma$ is the difference in conductivity ($\mathrm{ms{\cdot}cm^{-1}{\cdot}min^{-1}}$); Δt is the time (min); F is the dilution factor of urease solution, taken as 10 in this experiment; k is the relationship between solution conductivity and moles of ammonium ions, taken as 11.11 based on reference [34].

4.2.2. $CaCO_3$ Content and Conversion Rate Measurement

In this experiment, the urease activity was measured using the conductivity meter method, and the $CaCO_3$ content of the samples was determined via EDTA titration method. First, the treated soil specimen was rinsed with deionized water to remove the residual soluble substances. After that, the specimen was dried and placed in an excess amount of hydrochloric acid (HCl) solution with a concentration of 1 mol/L to dissolve all the generated $CaCO_3$ precipitates. The Ca^{2+} content dissolved in the hydrochloric acid solution was measured using titration method. Then, the $CaCO_3$ content in the specimen can be determined based on the measured Ca^{2+} content. $CaCO_3$ conversion rate was defined as the ratio of actual $CaCO_3$ production to theoretical $CaCO_3$ production.

4.2.3. Spraying Scheme

The recommended spraying volume of dust suppressor in sandy soil ranges from 3.66 to 4.00 L/m^2 [11]. Since silt particles are smaller than sand particles, it is necessary to determine the appropriate spraying volume for silt sand in Zhengzhou. For this experiment, the designed spray volume of EICP solution for this experiment was as follows: 1 L/m^2, 2 L/m^2, 3 L/m^2, 4 L/m^2, and 5 L/m^2.

The curing effect of EICP dust suppressor solution for silt soils will be influenced by the order of mixture and spraying. In the test, the order of spraying was, therefore, divided into three types, namely working conditions W1, W2, and W3, as shown in Table 2.

① Urease solution and urea solution first, followed by calcium chloride solution (W1);
② Calcium chloride solution and urea solution first, followed by urease solution (W2);
③ Direct mixing and spraying (W3).

4.2.4. Performance Tests

Performance tests include the unconfined compressive strength test, wind–rain resistance test, and friction test of plate samples.

1. Wind–rain resistance test

The wind force is typically classified into 13 levels, ranging from 0 to 12. Based on the wind data for Zhengzhou between 2011 and 2023, it can be observed that the prevailing wind conditions were predominantly at level 3, which corresponds to a wind speed of approximately 5.4 m/s. In order to simulate realistic wind erosion in this experiment, this experiment set the wind speeds at three different levels: 5 m/s (level 3), 10 m/s (level 5), and 15 m/s (level 7). Each experiment will last for a duration of 60 min.

According to data from the Central Meteorological Bureau, Figure 15 illustrates the monthly average rainfall and number of rainy days in Zhengzhou. The annual average precipitation in the city ranges from 477.08 to 1167.30 mm, with monthly averages of rainy days varying between 1.3 and 14.6 days. July and August have the highest precipitation levels, with recorded amounts of 146.2 mm and 138.9 mm, respectively. Therefore, a rainfall level of 40 mm is considered relatively high in the Zhengzhou area. This experiment simulated three different intensities of rainfall: 7 mm/h, 15 mm/h, and a heavy downpour at a rate of 40 mm/h for a duration of one hour.

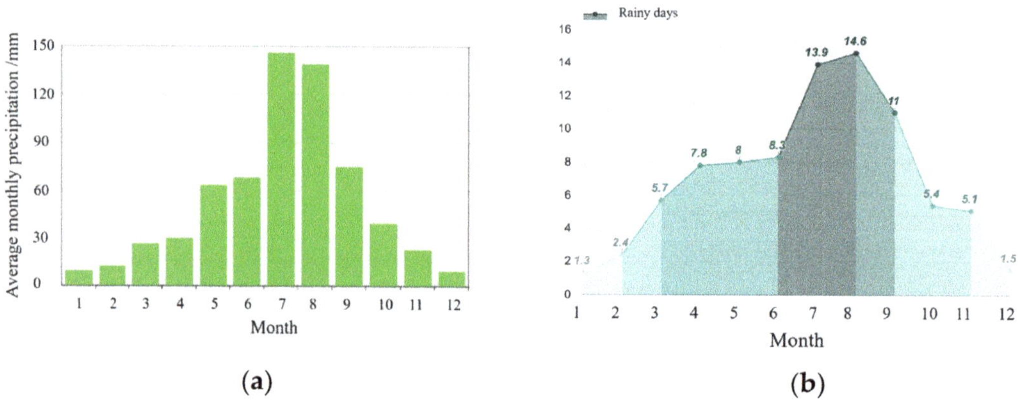

Figure 15. Precipitation date from Zhengzhou: (**a**) average monthly precipitation; (**b**) average rainy days.

This experiment involves a cyclic erosion process with wind–rain–wind action lasting 1 h each. The wind speeds were 5, 10, and 15 m/s (equivalent to Beaufort scale 3, 5, 7), while the precipitation rates were set at 7, 15, and 40 mm/h (representing heavy rain, rainstorm, and heavy rainstorm). Working conditions WR1 to WR3 represent increasing values of wind speed and precipitation rates from low to high. The untreated silt and specimens sprayed with deionized water were set as the control group, and the design plan is provided in Table 3.

Table 3. The design of wind–rain erosion test.

Working Conditions	Rotation 1		Rotation 2		Rotation 3	
	Wind Speed V_1/m·s^{-1}	Time t_1/min	Rainfall R_2/mm·h^{-1}	Time t_2/min	Wind Speed V_3/m·s^{-1}	Time t_3/min
WR1	5	60	7	60	15	60
WR2	10	60	15	60	15	60
WR3	15	60	40	60	15	60

A self-designed wind–rain erosion test device was utilized (Figure 16), comprising a blower, a water reservoir, a sample disk, an atomizing nozzle, a slope-adjusting platform, and a water-collecting tank. The atomizing nozzle is connected via the catheter, diaphragm pump, and flow meter to simulate various levels of rainfall intensity during testing. The water storage tank is positioned beneath the bottom plate for rainwater recycling purposes. Externally to the device, the blower and anemometer are employed to regulate different wind speeds.

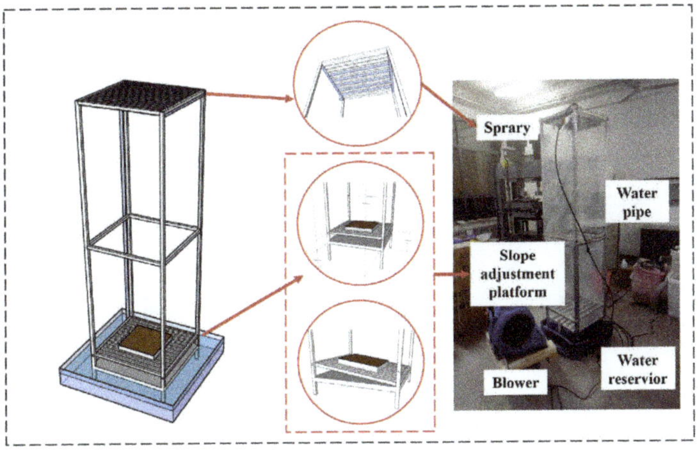

Figure 16. Self-designed wind–rain erosion test.

2. Friction test

In evaluating the abrasion resistance of the solidification layer by EICP, this study utilized the UMT-2 micro friction tester to simulate the friction caused by truck rubber tires on the ground. The UMT-2 (Universal Mechanical Tester-2, Bruker Corporation, Billerica, MA, USA), a tribological testing system, was employed to simulate rubber tire-ground friction under controlled loads and rotational speeds. Its reciprocating ball-on-disk configuration mimics real-world abrasion mechanisms, aligning with ASTM G133-22 standards [1]. The UMT-2′s precision (±0.1% load accuracy, ±1 rpm speed control) ensures reliable quantification of the solidification layer's wear resistance.

According to the site conditions, the maximum pressure exerted by fully loaded trucks on the road surface through tires is 80 kPa, equivalent to applying a load of 16.07 N on the lever arm of the micro friction tester. Meanwhile, the maximum driving speed of vehicles is 5 km/h when entering and leaving the factory or the production site, corresponding to a rotational speed of 2.19 r/s on the micro friction wear tester. Therefore, the rotate speed was set to 120 rpm, and the loads were 5 N, 10 N, and 15 N, with 10, 30, and 50 cycles for the wear tests, respectively. The details of the wear test design can be found in Table 4.

Table 4. The design of wear test.

Working Conditions	Load (N)	Pressure (kPa)	Revolution (r)
L5–r10	5	26.7	10
L5–r30	5	26.7	30
L5–r50	5	26.7	50
L10–r10	10	53.3	10
L10–r30	10	53.3	30
L10–r50	10	53.3	50
L15–r10	15	80	10
L15–r30	15	80	30
L15–r50	15	80	50

4.3. Microscopic Evaluation

In this study, the Hitachi Regulus 8230 field-emission scanning electron microscope (Hitachi Corporation, Japan, Tokyo) was used to observe the morphological characteristics of mineral precipitates in the silt after EICP treatment at different magnifications. The samples were ground into a fine powder using a mortar and pestle, and the crystalline phases of the powder were identified using the Malvern Panalytical Empyrean X-ray diffractometer (Global Headquarters, Malvern Panalytical, Malvern, UK), with a diffraction angle range from 10° to 80° and a scan rate of at least 10°/min.

Author Contributions: Conceptualization, J.Z.; data curation, H.J.; formal analysis, H.J. and J.L.; methodology, X.C.; project administration, S.W. and L.L.; validation, L.W.; writing—original draft, H.J.; writing—review and editing, J.L. All authors have read and agreed to the published version of the manuscript.

Funding: The research was funded by the Key Research and Development Special Program of Henan Province (241111322500), Support Plan for University Science and Technology Innovation Team of Henan Province (24IRTSTHN009) and Mechanism and process optimization of micro-grouting for reinforcement of silt soil foundation in yellow plain area (242102320219).

Institutional Review Board Statement: Not applicable.

Informed Consent Statement: Not applicable.

Data Availability Statement: The data used to support the findings of this study are available from the corresponding author upon request.

Acknowledgments: The authors appreciate the anonymous reviewers for their constructive comments and suggestions that significantly improved the quality of this manuscript.

Conflicts of Interest: Authors Shilong Wang and Lin Liu were employed by the company Zhengzhou City Construction Group Investment Co., Ltd. The remaining authors declare that the research was conducted in the absence of any commercial or financial relationships that could be construed as a potential conflict of interest.

References

1. Middleton, N.; Kang, U. Sand and dust storms: Impact mitigation. *Sustainability* **2017**, *9*, 1053. [CrossRef]
2. Wang, P.F.; Tan, X.H.; Zhang, L.Y.; Li, Y.J.; Liu, R.H. Influence of particle diameter on the wettability of coal dust and the dust suppression efficiency via spraying. *Process Saf. Environ. Prot.* **2019**, *132*, 189–199. [CrossRef]
3. Paul, S.; Chang, J.; Mukhopadhyay, S. Development of Coursework on Studying Fugitive Dust From Construction Site Using Optical-Type Dust Sensor. *IEEE Sens. J.* **2021**, *21*, 17318–17326.
4. Amato, F.; Querol, X.; Johansson, C.; Nagl, C.; Alastuey, A. A review on the effectiveness of street sweeping, washing and dust suppressants as urban PM control methods. *Sci. Total Environ.* **2010**, *408*, 3070–3084. [CrossRef]
5. Wang, H.X.; Sun, X.H.; Miao, L.C.; Zhang, J.Z.; Yin, W.H.; Wu, L.Y. Sand and dust storms control for sustainable anti-desertification: Large-scale eicp-pvac treatment field demonstration and insights. *Acta Geotech.* **2025**, *20*, 2201–2219. [CrossRef]
6. Miao, L.C.; Wang, H.X.; Sun, X.H.; Wu, L.Y. Biomineralization for Reducing and Controlling Sand-Dust Storms. *Adv. Sci.* **2024**, *11*, e2403961. [CrossRef]
7. Sun, X.H.; Miao, L.C.; Tong, T.Z.; Wang, C.C. Experimental study of solidifying sand using microbial-induced calcium carbonate precipitation. *Rock Soil Mech.* **2017**, *38*, 3225–3230, 3239. [CrossRef]
8. Khodadadi, T.H.; Kavazanjian, E.; Paassen, L.V.; Dejong, J. Bio-grout materials: A review. *Grouting* **2017**, 1–12. [CrossRef]
9. Li, C.; Li, S.; Xing, J.; Yao, D. On-site test of fixed mobile sand dunes using combined technology of sand plants and EICP in the Ulanbuh Desert, China. *Acta Geotech.* **2025**, *20*, 1921–1934. [CrossRef]
10. Cui, M.J.; Lai, H.J.; Hoang, T.; Chu, J. One-phase-low-pH enzyme induced carbonate precipitation (EICP) method for soil improvement. *Acta Geotech.* **2021**, *16*, 481–489. [CrossRef]
11. Sun, X.H.; Miao, L.C.; Yuan, J.H.; Wang, X.H.; Wu, L.Y. Application of enzymatic calcification for dust control and rainfall erosion resistance improvement. *Sci. Total Environ.* **2020**, *759*, 143468. [CrossRef] [PubMed]
12. Almajed, A.; Tirkolaei, H.K.; Kavazanjian, E.; Hamdan, N. Enzyme induced carbonate precipitation (EICP) for soil improvement: A review of material production methods. *J. Rock Mech. Geotech. Eng.* **2018**, *10*, 1131–1145. [CrossRef]
13. Arab, M.G.; Rohy, H.; Zeiada, W.; Almajed, A.; Omar, M. One-phase EICP biotreatment of sand exposed to various environmental conditions. *J. Mater. Civ. Eng.* **2021**, *33*, 04020489. [CrossRef]
14. Almajed, A. *Enzyme Induced Carbonate Precipitation (EICP) for Soil Improvement*; Arizona State University: Tempe, Arizona, 2017; p. 149.

15. Nam, I.H.; Chon, C.M.; Jung, K.Y.; Choi, S.G.; Choi, H.; Park, S.S. Calcite precipitation by ureolytic plant (*Canavalia ensiformis*) extracts as effective biomaterials. *KSCE J. Civ. Eng.* **2015**, *19*, 1620–1625. [CrossRef]
16. Park, S.S.; Choi, S.G.; Nam, I.H. Effect of plant-induced calcite precipitation on the strength of sand. *J. Mater. Civ. Eng.* **2014**, *26*, 06014017. [CrossRef]
17. Dilrukshi, R.A.N.; Nakashima, K.; Kawasaki, S. Soil improvement using plant-derived urease-induced calcium carbonate precipitation. *Soils Found.* **2018**, *58*, 894–910. [CrossRef]
18. Gao, Y.; He, J.; Tang, X.; Chu, J. Calcium carbonate precipitation catalyzed by soybean urease as an improvement method for fine-grained soil. *Soils Found.* **2019**, *59*, 1631–1637. [CrossRef]
19. Lee, S.; Kim, J. An experimental study on enzymatic-induced carbonate precipitation using yellow soybeans for soil stabilization. *KSCE J. Civ. Eng.* **2020**, *24*, 2026–2037. [CrossRef]
20. Liu, L.X.; Gao, Y.; Meng, H.; Pan, Q.W.; Wang, Z.B.; Zhou, Y.D.; Liu, B.; Cao, X.W. Pore-scale, mechanical, and hydraulic properties of EICP-treated sand using crude legume ureases with different protein contents. *Acta Geotech.* **2024**, *19*, 4747–4763. [CrossRef]
21. Jiang, N.J.; Wang, Y.J.; Chu, J. Bio-mediated soil improvement: An introspection into processes, materials, characterization and applications. *Soil Use Manag.* **2022**, *38*, 68–93. [CrossRef]
22. Phillips, A.J.; Gerlach, R.; Lauchnor, E.; Mitchell, A.C.; Cunningham, A.B.; Spangler, L. Engineered applications of ureolytic biomineralization: A review. *Biofouling* **2013**, *29*, 715–733. [CrossRef] [PubMed]
23. Cheng, L.; Shahin, M.A.; Mujah, D. Influence of key environmental conditions on microbially induced cementation for soil stabilization. *Geotech. Geoenviron. Eng.* **2017**, *143*, 04016083. [CrossRef]
24. Choi, S.G.; Park, S.S.; Wu, S.; Chu, J. Methods for calcium carbonate content measurement of biocemented soils. *J. Mater. Civ. Eng.* **2017**, *29*, 06017015. [CrossRef]
25. Gomez, M.G. *Field Scale Bio-Cementation for the Improvement of Loose Sands*; University of California, Davis: Davis, CA, USA, 2013.
26. Sun, X.H.; Miao, L.C.; Wu, L.Y. Applicability and theoretical calculation of enzymatic calcium carbonate precipitation for sand improvement. *Geomicrobiol. J.* **2020**, *37*, 389–399. [CrossRef]
27. Tang, C.S.; Yin, L.Y.; Jiang, N.J.; Zhu, C.; Zeng, H.; Li, H.; Shi, B. Factors affecting the performance of microbial-induced carbonate precipitation (MICP) treated soil: A review. *Environ. Earth Sci.* **2020**, *79*, 94. [CrossRef]
28. Xiao, Y.; He, X.; Stuedlein, A.W.; Chu, J.; Evans, T.M.; Van Paassen, L.A. Crystal growth of MICP through microfluidic chip tests. *Geotech. Geoenviron. Eng.* **2022**, *148*, 06022002. [CrossRef]
29. Almajed, A.; Khodadadi, H.; Kavazanjian, E. *Sisal Fiber Reinforcement of Eicp-Treated Soil*; American Society of Civil Engineers: Reston, VA, USA, 2018; pp. 29–36. [CrossRef]
30. Yuan, H.; Liu, K.; Zhang, C.; Zhao, Z. Experimental study on compressive strength of EICP technology solidifying silt in the Yellow River flooding area. *J. Henan Univ.* **2022**, *52*, 727–733. [CrossRef]
31. Carmona, J.P.S.F.; Venda Oliveira, P.J.; Lemos, L.J.L.; Pedro, A.M.G. Improvement of a sandy soil by enzymatic calcium carbonate precipitation. *Proc. Inst. Civ. Eng. Geotech. Eng.* **2018**, *171*, 3–15. [CrossRef]
32. Wen, K.; Li, Y.; Amini, F.; Li, L. Impact of bacteria and urease concentration on precipitation kinetics and crystal morphology of calcium carbonate. *Acta Geotech.* **2020**, *15*, 17–27. [CrossRef]
33. Whiffin, V.S.; van Paassen, L.A.; Harkes, M.P. Microbial carbonate precipitation as a soil improvement technique. *Geomicrobiol. J.* **2007**, *24*, 417–423. [CrossRef]
34. *ISO6058:1984*; ISO (1984) Water Quality: Determination of Calcium Content: EDTA Titrimetric Method. ISO: Geneva, Switzerland, 1984.

gels

MDPI

Article

Self-Healing and Tough Polyacrylic Acid-Based Hydrogels for Micro-Strain Sensors

Chuanjie Liu [1], Zhihong Liu [2,*] and Bing Lu [1,*]

[1] School of Chemistry and Chemical Engineering, Beijing Institute of Technology, Beijing 100081, China; 7520230176@bit.edu.cn
[2] School of Digital Media, Shenzhen Polytechnic University, Shenzhen 518055, China
* Correspondence: liuzhihong@szpu.edu.cn (Z.L.); blu@bit.edu.cn (B.L.)

Abstract: Self-healing hydrogels hold promise for smart sensors in bioengineering and intelligent systems, yet balancing self-healing ability with mechanical strength remains challenging. In this study, a self-healing hydrogel exhibiting superior stretchability was developed by embedding a combination of hydrogen bonding and dynamic metal coordination interactions, introduced by modified fenugreek galactomannan, ferric ions, and lignin silver nanoparticles, into a covalent polyacrylic acid (PAA) matrix. Synergistic covalent and multiple non-covalent interactions enabled the hydrogel with high self-healing ability and enhanced mechanical property. In particular, due to the introduction of multiple energy dissipation mechanisms, particularly migrative dynamic metal coordination interactions, the hydrogel exhibited ultra-high stretchability of up to 2000%. Furthermore, with the incorporation of lignin silver nanoparticles and ferric ions, the hydrogel demonstrated excellent strain sensitivity (gauge factor ≈ 3.94), with stable and repeatable resistance signals. Assembled into a flexible strain sensor, it effectively detected subtle human motions and organ vibrations, and even replaced conductive rubber in gaming controllers for real-time inputs. This study provides a versatile strategy for designing multifunctional hydrogels for advanced sensing applications.

Keywords: high strength and toughness; self-healing; micro-strain; sensing

1. Introduction

Flexible and wearable micro-sensors have attracted significant attention in recent years due to their vast potential in applications such as health monitoring, human–machine interfaces, and soft robotics [1–4]. To realize their full potential, the development of advanced sensing materials must seamlessly integrate mechanical flexibility with high sensitivity, ensuring reliable performance under dynamic and complex deformation conditions [5,6]. Hydrogels are three-dimensional (3D) network structures of chemically or physically crosslinked polymers with high water content, excellent flexibility and stretchability, making them potential candidates for bioengineering, expandable skin sensors, medical health monitoring, and soft robots [7–10]. However, conventional hydrogels often suffer from limitations such as poor mechanical robustness, low stretchability, and irreversible damage upon mechanical failure, which severely restrict their practical use in dynamic and demanding environments.

To address these challenges, recent research has focused on the development of tough and highly stretchable hydrogels with self-healing capabilities. Such hydrogels can maintain mechanical integrity under large deformations and autonomously restore their structure and functionality after damage without external stimuli, significantly enhancing device durability and lifespan [11,12]. This ability enables long-term, sustainable sensor operation, extends its service lifespan, and maintaining its strain sensitivity [13–15].

In recent years, non-covalent interactions, including metal–ligand, host–guest [16], hydrogen bonding [17], and hydrophobic interactions [18], have been introduced into the synthesis of self-healing hydrogels. In this context, metal–ligand interaction is an important dynamic non-covalent interaction and can be used as a physical cross-linker to prepare high-strength hydrogels. Through the dynamic ionic bonding and migration of metal ions, metal–ligand interactions can automatically heal, thereby preparing self-healing hydrogels [19,20]. Nevertheless, most previously reported self-healing sensors usually have difficulty in combining ideal mechanical properties, self-healing ability, and micro-strain sensing ability, which greatly limits the practical application of hydrogel sensors. Modified fenugreek galactomannan (OFG) is a natural polysaccharide derived from fenugreek seeds, chemically modified to enhance its solubility, water absorption, and mechanical properties [21,22]. When incorporated into hydrogels, OFG forms hydrogen bonds and dynamic non-covalent interactions with other components, such as PAA and metal ions, enabling the hydrogel to self-heal and improving its mechanical strength and flexibility.

In addition to mechanical resilience, the electrical sensitivity of hydrogels—particularly their resistance changes in response to mechanical stimuli—is critical for sensor performance. High gauge sensitivity allows for accurate and real-time monitoring of strain, pressure, and motion, which is essential for micro-scale sensing systems [23,24]. Therefore, developing multifunctional hydrogels that simultaneously integrate high toughness, large stretchability, self-healing ability, and pronounced piezoresistive responsiveness is of great significance.

In this study, a self-healing PAA/OFG-Fe^{3+} hydrogel (SPH) with excellent mechanical properties was developed by introducing multiple non-covalent interactions into a covalently crosslinked PAA network. Uniform and extensive H-bonding occurred between OFG, the PAA network, and lignin silver nanoparticles (Ag-NPs). In particular, dynamic metal coordination interactions played a key role in the development of the hydrogel, with Fe^{3+} forming coordination bonds with the carboxyl groups on the PAA/OFG matrix. The slippable dynamic metal coordination interactions allowed the hydrogel to achieve autonomous self-healing and exceptional mechanical strength (stretchability up to 2000%, fracture strength > 130 kPa). Furthermore, with the incorporation of conductive Ag-NPs and Fe^{3+}, the hydrogel demonstrated excellent strain sensitivity (gauge factor $\approx$ 3.94), along with repeatable and accurate resistance signal responses. Leveraging these advantages, the hydrogel was successfully assembled into a flexible strain sensor capable of monitoring subtle human motions and vocal vibrations of organs. This work offers a promising strategy for enriching the design and application of multifunctional hydrogels.

2. Results and Discussion

2.1. Characterization Results of the Hydrogel

The preparation mechanism of the hydrogel proposed in this paper is shown in Figure 1. A hydrogel with uniform texture and good performance was prepared by a one-pot polymerization method. The acrylic acid (AA) monomers undergo free radical polymerization under the action of the initiator ammonium persulfate (APS) and cross-linker N,N′-methylenebisacrylamide (MBA) to form covalent PAA network. The abundant carboxyl groups (–COOH) existing in PAA and OFG chains and hydroxyl (–OH) contributed to numerous H-bonds.

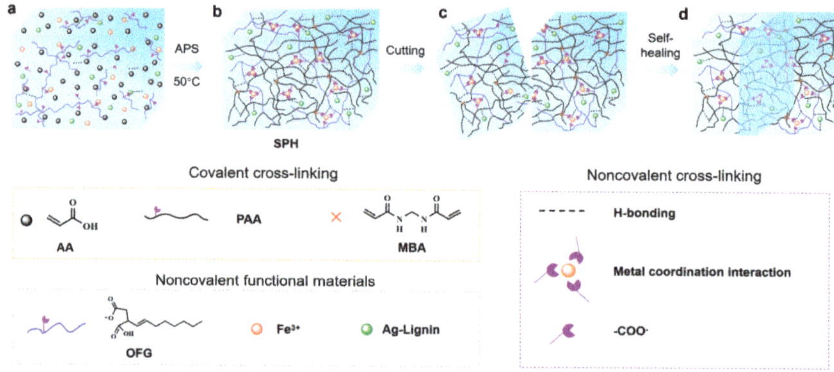

Figure 1. Synthesis and self-healing mechanism of the hydrogel. (**a**,**b**) Synthesis of the hydrogel. (**c**,**d**) Schematic diagram of the self-healing process of the hydrogel.

Meanwhile, the –COOH functionalities in the PAA and OFG chains engaged in dynamic and reversible coordination interactions with Fe^{3+} ions. Owing to the higher bonding energy compared to hydrogen bonds, metal coordination interaction can enhance the mechanical strength and performance stability of self-healing hydrogels. The self-healing ability and tensile properties of the hydrogel were studied by using hydrogels of different colors and observing their tensile images after recovery. As shown in Figure 2a, the dyed and undyed hydrogel samples were cut into two halves and then brought into contact with each other. After 24 h, the two pieces of hydrogel healed automatically, and the cut disappeared. During the self-healing process, the dye diffused from one piece of hydrogel to the other, resulting in a blurred contact interface between the two pieces of hydrogel, and the healed cut did not break after stretching Figure 2b.

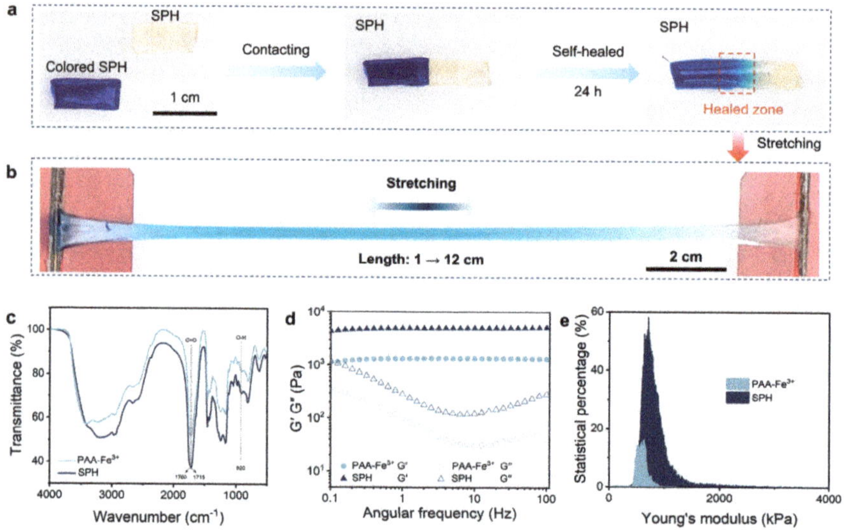

Figure 2. Characterization of PAA-Fe^{3+} and SPH. (**a**) Self-healing process of the hydrogel. Two hydrogels of different colors were placed at room temperature for 24 h. (**b**) The healed hydrogel being stretched. (**c**) FTIR. (**d**) Storage modulus (G′) and loss modulus (G″). (**e**) Distribution of Young's modulus.

As shown in Figure 2c, the absorption peak of the stretching vibration of the free carboxylic acid O-H is located at 3550 cm^{-1}. Due to the formation of the dimer, the carboxyl peak shifts to a lower wavenumber, forming a broad and dispersed peak in the range of 3200–2500 cm^{-1}. The formation of the dimer also affects the C=O stretching vibration of the free carboxylic acid, shifting it from 1760 cm^{-1} to 1715 cm^{-1}. A peak at 920 cm^{-1} is observed, which is a characteristic peak of the out-of-plane rocking vibration of the two-molecule association of the O-H group. The absorption band at 3424 cm^{-1} is attributed to the symmetric stretching vibration of the O-H stretching peak of the hydrogel, while the O-H stretching peak of SPH shifts to a lower wavenumber of 3400 cm^{-1}. According to previous reports [19], the obvious shift in the absorption band to a lower wavenumber indicates the formation of hydrogen bonds between PAA and OFG. Compared with PAA-Fe^{3+}, there is no obvious position change in SPH, indicating that the introduction of OFG does not significantly change the structure of the hydrogel. Figure S1 shows the X-ray diffraction pattern of the hydrogel. The X-ray diffraction spectrum of the hydrogel does not show an obvious crystalline phase, and there is a broad peak at about 20°, which is caused by the overall crystallinity of the hydrogel skeleton.

By comparing the rheological data of PAA-Fe^{3+} and SPH, the storage modulus G' of both hydrogels is higher than the loss modulus G'' during the rheological test (Figure 2d), and the loss factor is appropriate, indicating that their molecular chains have a certain degree of rigidity and flexibility, and an effective cross-linked network is formed between the molecular chains. The cross-linked structure may be relatively regular, enabling the material to exhibit good elasticity under dynamic stress. The dense entanglement of PAA and OFG chains around the cross-linking points of the SPH provides the mechanical strength for the hydrogel. The G' of SPH is significantly higher than that of PAA-Fe^{3+}, and its stress–strain data is discussed and analyzed in the following paragraphs. The change in Young's modulus of the hydrogel surface before and after the addition of OFG was measured by AFM (Figure 2e). The Young's modulus of the hydrogel after the addition of OFG increased significantly, which is consistent with the rheological data. Figure S2 shows the scanning electron microscope (SEM) images of the freeze-dried PAA-Fe^{3+} and SPHs; both hydrogels are composed of a cross-linked network and a uniform microporous structure, with a pore size range of 10–100 μm. However, the pore structure of the SPH network is more complex and the pore size is smaller, indicating that the structure of the hydrogel is denser. This is attributed to the formation process of the hydrogel; the strong hydrogen bonds between the functional groups and the metal–ligand interaction between Fe^{3+} and OFG increase the pore density of the hydrogel.

2.2. Mechanical Properties of the Hydrogel

We described a rationally designed topological molecular network. PAA and OFG chains are interconnected and entangled through abundant intermolecular hydrogen bonds, electrostatic interactions, and metal coordination interactions, serving as sacrificial conformations for energy dissipation during the deformation of the hydrogel (Figure 3a). As illustrated in Figure 3b, the fabricated hydrogel exhibits outstanding tensile properties, demonstrating the ability to undergo significant deformation, including uniaxial stretching, twisting under tension, and knotting while stretched, with an elongation exceeding ten times its original length. By comparing the rheological data (Figure 2c) and the tensile data (Figure 3), the hydrogel has a relatively high storage modulus and an appropriate loss factor during the rheological test, and the tensile Young's modulus conforms to Hooke's law, indicating that its molecular chains have a certain degree of rigidity and flexibility. In order to further explore the influence of the addition amount of each component in the preparation of the hydrogel on its mechanical properties, this paper discussed the influence of the addition amounts of OFG, Fe^{3+}, APS, and MBA on the stress–strain of the hydrogel.

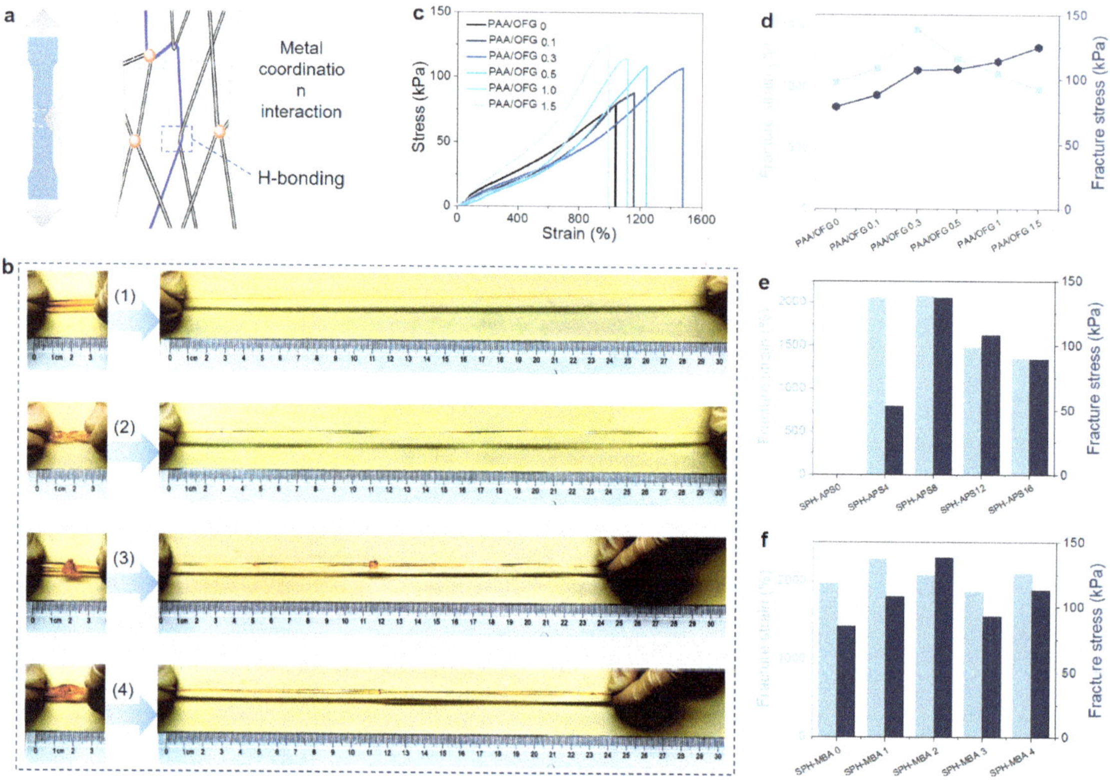

Figure 3. Tensile properties of the hydrogel. (**a**) A stretchable topological network structure composed of cross-linked molecular chains and entangled molecular chains. (**b**) The hydrogel can withstand different forms of stretching (knotting, crossing, and twisting). (**c**,**d**) Influence of the addition of OFG on the mechanical properties of the hydrogel. (**e**) Influence of the addition of APS on the mechanical properties of the hydrogel. (**f**) Influence of the addition of MBA on the mechanical properties of the hydrogel.

Figure 3c–f show the influence of different components on the mechanical properties of the hydrogel to evaluate the optimized content of each component. Firstly, the influence of the OFG content on the mechanical properties of the hydrogel was explored (Figure 3c). As the OFG content increased from 0 to 1.5%, the hydrogel exhibited a peak strain at 0.3% OFG, with a maximum breaking strength and elongation of 120 ± 10 kPa and 1000 ± 53% (n = 5), respectively. The highest stretchability and corresponding fracture strength reached 1450 ± 85% and 100 ± 13 kPa (n = 5). The mechanical strength of the SPH improved with increasing OFG content, likely due to enhanced hydrogen bonding and metal–ligand coordination. However, beyond 0.3% OFG, the elongation decreased, attributed to excessive non-covalent interactions restricting polymer chain mobility, thereby reducing flexibility and ductility.

Fe^{3+} ions coordinate with –COOH groups on PAA and OFG chains, forming a cross-linked network. Moderate Fe^{3+} addition increases cross-linking density, enhancing the hydrogel's strength and toughness by promoting uniform stress distribution. However, excessive Fe^{3+} leads to overly dense networks and possible aggregation, reducing chain mobility, increasing brittleness, and creating stress concentration points. As shown in Figure S3, PAA/OFG-Fe^{3+}0.10 shows the best mechanical performance.

Within a suitable range, increasing APS content promotes initiator decomposition, generating more free radicals that accelerate acrylic acid polymerization and enhance the cross-linking degree of the hydrogel. A higher cross-linking density contributes to a denser network, improving the hydrogel's strength, elasticity, and toughness (Figures 3e and S3c). However, excessive APS leads to an overly rapid reaction and high radical concentration, causing issues such as local overheating, uncontrolled polymerization, and structural defects. Moreover, an excessively cross-linked network may become too rigid, compromising flexibility and overall mechanical performance. Residual initiator may also negatively affect the hydrogel's properties.

Within a suitable range, increasing MBA content enhances the cross-linking density of the polyacrylic acid hydrogel, forming a denser three-dimensional network that improves stress transfer and restricts molecular chain slippage, thereby enhancing strength, hardness, and elastic modulus. Moderate MBA addition significantly improves tensile strength and deformation resistance (Figures 3f and S3d). However, excessive MBA leads to an overly rigid network, limiting chain mobility, reducing flexibility and toughness, and increasing the risk of brittle fracture. Additionally, a high MBA concentration may cause rapid gelation and uneven polymerization, resulting in local stress concentrations and compromised mechanical properties.

Overall, this study obtained an optimized formulation for the preparation of the hydrogel: (m (AA) 6.5 g, m (OFG) 0.09 g, m ($FeCl_3$) 0.10 g, m (APS) 8 mg, m (MBA) 2 mg), with stress and strain of 137 $\pm$ 17 kPa and 2076 $\pm$ 50% (n = 5), respectively. The excellent mechanical properties of SPH are derived from its COO^-/Fe^{3+} coordination network, H-bonding, PAA covalent network, high network density, and chain entanglement.

2.3. Self-Healing Properties of the Hydrogel

The hydrogel exhibits excellent self-healing capability, primarily attributed to its flexible polymer network and dynamic non-covalent interactions. On the one hand, the polymer chains possess intrinsic flexibility, allowing for rearrangement and entanglement after damage, which serves as a form of physical cross-linking to partially restore the network and mitigate further failure. On the other hand, dynamic and reversible interactions, such as hydrogen bonding between carboxyl groups and Fe^{3+} coordination, play a key role in healing. Upon fracture, these interactions dissociate at the damaged interface, generating active sites that can re-form under appropriate conditions through chain migration and reorientation. The synergistic effect of hydrogen bonding and metal–ligand coordination significantly enhances healing efficiency and network reconstruction, enabling the hydrogel to rapidly recover its structure and mechanical performance after damage.

In this study, the self-healing process of the hydrogel cut was observed using an inverted microscope. As shown in Figure 4a, the hydrogel sample was cut into two halves and then brought into contact with each other. After 24 h, the two pieces of hydrogel healed automatically, and the contact interface of the hydrogel became blurred. When stretching the hydrogel (Figure 4b), no cracks were observed, and the rupture site did not coincide with the wound healing site, indicating that the gel had been completely repaired. Generally, the area of the hysteresis loop represents the energy dissipation per unit volume during the deformation process. To evaluate the self-healing performance of SPH, loading and unloading tests were carried out on the prepared hydrogel. As shown in Figure 4c, the hysteresis loops of the hydrogel before and after self-healing were similar, further demonstrating that the hydrogel has remarkable self-healing properties.

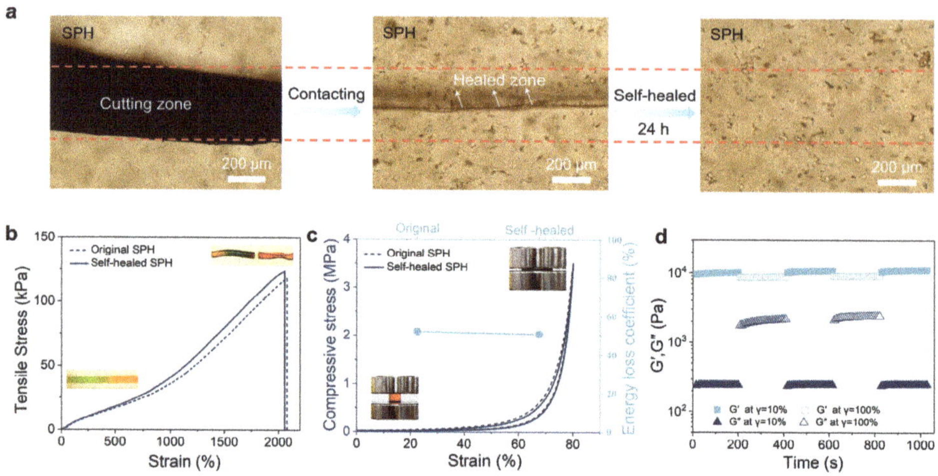

Figure 4. Self-healing properties of the hydrogel. (**a**) Optical microscope images show the changes in the cuts of two pieces of hydrogel over time at room temperature. (**b**) Tensile stress–strain curves of the original hydrogel and the self-healed hydrogel. (**c**) Compressive stress–strain curves and energy loss efficiency of the original hydrogel and the self-healed hydrogel. (**d**) The self-healing properties of the hydrogel are verified by measuring continuous step strains (10% strain→100% strain→10% strain→100% strain→10% strain).

The rheological experiment demonstrated that the hydrogel has stable mechanical strength and self-healing properties. Within a fixed time interval of 200 s, the hydrogel was subjected to alternating step strain tests (frequency = 1.0 Hz, strain = 10% or 100%), as shown in Figure 4d. The SPH oscillated under a small amplitude (frequency = 1.0 Hz, strain = 10%), with G' being approximately 10.0 kPa, G'' being approximately 0.24 kPa ($\text{Tan}\delta = G''/G' \approx 0.02$); when a large-amplitude oscillating force was applied to the hydrogel (frequency = 1.0 Hz, strain = 100%), the value of G' decreased from 10.0 kPa to approximately 8.7 kPa, and tanδ increased from 0.02 to 0.24. It can be seen from the rheological experiment that the mechanical stability of the hydrogel was somewhat lost, but the hydrogel system still existed, which was attributed to the stability of the hydrogel network structure. When the amplitude of the oscillating force was reduced (frequency = 1.0 Hz, strain = 10%), the G' and G'' of SPH could immediately return to their original values, which means that the internal network and mechanical properties of SPH were quickly restored.

2.4. Sensing Properties of the Hydrogel

Due to the presence of Fe^{3+} and lignin–Ag NPs, as well as the tensile strength and compressibility of PAA/OFG, it is speculated that the SPH can be used as a strain sensor. There is a correlation between the resistance change in the SPH and the mechanical strain, so a quantitative study was carried out on this sensor. As shown in Figure 5a, the addition of lignin–Ag NPs can improve the strain sensitivity of the hydrogel, and when the strain is 1200%, the gauge factor is 3.94. Ag NPs can construct nanoscale electronic conduction pathways, and lignin assists in electron transport through conjugate structures and interfacial interactions [22,25]. The Fe^{3+} dynamic network collaboratively regulates ion–electron mixed conductivity, breaking through the limitation of traditional hydrogels that only rely on ionic conduction, and providing a theoretical basis for the design of highly conductive and multifunctional intelligent soft materials. As shown in Figure 5g, the relative resistance change in the SPH can be intuitively observed by evaluating the change in the brightness of the LED light. An LED lamp, hydrogel, and external power supply are connected in series on a breadboard to form a complete conductive path. When the hydrogel deforms, dynamic adjustments in the conductive network structure, charge transport pathways, and interfacial interactions make the resistance positively correlated with the strain, thereby causing the brightness of the LED lamp to change in real time with the different stretching lengths of the hydrogel. As the strain increases, the resistance of the hydrogel increases, and the LED light gradually dims. Generally speaking, compared with traditional rigid strain sensors, stretchable strain sensors have the advantages of conformability and stretchability, solving the problem of mechanical mismatch between electronic devices and the human body. Although the sensitivity of SPH is lower than that of metal-based strain sensors, they still exhibit a large strain sensing range. Ten cycles of tensile loading–unloading measurements were carried out under different strains and speeds to evaluate the robustness of the sensing performance of SPH. The resistance response was stable in all cycles (Figure 5b,c), and SPH showed repeatability and durability.

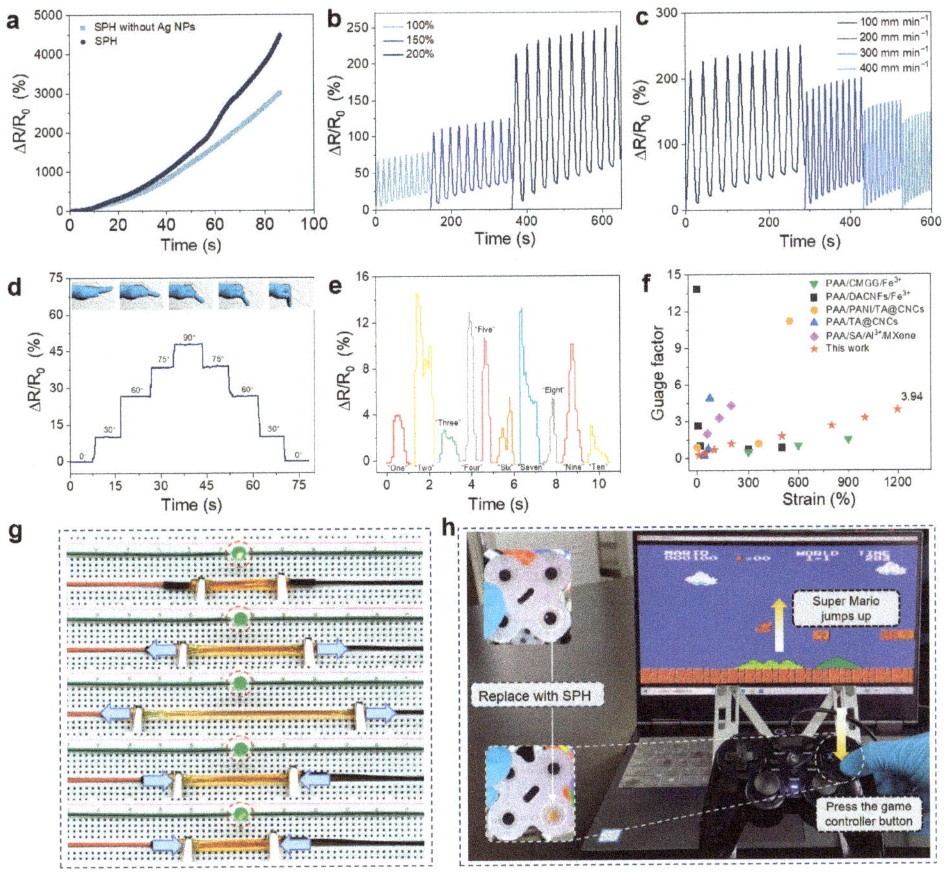

Figure 5. Sensing properties of the hydrogel. (**a**) Strain sensitivity of the hydrogel. (**b**) Curves of the relative resistance change under different strains. (**c**) Curves of the relative resistance change at different stretching speeds. (**d**) Monitoring the multi-angle movement of the finger. (**e**) Variation in the relative resistance over time when the human Adam's apple is speaking. (**f**) Comparison of the gauge factor between the sensor in this study and previously reported sensors [19,26–29]. (**g**) The brightness of the LED light changes with the deformation of the hydrogel. (**h**) The hydrogel replaces the conductive adhesive in the buttons of the game controller and successfully controls the computer game.

Since the prepared SPH have high tensile strength and self-healing ability, they were directly used as strain sensors to identify joint movements and vocalizations of organs, so as to construct wearable strain sensors. The SPH sensors were connected to wires, and an electrochemical workstation was used to record the corresponding signals. Figure 5d,e show that the PAA-based sensors are used to detect finger movements and Adam's apple movements. When the finger connected to the hydrogel sensor bends from the straight state to 0°, 30°, 60°, 75° and 90°, the relative resistance change rate presents a stepped curve (Figure 5d). This indicates that the PAA-based sensor can also be used for data collection and storage of finger movements. At the same time, when the volunteer successively pronounced different Arabic numerals, including "one" to "nine" and "zero", the hydrogel sensor was able to detect the vibration of the vocal cords (Figure 5e). These results show that the PAA-based hydrogel sensor has excellent micro-strain sensing potential and can be used for precise observation of human movements with a rapid response. To further explore and expand the application field of the hydrogel, the game controller was modified, and the hydrogel was used to replace the conductive adhesive in the controller buttons. After the modification, the game controller can still work normally without delay, further confirming the feasibility of the hydrogel as a conductive material (Figure 5h and Video S1). In addition, the preparation of the multifunctional self-healing hydrogel sensor was compared with the previously reported hydrogel sensors [19,26–29] in terms of the GF (Figure 5f), which indicates that the PAA hydrogel has superior performance and has great potential in human activity monitoring and personal health diagnosis.

3. Conclusions

In summary, a PAA-based hydrogel with superior stretchability and self-healing properties was synthesized by constructing a polymer network incorporating both covalent and multiple non-covalent interactions. The hydrogel demonstrates remarkable mechanical properties, including a stretchability of up to 2000% and a fracture strength of 130 kPa, facilitated by dynamic and reversible metal–ligand coordination interactions. In addition, the reversibility (dissociation and reconstruction) of various non-covalent bonds (H-bonding and metal coordination interaction) endows the hydrogel with excellent self-healing properties (approximately 100%). Furthermore, the incorporation of Fe^{3+} and Ag NPs imparts ionic conductivity, enabling the hydrogel to sense various human movements, including finger gestures and subtle vibrations from the Adam's apple, and to function as a conductive adhesive in gaming controllers for computer interface control. Therefore, PAA hydrogels exhibit application potential in multiple fields due to their excellent mechanical strength, self-healing ability, and micro-strain sensitivity: in biomedicine, they can serve as advanced wound dressings to monitor healing in real time; in soft robotics, they are suitable for manufacturing high-precision actuators to reduce maintenance requirements; in environmental monitoring, they can be made into highly sensitive sensors adaptable to harsh conditions; and in wearable electronics, they enable the creation of comfortable skin-friendly devices for accurate physiological signal tracking. In the future, further optimization of their properties and functional integration can expand their application prospects.

4. Materials and Methods

4.1. Materials

AA, $FeCl_3 \cdot 6H_2O$, APS, and MBA were all purchased from Aladdin Reagent (Shanghai) Co., Ltd. (Shanghai China), with analytical-grade purity. Modified fenugreek galactomannan (OFG) and lignin–Ag NPs (Ag NPs) were prepared according to the methods described in our previously published articles [21,22]. Deionized water was used as the solvent in this study.

4.2. Preparation of Hydrogels

The synthesis of PAA/OFG–Fe^{3+} hydrogels involved in situ radical polymerization of AA monomer within an aqueous OFG suspension, using MBA and Fe^{3+} as cross-linkers, and APS as the initiator. Initially, OFG was dissolved in deionized water under room-temperature stirring to form a homogeneous solution with a 0.3% mass fraction. Subsequently, 3.25 g of AA, 0.11 g of $FeCl_3$, and 8 mg of APS were added and mixed until uniform. Following this, 2 mg of MBA cross-linker and 200 μL of Ag NPs solution (25 mg/mL) were introduced, and the mixture was rapidly stirred. Oxygen was purged with nitrogen for 1 min before the solution was injected into a custom-made mold composed of two glass plates separated by 2 mm rubber gaskets. The molds were then subjected to polymerization at 50 °C for 2 h to yield the composite hydrogels.

To optimize the influence of various factors on the mechanical properties of hydrogels, different compositions of hydrogels were prepared. In the experiment, the prepared composite hydrogels were named PAA/OFGa ("a" representing the mass percentage of OFG), PAA/OFG-Fe^{3+}b ("b" represents the mass content of $FeCl_3$), SPH-APSc ("c" represents the mass content of APS), and SPH-MBAd ("d" represents the mass content of the MBA). The total volume of the solution mixture was fixed at 30 mL with deionized water. Tables S1–S4 (Supplementary information) list the detailed components.

4.3. Characterization

A Fourier Transform Infrared Spectrometer (FT-IR, Model: Bruker Optics Ltd., Ettlingen, Germany) was employed for qualitative analysis of chemical structure changes in PAA-Fe^{3+} and SPH, with the spectral range set at 400–4000 cm^{-1}. X-ray diffraction (XRD) patterns of PAA-Fe^{3+} and SPH were obtained using a Bruker D8 ADVANCE diffractometer (Ettlingen, Germany) under operating conditions of 80 mA and 60 kV, with the diffraction angle (2θ) scanned from 5° to 60°. Young's modulus data were acquired via a Bruker Icon atomic force microscope (AFM, Bruker Corp., Ettlingen, Germany). The surface morphology of PAA-Fe^{3+} and SPH particles was characterized by a scanning electron microscope (SEM, Model: S-3400 N II, Hitachi, Japan). Prior to testing, samples were dispersed on a metal sample holder using conductive silver paste and subjected to gold sputtering.

The rheological behaviors of PAA-Fe^{3+} and SPHs were investigated using a rotational rheometer (Model: Ares G2, New Castle, DE, USA) with a parallel plate geometry (diameter: 25 mm). The storage modulus (G′) and loss modulus (G″) were measured as functions of angular frequency (ω) within 0.1–100 rad/s. Additionally, the recovery properties of the hydrogels under applied shear forces were tested at ω = 1.0 Hz following the procedure: 10% strain (200 s) → 100% strain (200 s) → 10% strain (200 s) → 100% strain (200 s) → 10% strain (200 s).

4.4. Mechanical Testing

Tensile tests were performed using a HESON HS-3004B-S (Shanghai, China) machine equipped with a 100-N load cell. Hydrogel samples with dimensions of 12 mm × 3 mm × 2 mm were tested at a tensile speed of 100 mm/min. The energy dissipation (ΔE) of the self-recovery hydrogel was calculated from the area between loading–unloading curves of cyclic tensile loads, as defined by

$$\Delta E = \int \text{loading } S(\mu)d\mu - \int \text{unloading } S(\mu)d \quad (1)$$

where S(μ) and μ denote tensile stress and strain, respectively.

The experimental data were independently repeated at least 3 times ($n \geq 3$), and the sample size (n) and standard deviation (SD) of each group of experiments were marked in the Section 2.

4.5. Self-Healing Testing

The self-repairing properties of hydrogels were examined by cutting the origin hydrogel and dyeing the hydrogel (blue) into small fragments. With the mold, the size of the hydrogel block was rapidly reconstructed, and the self-healing process of the hydrogel was employed at room temperature without any external force or stimulation. The microscopic morphology of the original hydrogel and the healing hydrogel was observed with a camera.

4.6. Fabrication Strain Sensors

An electrochemical workstation (CHI 800 D, Shanghai, China) was used to record relative resistance changes in hydrogel sensors at a constant voltage of 2 V during finger and throat movements. For cyclic strain sensing measurements, the electrochemical workstation was coupled with a tensile testing machine to synchronously record resistance changes during loading. The feasibility of using the hydrogel as a sensor was verified by the brightness variation in an LED lamp and side reactions of a game handle: the LED lamp, hydrogel, and external power supply were connected in series on a breadboard to form a conductive path, and LED brightness was observed by controlling hydrogel deformation. The relative resistance change is defined by Equation (2), and the gauge factor (GF) of the hydrogel is calculated by Equation (3):

$$\Delta R/R_0\ (\%) = (R - R_0)/R_0 \times 100\% \tag{2}$$

$$GF = (\Delta R/R_0)/\varepsilon \text{ with } \varepsilon = (l_T - l_0)/l_0 \tag{3}$$

where R_0 and R are the initial resistance at 0% strain and the real-time resistance at specific strain, respectively; l_0 and l_T are the initial length and the length at time T of the hydrogel.

Supplementary Materials: The following supporting information can be downloaded at: https://www.mdpi.com/article/10.3390/gels11070475/s1, Figure S1: XRD curves of PAA-Fe^{3+} and SPH. Figure S2: SEM images of PAA-Fe^{3+} and SPH. [Scale bar: 500 μm]. Figure S3: Tensile properties of the hydrogel. (a and b) Influence of the addition of Fe^{3+} on the mechanical properties of the hydrogel. (c) Influence of the addition of APS on the mechanical properties of the hydrogel. (d) Influence of the addition of MBA on the mechanical properties of the hydrogel; Table S1: Schemes of optimized experiment (OFG). Table S2: Schemes of optimized experiment (Fe^{3+}). Table S3: Schemes of optimized experiment (APS). Table S4: Schemes of optimized experiment (MBA).; Video S1: Playing games with a controller.

Author Contributions: Data curation, C.L., Z.L. and B.L.; formal analysis, C.L.; investigation, C.L.; methodology, C.L.; resources, Z.L. and B.L.; validation, Z.L. and B.L.; writing—original draft, C.L.; writing—review and editing, Z.L. and B.L. All authors have read and agreed to the published version of the manuscript.

Funding: This work was financially supported by the National Natural Science Foundation of China (22205129) and the Research Projects of Department of Education of Guangdong Province (2024CJPT002).

Institutional Review Board Statement: Not applicable.

Informed Consent Statement: Not applicable.

Data Availability Statement: The original contributions presented in this study are included in the article. Further inquiries can be directed to the corresponding author.

Conflicts of Interest: The authors declare no conflicts of interest.

Abbreviations

The following abbreviations are used in this manuscript:

OFG	Modified fenugreek galactomannan
PAA	Polyacrylic acid
Ag-NPs	Lignin–silver nanoparticles
SPH	Self-healing PAA/OFG-Fe^{3+} hydrogel

References

1. Chen, K.Y.; Xu, Y.T.; Zhao, Y.; Li, J.K.; Wang, X.P.; Qu, L.T. Recent progress in graphene-based wearable piezoresistive sensors: From 1D to 3D device geometries. *Nano Mater. Sci.* **2023**, *5*, 247–264. [CrossRef]
2. Liang, Y.; Zhao, F.; Cheng, Z.H.; Deng, Y.; Xiao, Y.; Cheng, H.; Zhang, P.; Huang, Y.; Shao, H.; Qu, L. Electric power generation via asymmetric moisturizing of graphene oxide for flexible, printable and portable electronics. *Energy Environ. Sci.* **2018**, *11*, 1730–1735. [CrossRef]
3. Wu, M.; Qiao, C.Y.; Sui, P.F.; Luo, J.; Li, Z.; Cao, Y.; Pei, R.; Peng, X.; Zeng, H. Stratum corneum-inspired zwitterionic hydrogels with intrinsic water retention and anti-freezing properties for intelligent flexible sensors. *Adv. Funct. Mater.* **2025**, 2422755. [CrossRef]
4. Liu, T.; Zhang, M.Y.; Li, Z.H.; Dou, H.; Zhang, W.; Yang, J.; Wu, P.; Li, D.; Mu, X. Machine learning-assisted wearable sensing systems for speech recognition and interaction. *Nat. Commun.* **2025**, *16*, 2363. [CrossRef]
5. Tchantchane, R.; Zhou, H.; Zhang, S.; Alici, G. Fabrication and characterization of a soft and stretchable capacitive strain sensor for hand gesture recognition. *IEEE Sens. J.* **2025**, *25*, 601–612. [CrossRef]
6. Zhou, X.L.; Chen, X.L.; Yang, B.; Luo, S.; Guo, M.; An, N.; Tian, H.; Li, X.; Shao, J. Advancements in functionalizable metal-organic frameworks for flexible sensing electronics. *Adv. Funct. Mater.* **2025**, 2501683. [CrossRef]
7. Kovacevic, B.; Jones, M.; Ionescu, C.; Walker, D.; Wagle, S.; Chester, J.; Foster, T.; Brown, D.; Mikov, M.; Mooranian, A.; et al. The emerging role of bile acids as critical components in nanotechnology and bioengineering: Pharmacology, formulation optimizers and hydrogel-biomaterial applications. *Biomaterials* **2022**, *283*, 121459. [CrossRef] [PubMed]
8. Yang, D.; Ni, Y.; Kong, X.; Li, S.; Chen, X.; Zhang, L.; Wang, Z.L. Self-healing and elastic triboelectric nanogenerators for muscle motion monitoring and photothermal treatment. *ACS Nano* **2021**, *15*, 14653–14661. [CrossRef]
9. Li, H.; Liang, Y.; Gao, G.; Wei, S.; Jian, Y.; Le, X.; Lu, W.; Liu, Q.; Zhang, J.; Chen, T. Asymmetric bilayer CNTs-elastomer/hydrogel composite as soft actuators with sensing performance. *Chem. Eng. J.* **2021**, *415*, 128988. [CrossRef]
10. Li, Z.; Liu, P.; Ji, X.; Gong, J.; Hu, Y.; Wu, W.; Wang, X.; Peng, H.; Kwok, R.T.K.; Lam, J.W.Y.; et al. Bioinspired simultaneous changes in fluorescence color, brightness, and shape of hydrogels enabled by AIEgens. *Adv. Mater.* **2020**, *32*, 1906493. [CrossRef]
11. Tan, Y.; Yan, M.X.; Dong, H.Q.; Wang, C.; Shao, L.; Xiao, X.; Li, W.; Ji, Z.; Ling, Z. Biomimetic construction of adhesive, self-healing and antifatigue hydrogels via galactomannan-induced double-network cross-linking for flexible strain sensors. *ACS Appl. Polym. Mater.* **2025**, *7*, 2517–2528. [CrossRef]
12. Tian, Y.S.; Wei, Y.; Wang, M.; Wang, J.; Li, X.; Qin, X.; Zhang, L. Ultra-stretchable, tough, and self-healing polyurethane with tunable microphase separation for flexible wearable electronics. *Nano Energy* **2025**, *139*, 110908. [CrossRef]
13. Robby, A.I.; Lee, G.; Park, S.Y. NIR-induced pH-reversible self-healing monitoring with smartphone by wireless hydrogel sensor. *Sens. Actuators B-Chem.* **2019**, *297*, 126783. [CrossRef]
14. Rao, V.K.; Shauloff, N.; Sui, X.; Wagner, H.D.; Jelinek, R. Polydiacetylene hydrogel self-healing capacitive strain sensor. *J. Mater. Chem. C* **2020**, *8*, 6034–6041. [CrossRef]
15. Zhang, J.; Chen, L.; Shen, B.; Mo, J.; Tang, F.; Feng, J. Highly stretchable and self-healing double network hydrogel based on polysaccharide and polyzwitterion for wearable electric skin. *Polymer* **2020**, *194*, 122381. [CrossRef]
16. Ren, Z.; Ke, T.; Ling, Q.; Zhao, L.; Gu, H. Rapid self-healing and self-adhesive chitosan-based hydrogels by host-guest interaction and dynamic covalent bond as flexible sensor. *Carbohydr. Polym.* **2021**, *273*, 118533. [CrossRef] [PubMed]
17. Wu, L.; Li, L.; Pan, L.; Wang, H.; Bin, Y. MWCNTsreinforced conductive, self-healing polyvinyl alcohol/carboxymethyl chitosan/oxidized sodium alginate hydrogel as the strain sensor. *J. Appl. Polym. Sci.* **2021**, *138*, 49800. [CrossRef]
18. Wang, J.; Tang, F.; Wang, Y.; Lu, Q.; Liu, S.; Li, L. Self-healing and highly stretchable gelatin hydrogel for self-powered strain sensor. *ACS Appl. Mater. Interfaces* **2020**, *12*, 1558–1566. [CrossRef]
19. Chen, W.; Bu, Y.H.; Li, D.L.; Liu, Y.; Chen, G.; Wan, X.; Li, N. Development of high-strength, tough, and self-healing carboxymethyl guar gum-based hydrogels for human motion detection. *J. Mater. Chem. C* **2020**, *8*, 900–908. [CrossRef]

20. Chen, W.; Bu, Y.H.; Li, D.L.; Liu, C.; Chen, G.; Wan, X.; Li, N. High-strength, tough, and self-healing hydrogel based on carboxymethyl cellulose. *Cellulose* **2019**, *27*, 853–865. [CrossRef]
21. Liu, C.J.; Ning, R.X.; Lei, F.H.; Li, P.; Wang, K.; Jiang, J. Study on the structure and physicochemical properties of fenugreek galactomannan modified via octenyl succinic anhydride. *Int. J. Biol. Macromol.* **2022**, *214*, 91–99. [CrossRef]
22. Liu, C.J.; Cheng, X.C.; Zhang, F.L.; Lei, F.; Li, P.; Wang, K.; Jiang, J. Preparation and application of galactomannan-based green hydrogels initiated by lignin-Ag NPs. *Mater. Today Commun.* **2023**, *34*, 105256. [CrossRef]
23. Hu, F.H.; Yu, D.H.; Gong, X.; Li, Z.; Zhao, R.; Wang, Q.; Zhang, F.; Li, G.; Wang, H.; Liu, W.; et al. Amylopectin-enhanced MXene/gallium hydrogels: High-performance flexible conductive materials for multifunctional sensing, EMI shielding, and energy storage applications. *Chem. Eng. J.* **2025**, *510*, 161793. [CrossRef]
24. Liu, X.; Chen, L.Z.; Sufu, A.; Liu, F.F. Stretchable and self-healing carboxymethyl cellulose/polyacrylic acid conductive hydrogels for monitoring human motions and electrophysiological signals. *Int. J. Biol. Macromol.* **2025**, *293*, 138900. [CrossRef]
25. Gan, D.; Xing, W.; Jiang, L.; Fang, J.; Zhao, C.; Ren, F.; Fang, L.; Wang, K.; Lu, X. Plant-inspired adhesive and tough hydrogel based on Ag-Lignin nanoparticles-triggered dynamic redox catechol chemistry. *Nat. Commun.* **2019**, *10*, 1487. [CrossRef] [PubMed]
26. Wang, Y.; Zhang, H.; Zhang, H.; Chen, J.; Li, B.; Fu, S. Synergy coordination of cellulose-based dialdehyde and carboxyl with Fe^{3+} recoverable conductive self-healing hydrogel for sensor. *Mater. Sci. Eng. C-Mater. Biol. Appl.* **2021**, *125*, 112094. [CrossRef]
27. Shao, C.Y.; Meng, L.; Cui, C.; Yang, J. An integrated self-healable and robust conductive hydrogel for dynamically self-adhesive and highly conformable electronic skin. *J. Mater. Chem. C* **2019**, *7*, 15208–15218. [CrossRef]
28. Shao, C.; Wang, M.; Meng, L.; Chang, H.; Wang, B.; Xu, F.; Yang, J.; Wan, P. Mussel-inspired cellulose nanocomposite tough hydrogels with synergistic self-healing, adhesive, and strain-sensitive properties. *Chem. Mater.* **2018**, *30*, 3110–3121. [CrossRef]
29. Fan, C.H.; Wang, D.; Huang, J.Y.; Ke, H.Z.; Wei, Q.F. A highly sensitive epidermal sensor based on triple-bonded hydrogels for strain/pressure sensing. *Compos. Commun.* **2021**, *28*, 100951. [CrossRef]

gels

MDPI

Article

Study on Road Performance and Ice-Breaking Effect of Rubber Polyurethane Gel Mixture

Yuanzhao Chen [1,2,3,4], Zhenxia Li [1,2,3,4], Tengteng Guo [1,2,3,4,*], Chenze Fang [1,2,3,4], Jingyu Yang [1,2,3,4], Peng Guo [5], Chaohui Wang [6], Bing Bai [1], Weiguang Zhang [7], Deqing Tang [1] and Jiajie Feng [1]

1 School of Civil Engineering and Transportation, North China University of Water Resources and Electric Power, Zhengzhou 450045, China; cyz740513@ncwu.edu.cn (Y.C.); zhenxiali2009@ncwu.edu.cn (Z.L.); fangchenze@126.com (C.F.); yangjingyu@ncwu.edu.cn (J.Y.); baibing7777@ncwu.edu.cn (B.B.); tdq18738952643@163.com (D.T.); 18027459877@163.com (J.F.)

2 Henan Province Engineering Technology Research Center of Environment Friendly and High-Performance Pavement Materials, Zhengzhou 450045, China

3 Technology Innovation Center of Henan Transport Industry of Utilization of Solid Waste Resources in Traffic Engineering, North China University of Water Resources and Electric Power, Zhengzhou 450045, China

4 Henan Province University-Enterprise Research and Development Center for Green, Low-Carbon and High-Performance Road Materials, Zhengzhou 450045, China

5 National and Local Joint Engineering Laboratory of Traffic Civil Engineering Materials, Chongqing Jiaotong University, Chongqing 400074, China; guopeng@cqjtu.edu.cn

6 School of Highway, Chang'an University, Xi'an 710064, China; wchh0205@chd.edu.cn

7 School of Transportation, Southeast University, Nanjing 210096, China; wgzhang@seu.edu.cn

* Correspondence: guotth@ncwu.edu.cn; Tel.: +86-13673359605; Fax: +86-0371-69127209

Abstract: Aiming at the problems of serious pavement temperature diseases, low efficiency and high loss of ice-breaking methods, high occupancy rate of waste tires and the low utilization rate and insufficient durability of rubber particles, this paper aims to improve the service level of roads and ensure the safety of winter pavements. A pavement material with high efficiency, low carbon and environmental friendliness for active snow melting and ice breaking is developed. Firstly, NaOH, NaClO and KH550 were used to optimize the treatment of rubber particles. The hydrophilic properties, surface morphology and phase composition of rubber particles before and after optimization were studied, and the optimal treatment method of rubber particles was determined. Then, the optimized rubber particles were used to replace the natural aggregate in the polyurethane gel mixture by the volume substitution method, and the optimum polyurethane gel dosages and molding and curing processes were determined. Finally, the influence law of the road performance of RPGM was compared and analyzed by means of an indoor test, and the ice-breaking effect of RPGM was explored. The results showed that the contact angles of rubber particles treated with three solutions were reduced by 22.5%, 30.2% and 36.7%, respectively. The surface energy was improved, the element types on the surface of rubber particles were reduced and the surface impurities were effectively removed. Among them, the improvement effect of the KH550 solution was the most significant. With the increase in rubber particle content from 0% to 15%, the dynamic stability of the mixture gradually increases, with a maximum increase of 23.5%. The maximum bending strain increases with the increase in its content. The residual stability increases first and then decreases with the increase in rubber particle content, and the increase ranges are 1.4%, 3.3% and 0.5%, respectively. The anti-scattering performance increases with the increase in rubber content, and an excessive amount will lead to an increase in the scattering loss rate, but it can still be maintained below 5%. The fatigue life of polyurethane gel mixtures with 0%, 5%, 10% and 15% rubber particles is 2.9 times, 3.8 times, 4.3 times and 4.0 times higher than that of the AC-13 asphalt mixture, respectively, showing excellent anti-fatigue performance. The friction coefficient of the mixture increases with an increase in the rubber particle content, which can be

 https://doi.org/10.3390/gels11070505

increased by 22.3% compared with the ordinary asphalt mixture. RPGM shows better de-icing performance than traditional asphalt mixtures, and with an increase in rubber particle content, the ice-breaking ability is effectively improved. When the thickness of the ice layer exceeds 9 mm, the ice-breaking ability of the mixture is significantly weakened. Mainly through the synergistic effect of stress coupling, thermal effect and interface failure, the bonding performance of the ice–pavement interface is weakened under the action of driving load cycle, and the ice layer is loosened, broken and peeled off, achieving efficient de-icing.

Keywords: pavement materials; rubber particles; polyurethane gels; ice-breaking effect; road performance; ice breaking mechanism

1. Introduction

Pavement needs to withstand the test of a complex natural environment during service, and the temperature disease caused by extreme temperature accounts for a significant proportion of all kinds of pavement diseases. These diseases will lead to pavement structure damage and performance degradation, seriously affecting the service life of the road and driving safety [1,2]. Most parts of China belong to seasonal frozen areas, and the low-temperature period in winter is long, which is often accompanied by rain and snow weather [3]. Snow and ice can easily lead to a significant reduction in road surface adhesion, causing vehicle tire slip and loss of control, resulting in casualties and traffic accidents, which seriously threaten the safety of public transportation [4–6]. In this regard, researchers have proposed many ways to melt ice and snow, such as spreading snow-melting agent, artificial-mechanical de-icing, and electrothermal snow-melting pavement. However, the above methods occupy traffic resources to varying degrees and reduce the level of road services. In this context, road active snow melting and de-icing technology has received extensive attention. Through the application of new materials, new ideas and new technologies, this technology gives the road surface the ability to melt ice and snow independently, which significantly improves the safety of road operation in winter. The low freezing point pavement [7,8] achieves ice melting and snow melting by improving the interfacial adhesion between the pavement and the ice and snow layer, but its snow-melting components are still dominated by chloride salts, resulting in the possibility that the salt residue in the lower part of the salt storage pavement cannot be released, which is difficult to meet the actual needs of environmental protection and practicality. As a branch of active ice and snow removal technology, energy conversion ice and snow removal pavement [9–11] has high snow-melting efficiency, but there are problems such as high construction cost and easy aging of materials. The construction technology of self-stress elastic pavement [12,13] is relatively simple, has better economy, avoids the negative impact of traditional ice and snow melting technology and has a certain environmental protection value. Therefore, it is necessary to study this aspect.

Under the premise of confirming the feasibility of ice melting and snow melting of rubber asphalt pavement, most of the relevant research focuses on the forming process, ice-breaking mechanism, snow-melting and ice-melting characteristics and influencing factors, mixture composition design and the performance improvement of rubber asphalt ice-melting pavement. Liang et al. [14] combined diatomite and crumb rubber particles to prepare a modified asphalt mixture. It was found that the incorporation of rubber particles and diatomite significantly improved the high-temperature stability and low-temperature crack resistance of the asphalt mixture. Chen Yuanzhao [13] proposed a prediction method of elastic modulus by establishing a multi-step, multi-phase micromechanical model. The research shows that an increase in rubber particles will reduce the elastic modulus of the mixture, and the elastic modulus of the mixture will increase significantly under low-temperature conditions, resulting in the weakening of the de-icing effect. The monitoring data of the test road by American researchers show that there is a problem of particle peeling in the practical application of rubber asphalt pavement, which leads to the road performance of the test section not being up to expectations, and the effect of ice and snow removal is limited. Li et al. [15] tested the aging performance of three typical rubber materials—ethylene propylene rubber, liquid silicone rubber and fluorine rubber—under different high- and low-temperature cycling aging conditions. The experimental results showed that repeated temperature cycling can cause fatigue failure, which may lead to a permanent increase in rubber compression deformation. Ma et al. [16] proposed a new comprehensive evaluation index (snowmelt performance coefficient; SMPC) and optimized the design parameters of the conductive rubber snowmelt bridge deck through the I-PSO algorithm. Shan et al. [17] found that the incorporation of terminal carboxylated nitrile rubber significantly improved the mechanical properties and low-temperature crack resistance of asphalt without changing the curing time. Although the high-temperature rutting resistance of asphalt itself is reduced, the high-temperature, low-temperature and water stability of porous asphalt concrete are improved. It can be seen that although rubber asphalt pavement can effectively alleviate the ice and snow problem of pavement in ice and snow weather, there are still some technical limitations. In engineering applications, rubber will age over time due to the influence of natural and artificial environments, lose elasticity, and decrease mechanical properties, resulting in cracked asphalt pavement. This causes great harm to the performance and service life of the road, and also means that the anti-icing function of asphalt pavement mixed with rubber particles will be weakened. Therefore, how to make up for the deficiency of rubber particle asphalt mixture in terms of strength and durability has become more and more difficult.

Polyurethane gels are a new type of polymer. It can be used to obtain a variety of products by adjusting the synthetic materials and preparation process. Because of its good performance, it has been widely used in various fields at home and abroad [4,18–21]. Polyurethane-modified asphalt mixture is mainly committed to improving the performance of asphalt. However, this does not completely make up for the shortcomings of the asphalt material itself. Therefore, researchers began to use it as a binder to completely replace asphalt in the development of polyurethane mixtures. Zheng et al. [22] found that the optimum molding time window for PERS is 40 to 50 min after the curing of polyurethane, balancing mechanical properties and minimizing springback. Gao et al. [23] found that the direct tensile change process of a polyurethane rubber particle mixture is divided into four stages. The mixture of polyurethane rubber particles and F2 polyurethane has high tensile properties at 18% content. Chen et al. [24,25] prepared a polyurethane mixture according to the gradation specification of an asphalt mixture. According to the research, it is found that polyurethane binder has outstanding performance in thermal conductivity, and its thermal conductivity is much higher than that of asphalt, so polyurethane gel mixtures can effectively shorten the time required for road icing in road laying applications and have excellent anti-icing and de-icing performance. Zou et al. [26] found optimal toughness at a 0.70 water–cement ratio with 6% rubber content, meeting mechanical pumping specifications while maintaining structural performance. Agavriloaie et al. [27] developed a polymer concrete with acrylate as the main component by implementing the polymerization reaction of acrylate. The results show that, compared with ordinary concrete, acrylate polymer concrete exhibits superior mechanical properties. The research results of Min Sun et al. [28] pointed out that the adhesion performance between basalt and polyurethane gels is better than that of limestone in the consideration of aggregate lithology and the selection of gradation, which has a positive effect on improving water stability. Li et al. [29] studied the physical and rheological properties of ACR/TPU composite modified asphalt, characterized the microscopic mechanism of active rubber powder and found that the choice of modifier dosage can be verified by digital fluorescence microscope. Wang et al. [30] found that the strain value of a polyurethane porous elastic pavement layer was significantly higher than that of ordinary porous asphalt pavement through indoor testing and numerical simulation. This phenomenon strongly confirmed the applicability and engineering advantages of polyurethane porous elastic pavement in urban road applications in cold regions.

In summary, polyurethane gel binder has the advantages of high viscoelasticity, strong chemical corrosion resistance and strong wear resistance, and it has broad application prospects in the field of road engineering. However, it is rare to study the application of polyurethane gels as a binder in the ice breaking of road pavement. Due to the poor adhesion between rubber particles and asphalt, rubber particles are prone to fall off under vehicle load, resulting in insufficient stability of the pavement structure, which, in turn, affects the durability and performance of the pavement. The emergence of polyurethane gels provides a new direction and idea for the lack of structural stability of rubber particle mixtures. Therefore, in this paper, polyurethane gels are used as the binder of new pavement. Through economical, simple and feasible modification methods, rubber particles with good bonding performance are developed and incorporated into a polyurethane gel mixture. By using the overall elastic deformation of pavement, the effect of active snow and ice breaking is realized, and the anti-skid performance and driving safety of pavement under cold weather conditions are improved, thus effectively improving the operation efficiency and traffic capacity of pavement. At the same time, it avoids the damage to infrastructure and environmental pollution caused by traditional de-icing methods and prolongs the service life of the road. It is of great significance to promote the development of green pavement materials and improve the service life of roads.

2. Results and Discussion

2.1. *Performance Analysis of Modified Rubber Particles*

2.1.1. Analysis of Hydrophilic Properties of Modified Rubber Particles

The contact angle test results of the rubber particle surface under different treatment methods are shown in Table 1.

Table 1. Contact angle test results of rubber particles–water surface.

Surface Modification Methods	Without Modification	NaOH Modification	NaClO Modification	KH550 Modification
contact angle (°)	125.5	88.6	79.8	72.3

It can be seen from Table 1 that the contact angle between the surface of rubber particles and water decreased after different solution treatments; that is, the hydrophilicity of the surface of rubber particles was improved. The contact angle of the unmodified rubber particles was 125.5°, showing obvious hydrophobicity. After 30 min of treatment, the contact angle of the rubber particles showed a decreasing trend. The contact angle of the rubber particles treated with NaOH solution decreased from 125.5° to 88.6°, which was reduced by 29.6%. The contact angle of the rubber particles modified by NaClO solution decreased to 79.8°, which was reduced by 36.4%. The contact angle of rubber particles after immersion in KH550 solution was 72.3°, which was reduced by 42.4%. The surface of the rubber material changed from hydrophobic to hydrophilic, indicating that the surface properties of the rubber particles were significantly changed by the modification treatment: from the original hydrophobic state to partial hydrophilic characteristics, the surface wetting angle was significantly reduced, and the water contact performance was significantly improved. This change in surface properties is due to the synergistic effect of two aspects in the modification process: on the one hand, it effectively removes the hydrophobic impurity phase on the surface, and on the other hand, polar functional groups such as hydroxyl (-OH) and carboxyl (-COOH) were successfully introduced, which significantly improved the surface energy characteristics of the material. It can be seen that the improvement of the surface hydrophilicity of the rubber particles by the three modifiers is KH550 solution > NaClO solution > NaOH solution. After modification, the surface polarity and surface energy of the rubber particles are significantly improved, resulting in a decrease in the contact angle with the liquid and a significant improvement in the wettability. The optimization of this surface characteristic shows that the modified rubber particles have enhanced interfacial affinity, thereby improving their compatibility with the matrix material. This improvement is conducive to the full penetration of the polar adhesive at the interface and ultimately significantly improves the adhesion strength between the two-phase materials.

2.1.2. Fine Microstructure Analysis of Modified Rubber Particles

SEM tests were carried out on the surface morphology of rubber particles with different modification methods, and the microscopic morphology of different multiples is shown in Figures 1–4.

It can be seen from Figure 1 that as the magnification increases, the microstructure of the rubber particles becomes clearer and clearer. From the microscopic perspective, the surface of the rubber particles presents a rough and uneven state, and the surface is scattered with micropores. When the magnification reaches 2000 times, the bulge on the surface shows a multi-edged and sharp shape, and there is no specific regular shape. At the same time, it contains more impurity phases. These impurities are not only adsorbed dust but are also due to waste tires in the process of production and storage, as well as additives such as fatty acids and zinc oxide.

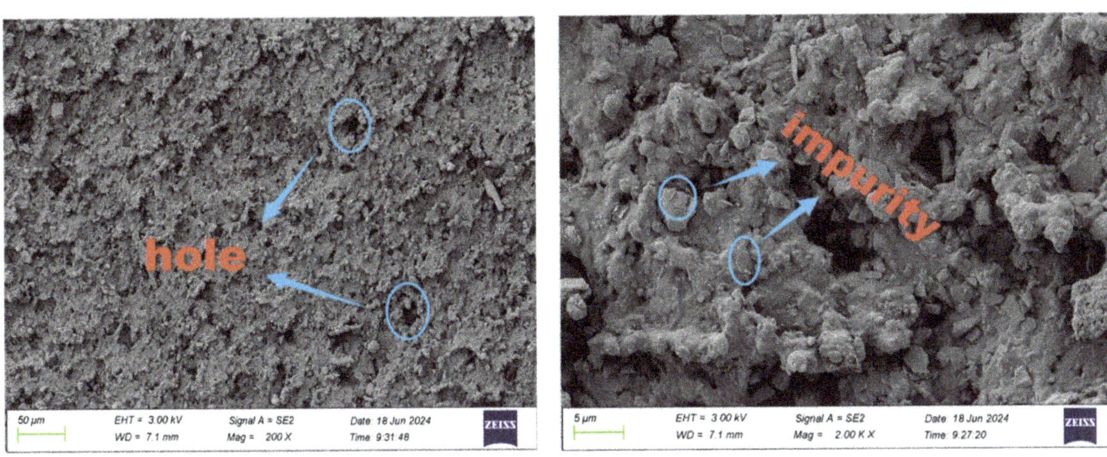

(**a**) 200 times (**b**) 2000 times

Figure 1. Microstructure of unmodified rubber particles.

It can be seen from Figure 2 that when the magnification is 200 times, the surface microstructure of the rubber particles modified by NaOH solution changes significantly: the number of corroded micropores increases greatly, the pore size increases and the surface roughness increases significantly. At a high magnification of 2000 times, the surface impurity phase of the modified rubber particles was significantly reduced, and the surface convex structure showed round and smooth morphological characteristics. NaOH modification not only improves the porosity of rubber particles through water washing but also makes the pore structure clearer, the pore size distribution more uniform and the surface morphology more rough and uneven.

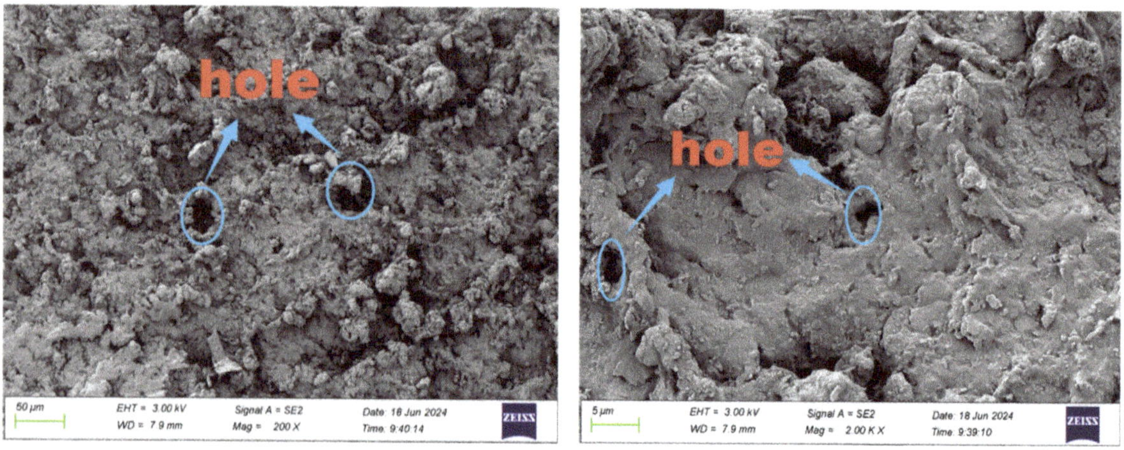

(**a**) 200 times (**b**) 2000 times

Figure 2. Microstructure of NaOH-modified rubber particles.

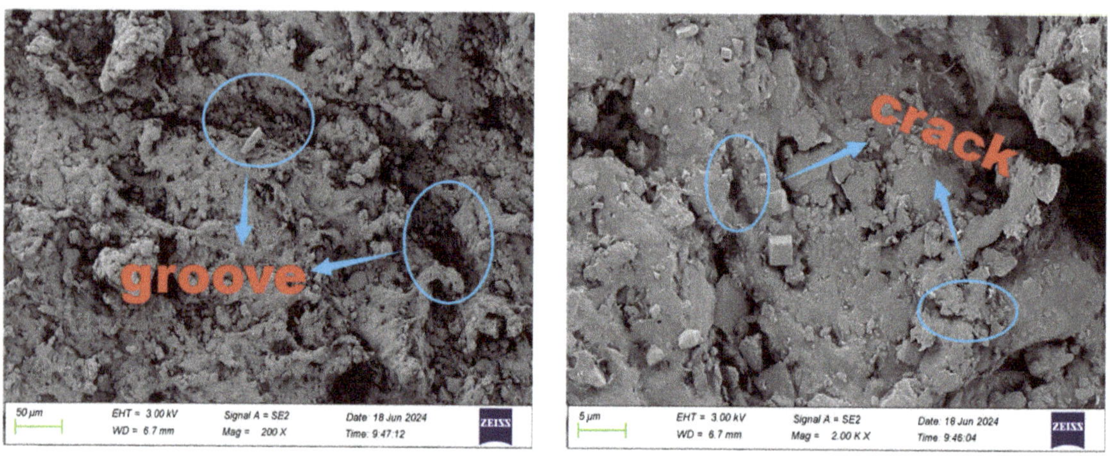

(**a**) 200 times (**b**) 2000 times

Figure 3. Microstructure of NaClO-modified rubber particles.

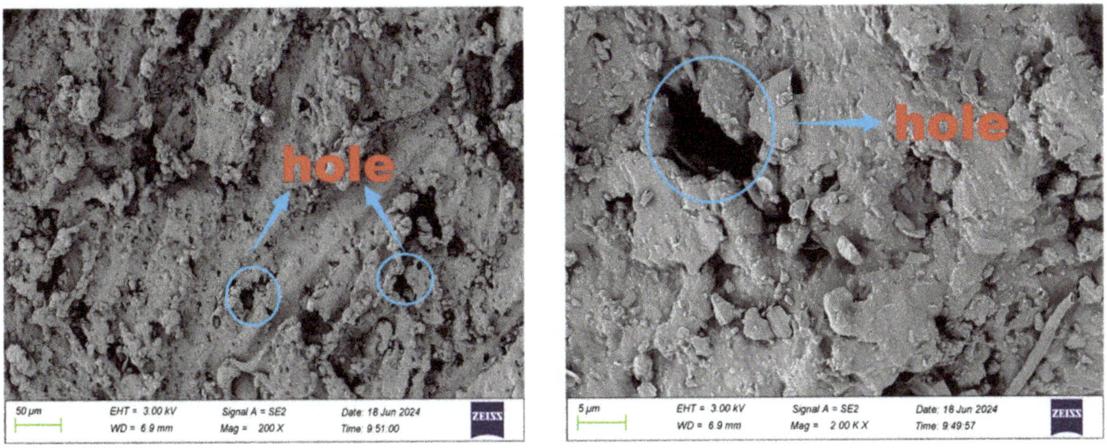

(**a**) 200 times (**b**) 2000 times

Figure 4. Microstructure of KH550-modified rubber particles.

This significant change in surface morphology is mainly attributed to the removal effect of residual additives in rubber particles. The surface pretreatment with NaOH solution can effectively remove the zinc stearate coating layer on the surface of rubber particles through saponification reaction, remove the residual solvent on the surface, and form a porous structure on the surface of rubber particles. This surface modification significantly improves the roughness and porosity of the rubber particles, which is conducive to enhancing the interfacial bonding performance between the cementitious material and the rubber particle interface and improving the overall strength of the mixture.

It can be seen from Figure 3 that after NaClO solution treatment, the surface wrinkles of rubber particles increased significantly, and a large number of grooves and pores were formed, which significantly improved the unevenness of the surface. The main reason for the change in surface morphology is that NaClO solution can effectively remove the residual solvent and low molecular weight organic matter on the surface of rubber particles, thus forming a porous structure on the surface. Compared with the untreated rubber particles, the surface roughness of the modified rubber particles was significantly improved, and a large number of micron-sized voids and microcracks were generated.

According to the mechanical meshing theory, the increase in the surface roughness of the clay provides more permeation channels and anchoring points for the binder molecules. During the curing process, the adhesive can fully penetrate into the surface pores and microcracks to form a three-dimensional interlocking structure, thereby significantly improving the interfacial bonding strength. This surface modification method provides an effective technical way to improve the interfacial compatibility between rubber particles and cementitious material matrix.

After being modified by the KH550 silane coupling agent, the surface morphology of rubber particles obviously changed. Due to the chemical adsorption and self-assembly of the coupling agent molecules on the surface of the rubber particles, the surface morphology of the rubber particles develops in the direction of flattening, and the continuity of the surface protrusions is significantly enhanced. At the same time, a large number of villous protrusions were formed on the surface of rubber particles, which further improved the surface roughness. As shown in Figure 4, the surface roughness of the rubber particles modified by KH550 is higher, the porosity is larger and the surface structure is looser. The number and continuity of surface corrosion pores increase significantly, which provides more anchorage points for interface bonding. The increase in surface roughness enhances the mechanical meshing effect. The three-dimensional fluffy topology formed on the surface of rubber particles increased significantly after modification. The synergistic effect of these surface characteristics significantly enhances the interfacial bonding strength between the rubber particles and the cementitious material matrix, thereby effectively improving the working performance of the rubber particle mixture.

2.1.3. Phase Composition Analysis of Modified Rubber Particles

Table 2 summarizes the results of energy spectrum composition analysis on the surface of rubber particles after different modification methods.

Table 2. Energy spectrum composition table of rubber particles with different modification methods.

Without Modification			NaOH Modification			NaClO Modification			KH550 Modification		
ele.	Wt%	At%	ele.	Wt%	At%	ele.	Wt%	At%	ele.	Wt%	At%
C	59.3	69.7	C	67.2	74.9	C	60.1	70.2	C	61.4	70.7
O	17.2	18.8	O	21.9	21.4	O	26.3	25.3	O	21.1	20.8
Zn	17.9	6.7	Zn	6.3	1.4	Zn	9.2	2.1	Zn	7.6	2.2
Cl	1.5	2.6	Cl	1.9	1.0	Cl	3.5	1.7	Cl	1.8	1.7
Zr	0.6	0.3	Zr	0.2	0.2	Zr	0.3	0.1	Si	4.3	2.8
S	0.2	0.3	S	1.1	0.4	S	0.2	0.4	Ca	0.2	0.1
K	0.3	0.1	Ca	1.2	0.4	Al	0.1	0.1	N	3.6	1.7
Ca	2.5	0.4	Al	0.2	0.3	Ca	0.3	0.1	—		
Al	0.5	1.1	—			—			—		

It can be seen from Table 2 that the types of surface elements of rubber particles treated by three modification methods are reduced, indicating that the surface impurity phase is effectively removed. Among them, the content of Zn element is significantly reduced, which confirms that the removal effect of zinc stearate is obvious. The mass fraction of Zn element on the surface of rubber particles modified by NaOH decreased by 84%, which was mainly attributed to the fact that NaOH solution could effectively dissolve the zinc stearate layer remaining on the surface of rubber particles during the crushing process of waste tires. The modification of NaClO led to a significant increase in the content of O element on the surface of rubber particles, indicating that NaClO successfully achieved surface activation and introduced more oxygen-containing functional groups, such as hydroxyl (-OH) and carboxyl (-COOH). This chemical modification changed the surface morphology of rubber particles from relatively smooth to wrinkles and grooves. In contrast, the KH550 silane coupling agent treatment formed a uniform silane layer on the surface of the rubber particles. This interface transition layer effectively filled the surface grooves and wrinkles, making the surface morphology tend to be flat. This modification not only improved the surface characteristics but also enhanced the interface compatibility between the rubber particles and the matrix material.

Compared with unmodified and NaOH- and NaClO-modified rubber particles, the mass fraction of Si element on the surface of rubber particles increased significantly after KH550 modification. This phenomenon is attributed to the chemical grafting reaction between the KH550 silane coupling agent and the surface of rubber particles. The silanol group (-SiOH) generated after the hydrolysis of KH550 undergoes a dehydration condensation reaction with the oxygen-containing functional groups (such as -OH, -COOH) on the surface of the rubber particles. At the same time, the adjacent R group forms a stable Si-O-Si covalent bond through condensation, thus constructing a uniform silane coupling agent structure layer on the surface of the rubber particles. The organic functional groups in the molecular structure form chemical bonds with the surface of the rubber particles and play a molecular bridging role at the inorganic–organic interface. This interfacial modification significantly improves the interfacial compatibility between rubber particles and cementitious materials, enhances the interfacial bonding strength and further optimizes the mechanical properties of the mixture.

2.2. Polyurethane Gel Dosage Test Analysis

According to the relevant specifications [31], the freeze–thaw splitting test was carried out. The relationship between the splitting strength and the splitting strength ratio and the amount of polyurethane gels was shown in Figure 5.

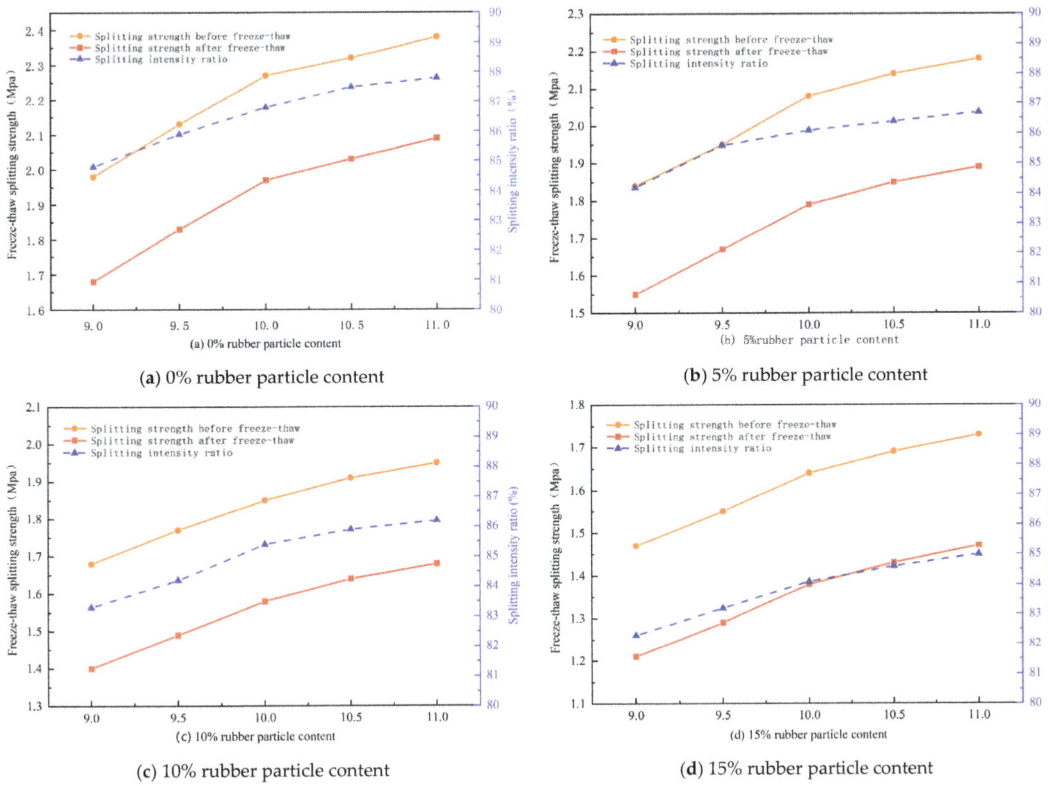

(**a**) 0% rubber particle content (**b**) 5% rubber particle content (**c**) 10% rubber particle content (**d**) 15% rubber particle content

Figure 5. Freeze–thaw splitting strength–polyurethane gel change curve of mixtures with different rubber particle contents.

It can be found from Figure 5 that the splitting strength ratio of the mixture prepared by replacing the fine aggregate with four kinds of rubber particles of 0%, 5%, 10% and 15% meets the technical requirements of the specification, which indicates that the polyurethane gel mixture shows good water damage resistance under different rubber particle content conditions. The freeze–thaw splitting strength of the mixture is positively correlated with the amount of polyurethane gels, but with an increase in the amount, the strength growth shows obvious stage characteristics. Under the same rubber particle content, when the amount of polyurethane gels increased from 9–9.5% and then to 10%, the freeze–thaw splitting strength of the specimen showed a rapid upward trend; however, when the amount of polyurethane gels continued to increase from 10% to 10.5% and then to 11%, the strength growth rate significantly slowed down. Taking RPGM mixed with 10% rubber particles as an example, when the amount of polyurethane gels increased from 9–9.5% and then to 10%, the freeze–thaw splitting strength ratio of the specimens increased by 1.1% and 1.4%, respectively; while the amount increased from 10–10.5%, the strength only increased by 0.5%. This is because the strength of the mixture mainly depends on the bonding force formed by the polyurethane gel binder at the aggregate interface. Therefore, increasing the amount of glue at the initial stage can significantly improve the interface bonding effect. However, due to the limited contact surface of rubber particles in the mixture, the excessive amount of glue only leads to the thickening of the adhesive film on the aggregate surface, which has a limited effect on the overall strength improvement, thus making the strength growth trend gradually flatten out.

In summary, when the amount of polyurethane gels increases to 10%, the strength of the RPGM increases most significantly, and then the growth rate gradually slows down, and the water damage resistance of the mixture fully meets the use requirements. From the perspective of engineering economy and performance, in order to ensure that the mixture has sufficient water damage resistance reserve and to avoid cost waste caused by excessive use, the optimal polyurethane gel dosage of the mixture is determined to be 10%.

2.3. Road Performance Analysis of Mixture

2.3.1. Elevated Temperature Property

As the evaluation index of the rutting test indicates, dynamic stability is positively correlated with the high-temperature performance of the mixture. The results after three tests are shown in Figure 6.

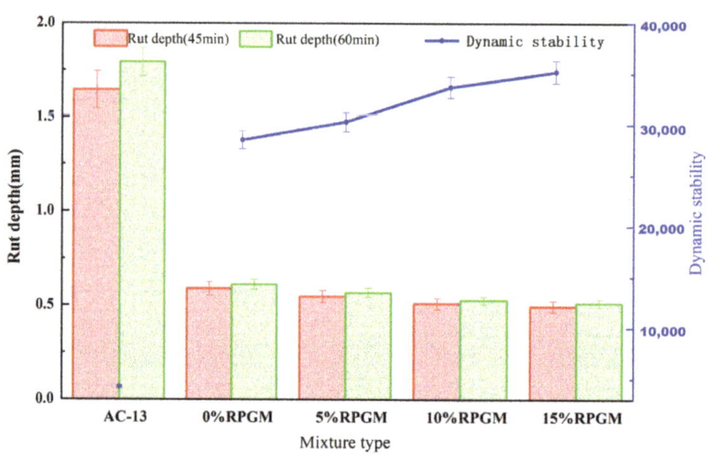

Figure 6. Rutting deformation and dynamic stability change curve.

It can be seen from Figure 6 that the deformation of RPGM is significantly lower than that of the ordinary asphalt mixture. The dynamic stability of the AC-13 asphalt mixture is 4229 times/mm, and the dynamic stability of RPGM with 0% rubber particle content is 28,507 times/mm, which is more than 7 times that of the former, and shows an upward trend with an increase in rubber particle content. It can be seen that RPGM has an absolute advantage in terms of high-temperature stability. This performance advantage is due to the essential difference between the two binders: asphalt binder is highly sensitive to temperature, and it is easy to soften and flow under high-temperature conditions, resulting in insufficient high-temperature stability of the asphalt mixture. Polyurethane gel binder is a kind of thermosetting material, and its two components form cross-linking solidification through a chemical reaction, resulting in excellent thermal stability, so that the polyurethane gel mixture has excellent high-temperature rutting resistance.

Compared with RPGM without rubber particle content, the dynamic stability of RPGM with 5% rubber particle content increased by 6.2%. The dynamic stability of RPGM with 10% dosage increased by 18.2%. The dynamic stability of RPGM with 15% rubber particle content increased by 23.5%. This shows that rubber particles have a significant effect on enhancing the anti-rutting performance of the mixture. This is because the rubber particles have a low elastic modulus, and the external load is converted into internal elastic potential energy through elastic deformation. Under the action of wheel load, the rubber particles undergo recoverable deformation, thus effectively dispersing the stress concentration and reducing the strain concentration of the mixture. Due to the excellent elastic recovery performance of rubber particles, they can be quickly restored to the original state after unloading, thereby reducing the permanent deformation of the mixture.

2.3.2. Low-Temperature Performance

The maximum flexural tensile strain at the bottom of the beam was selected to characterize the low-temperature performance of the rubber polyurethane gel mixtures. The results after four tests are shown in Figure 7.

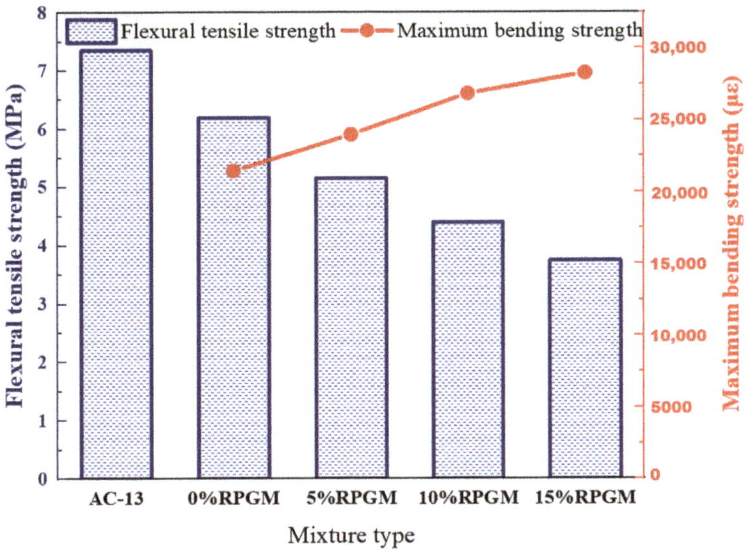

Figure 7. Low-temperature bending test results.

It can be seen from Figure 7 that the addition of rubber particles significantly increased the maximum bending strain of RPGM. When the content was 5%, 10% and 15%, the maximum bending strain was 11.8%, 25.1% and 31.7% higher than that of RPGM with 0% rubber particles. However, the incorporation of rubber particles has a negative impact on the flexural tensile strength. The flexural tensile strength of RPGM with 5%, 10% and 15% rubber particles decreased by 16.6%, 28.9% and 39.6%, respectively, compared with RPGM without rubber particles. This is mainly due to the introduction of rubber particles, which reduces the overall strength of the mixture and makes the material more prone to cracking when stressed.

Although the flexural strength of RPGM is slightly lower than that of the traditional asphalt mixture, its maximum flexural strain value is much higher than that of the latter, which is more than 7 times that of the asphalt mixture. With an increase in rubber particle content, the elastic deformation ability of the mixture is significantly enhanced, which further verifies that RPGM has good deformation ability, so that it can effectively absorb and disperse stress under complex load conditions, thereby improving the durability of the pavement. It can be seen that the introduction of rubber particles improves the low-temperature performance of the mixture, mainly due to its excellent stress relaxation characteristics, so that RPGM can still maintain good deformation adaptability when the temperature drops sharply, inhibiting the generation of low-temperature shrinkage cracks and prolonging the service life of the pavement.

2.3.3. Water Stability

The water stability of RPGM was evaluated by the immersion Marshall test and the immersion dispersion test. The test results are shown in Figures 8 and 9.

It can be seen from Figure 8 that the residual stability of RPGM is much higher than that of the AC-13 asphalt mixture under four kinds of rubber particle substitution, indicating that RPGM has better water damage resistance under different rubber particle contents. Moreover, with the increase in rubber particle content, the residual stability of RPGM showed a trend of increasing first and then decreasing. Compared with the polyurethane gel mixture without rubber particles, the residual stability of RPGM increased by 1.4%, 3.3% and 0.5%, respectively, indicating that increasing the content of rubber particles can improve the water stability of the mixture. This is due to the fact that the polarity of the optimized rubber particles and polyurethane gel molecules is relatively close, which strengthens the bonding force between polyurethane gels and rubber particles. The optimized rubber particles can fully fill the voids in the mixture, improve the compactness, reduce water intrusion and form a more stable and water-resistant structure. The higher the rubber particle content, the better the water stability of the mixture. However, when the content of rubber particles increases from 10–15%, the residual stability of the mixture shows a decreasing trend, but it is still higher than that of the ordinary asphalt mixture. This is because too many rubber particles may lead to insufficient encapsulation of polyurethane gel binder, uneven dispersion, increased porosity and other problems, affecting its bearing capacity and stability. Therefore, with the increase in rubber particle substitution, the residual stability of the polyurethane gel mixture increases first and then decreases.

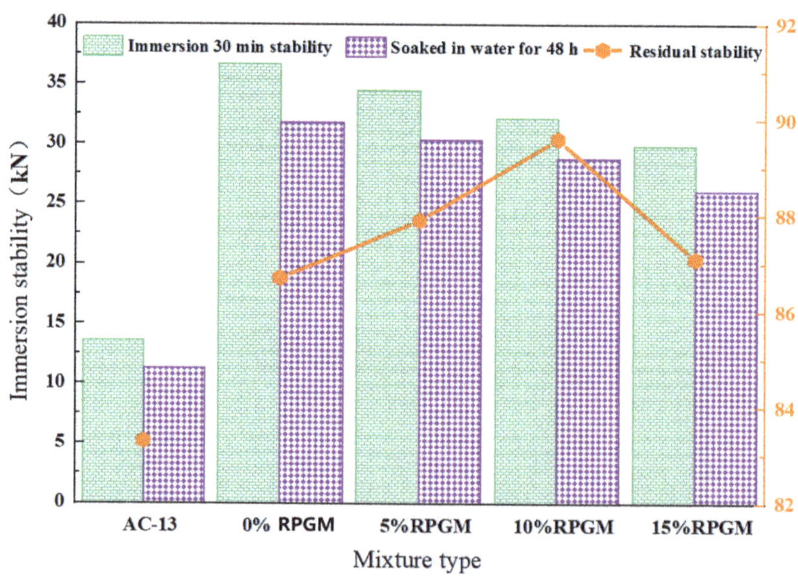

Figure 8. Results of Marshall immersion test.

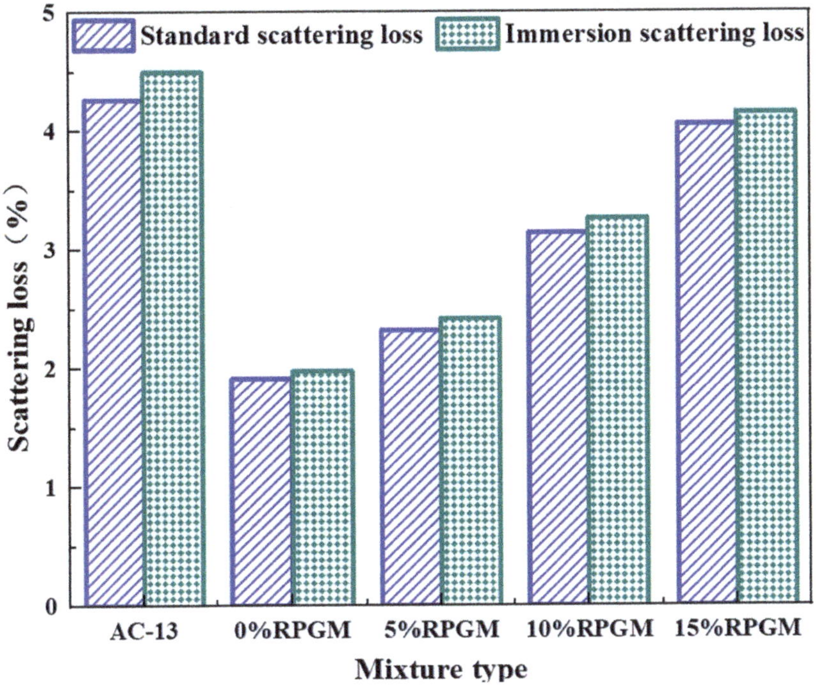

Figure 9. Results of immersion scattering test.

Compared with the AC-13 asphalt mixture, the scattering loss rate of the mixtures with four kinds of rubber particle content decreased by 56.2%, 46.3%, 27.5% and 7.7%, showing stronger wear resistance, and the scattering resistance of the specimen was improved. In addition, the mass loss of RPGM before and after soaking is less than 5%, and it does not have a great impact with the change in rubber particle content. This shows that under the action of water, the polyurethane gel binder and aggregate still maintain a good bond strength and have good water stability. However, when the content of rubber particles continues to increase, the scattering loss rate will show a continuous upward trend. The scattering loss rate of the mixture with 5%, 10% and 15% rubber particles is 22.6%, 65.4% and 110.6% higher than that of the mixture with 0% rubber particles, respectively. This is because the bonding performance between rubber particles and polyurethane gels is worse than that of stone, which leads to the formation of a large number of 'rubber–rubber' contact points in the aggregate when the content of rubber particles is too high. Under the action of collision, these contact points easily lead to the separation of the aggregate, thus reducing the overall strength of the specimen and ultimately leading to an increase in the scattering loss, but it still meets the requirements. This shows that the urethane adhesive can still maintain good bonding strength under soaking conditions, and the aggregate does not easily fall off the surface of the specimen, which ensures the overall structural stability and high strength of the mixture.

2.3.4. Fatigue Property

The fatigue test results of RPGM are shown in Figure 10.

According to Figure 10, the fatigue resistance of the polyurethane gel mixture is much higher than that of the ordinary asphalt mixture. When the stress ratio is 0.3, the fatigue life of polyurethane gel mixtures with 0%, 5%, 10% and 15% rubber particles is 3.6 times,

3.4 times, 3.2 times and 2.8 times that of the AC-13 asphalt mixture, respectively. This is because polyurethane gels have excellent bonding performance and high strength, which can firmly bond rubber particles together to form a network structure with certain flexibility and strength. This structure makes the RPGM bear the load. Through the synergistic effect of the elastic deformation of rubber particles and the polyurethane gel network, the stress can be effectively dispersed and transmitted, and the local stress concentration can be reduced, thereby improving the fatigue resistance of the material.

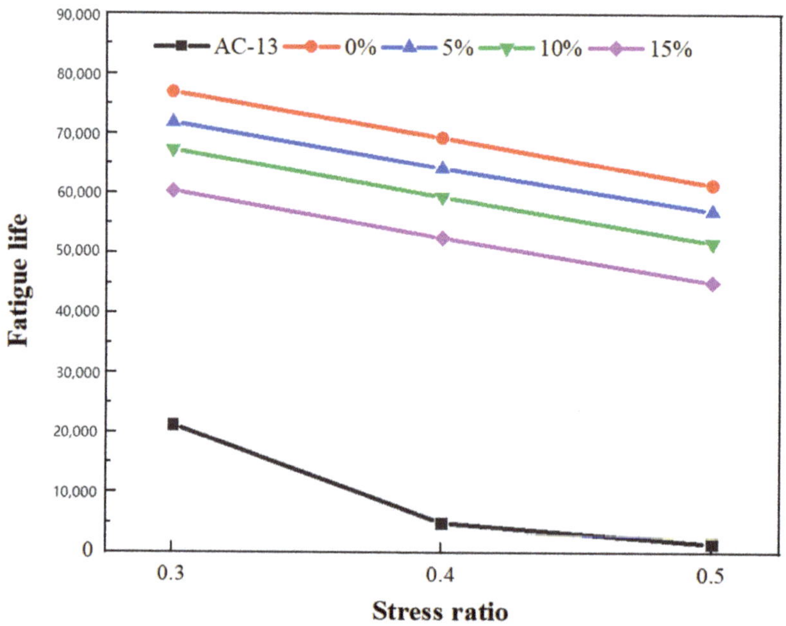

Figure 10. Fatigue life curve of RPGM.

When the stress level is the same and the content is different, the fatigue life of the mixture gradually decreases with the increase in the content of rubber particles, indicating that the incorporation of rubber particles reduces the fatigue performance of the polyurethane gel mixture. Under the 0.3 stress ratio, compared with the polyurethane gel mixture with 0% rubber particle content, the fatigue life of the mixture with 5%, 10% and 15% rubber particle content decreased by 6.6%, 12.5% and 21.5%, respectively. When the content is the same and the stress ratio is different, the fatigue life of the RPGM gradually decreases with the increase in the stress ratio. Taking the content of 10% as an example, the logarithmic fatigue life of RPGM at 0.4 and 0.5 stress ratios was 4.7741 and 4.7144, respectively, and the logarithmic fatigue life at 0.3 stress ratio decreased by 4.17%, 7.03% and 8.18%, respectively. It can be seen that rubber particles have a certain negative effect on the fatigue performance of the polyurethane gel mixture, and the degree of influence gradually increases with the increase in content. This is because the modulus of rubber is lower than that of polyurethane gels. Excessive incorporation will reduce the overall stiffness of the mixture, resulting in increased strain amplitude and accelerated fatigue damage.

According to Formula (1), the fatigue life of RPGM under different stress levels is analyzed by regression fitting, and the results are shown in Figure 11.

$$\log N_f = C - D\sigma \tag{1}$$

where N_f is the number of load action. σ is the stress level, and C and D are characteristic parameters of fatigue test.

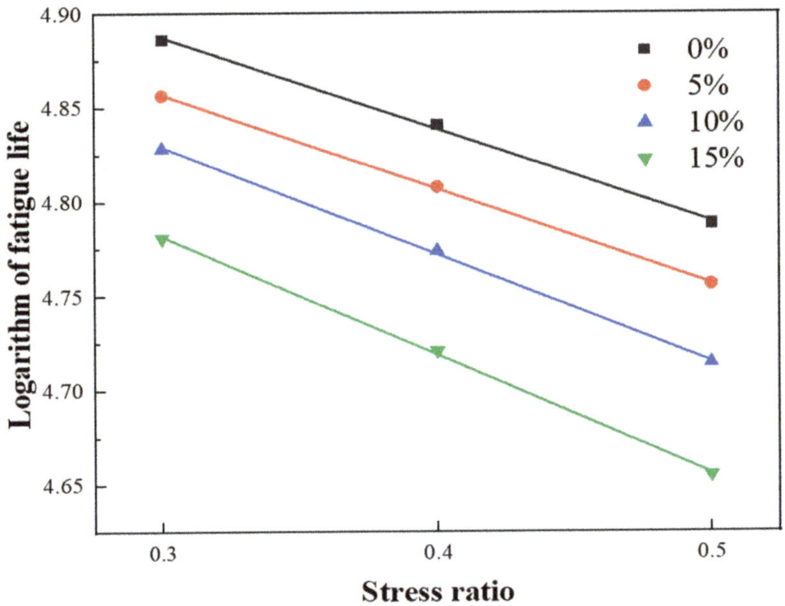

Figure 11. RPGM logarithmic fatigue life curve fitting results.

It can be seen from Figure 11 that after the logarithm of fatigue life is linearly fitted, the fatigue life of RPGM with different contents shows good linear regression characteristics at a 0.3~0.5 stress ratio. The correlation coefficient R^2 obtained after fitting reached more than 99.0%, indicating that the linear equation can effectively fit the test data, so the equation can be used for the regression analysis of RPGM. Among them, the coefficient D value represents the sensitivity of the fatigue life of the RPGM to the stress level. The larger the D value, the higher the sensitivity of the fatigue life to the stress level. The C value represents the intercept of the fatigue curve on the coordinate axis. The larger the C value, the better the fatigue resistance of the RPGM. The C value decreases with the increase in rubber particle content, indicating that the fatigue performance of polyurethane gel mixtures becomes worse with the increase in rubber particle content.

2.3.5. Slip Resistance

Research on the anti-skid properties of icy and snowy road surfaces is of great significance for ensuring traffic safety, economically efficient winter maintenance and energy conservation. Skid resistance is a key factor in ensuring vehicle safety on road surfaces, and excellent skid resistance is a prerequisite for safe vehicle operation. This chapter follows the method outlined in the "Field Testing Procedures for Highway Subgrade and Pavement" [31] (JTG 3450-2019), recording test temperatures and measured swing values and applying temperature corrections according to Equation (2). The test results are presented in Table 3 and Figure 12.

$$BPN_{20} = BPN_T + \Delta BPN \tag{2}$$

In the formula: BPN_{20}—Converted to the pendulum value at a standard temperature of 20 °C;

BPN_T—Swing value at road surface temperature T;

ΔBPN—temperature correction value; see Table 3.

Table 3. Temperature correction value.

Temperature (°C)	0	5	10	15	20	25	30	40
temperature correctionΔBPN	−6	−4	−3	0	+2	+3	+5	+7

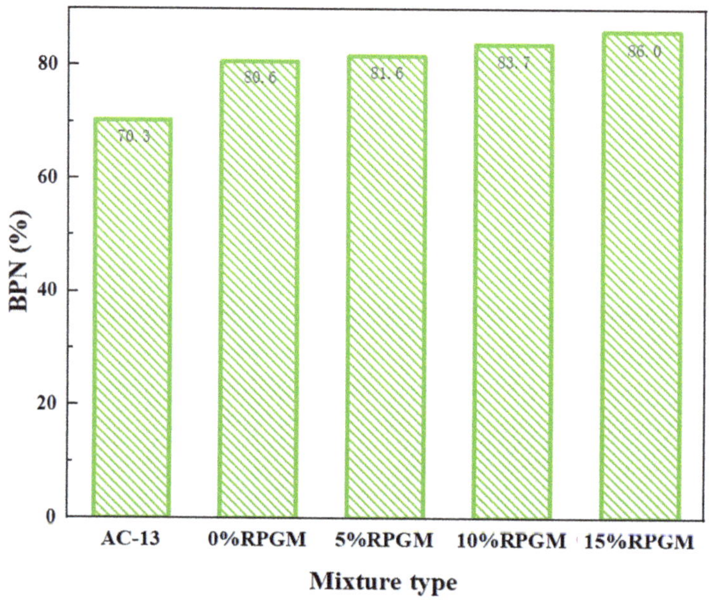

Figure 12. Friction coefficient test results.

It can be seen from Table 4 and Figure 12 that with an increase in rubber particle content, the pendulum value of RPGM continues to increase and is greater than that of the asphalt mixture. Compared with the AC-13 asphalt mixture, the BPN value increased by 14.7 units, 16.1 units, 19.1 units and 22.3 units, respectively. Note that BPN is a relative index reflecting surface friction characteristics and does not linearly correlate with the actual friction coefficient when exceeding 70. Compared with the RPGM with 0% rubber particles, the friction coefficients of RPGM with different rubber particles increased by 1.2%, 3.8% and 6.7%, respectively. This is because the rubber particles themselves have a high friction coefficient and a small modulus. When it is combined with a polyurethane gel mixture, it can improve the friction performance of the mixture surface, thereby improving the surface friction coefficient of the mixture. In addition, the optimized rubber particles have better adhesion performance with the polyurethane gel binder. After the mixture is fully mixed, the rubber particles are evenly distributed on the surface of the rutting plate of the RPGM. The surface of the rubber particles is rough, the wear resistance is good and it has good elasticity and toughness. When impacted by the pendulum, it can effectively absorb the impact energy and can quickly recover the deformation and maintain its friction coefficient. Therefore, the more rubber particles are added, the greater the friction coefficient of the RPGM and the higher the skid resistance.

Table 4. BPN test results.

Mix Type	BPN Value 1	BPN Value 2	BPN Value 3	Mean Value	Standard Deviation	Coefficient of Variation
AC-13 Asphalt mixture	71.2	70.4	69.4	70.3	0.90	1.28
0% RPGM	79.4	81.8	80.5	80.6	1.20	1.49
5% RPGM	81.6	82.3	80.9	81.6	0.70	0.86
10% RPGM	83.4	84.9	82.7	83.7	1.12	1.34
15% RPGM	85.9	85.4	86.8	86.0	0.71	0.82

2.4. Analysis of Ice-Breaking Effect and Mechanism of Mixture

2.4.1. Phenomenon Analysis of Ice-Breaking Test

The test was carried out at room temperature in January, during the winter in Zhengzhou City. The temperature was about 0 °C. The thickness of the ice layer of the specimen was controlled to be 4 mm. After 20 min of rolling, the phenomenon before and after the ice-breaking test of different rutting specimens is shown in Figures 13 and 14.

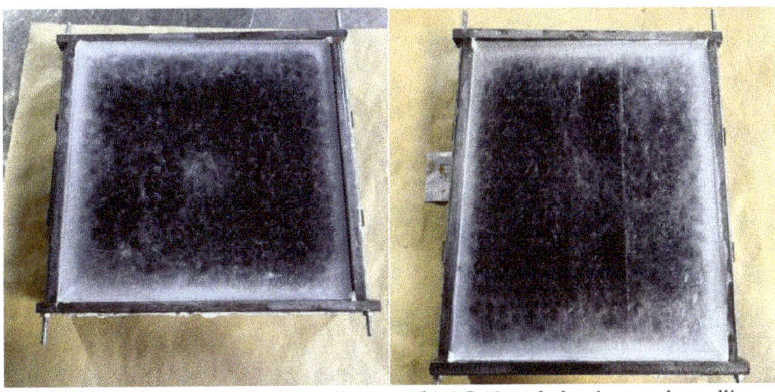

(**a**) AC-13 asphalt mixture before rolling (**b**) AC-13 asphalt mixture after rolling

Figure 13. Ice-breaking rutting test.

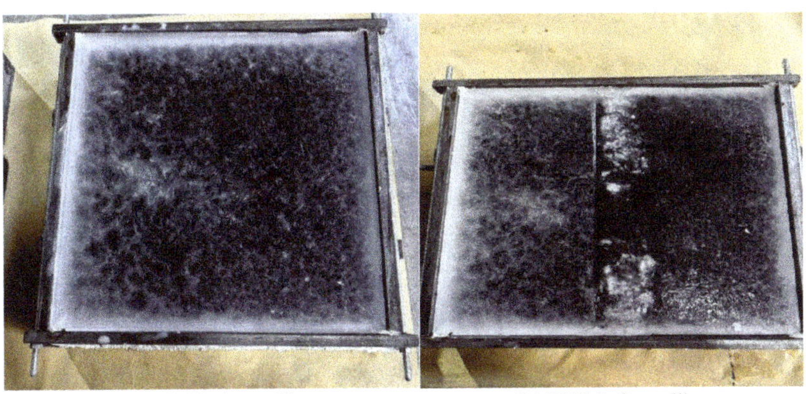

(**a**) RPGM before rolling (**b**) RPGM after rolling

Figure 14. Ice-breaking rutting test.

As shown in Figures 13 and 14, during the test, the rutting test piece was rolled for 20 min. The ordinary AC-13 asphalt mixture test piece did not change significantly under the reciprocating motion of the wheel, but it formed a wheel track belt. There were some fine cracks, and the ice layer did not fall off. For the rubber particle polyurethane gel mixture specimen, cracks appear on the ice surface. The ice layer at both ends of the wheel track is first broken, and then a large crack is formed. With the increase in the number of round trips of the wheel, the cracks continue to expand, and the ice layer gradually falls off, exposing the RPGM specimen. The wheel changes direction at both ends of the wheel track while applying a large tangential force to the ice layer. Due to the high elasticity of rubber particles and polyurethane gel binders, under the wheel load, the rubber particles undergo elastic deformation, while the surrounding stone deformation is small, resulting in stress concentration in the edge area of the rubber particles. This stress concentration phenomenon causes cracks in the ice and snow layer under shear failure. As the load continues to be applied, the ice and snow layer gradually forms large cracks, which eventually leads to the shedding of the ice and snow layer. In addition, during the test, it was found that the broken ice layer was more likely to fall off the rutting surface of the RPGM. This is due to the fact that the surface of the rutting plate is covered with a layer of polyurethane gel film. Polyurethane gels have the characteristics of low surface energy and high flexibility, resulting in a low interface adhesion with ice, thereby promoting the ice layer from the surface. In summary, the rubber particle polyurethane gel mixture shows better ice and snow removal performance than the traditional asphalt mixture.

2.4.2. The Effect of Rubber Particle Content on Ice-Breaking Effect

In this study, 10% polyurethane gel was selected to form the rut board specimen, and the thickness of the ice layer was initially controlled at 3 mm. Through the indoor icebreaking test of RPGM with different rubber particle contents, the BPN change values were measured, respectively, and the results are shown in Figure 15.

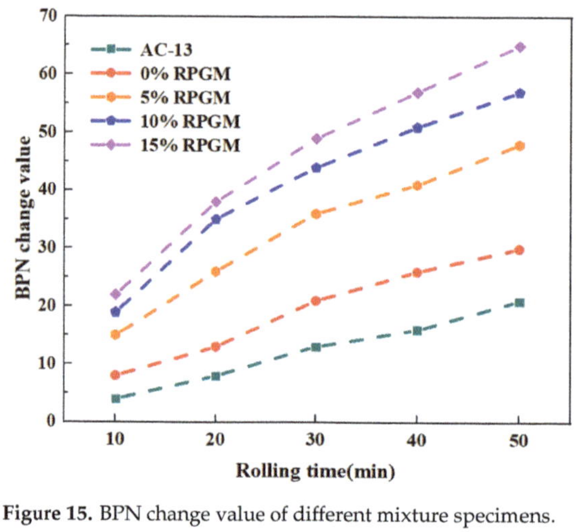

Figure 15. BPN change value of different mixture specimens.

The test results show that with the extension of rolling time, the BPN variation of the rut plate specimens shows a positive correlation trend. Compared with the AC-13 asphalt mixture specimens, the BPN variation value of RPGM increases significantly. When the rolling time is 30 min, the polyurethane gel mixture with rubber particle content of 0%, 5%, 10% and 15% increases the BPN variation value by 0.6 times, 1.8 times, 2.4 times and 2.8 times, respectively, which indicates that the ice-breaking effect of RPGM is obviously better than that of the traditional asphalt mixture. It should be noted that the growth rate of the BPN change value of the AC-13 asphalt mixture specimen will increase with the increase in rolling time. The reason for this phenomenon is that the test temperature is higher than the melting point of ice. As the rolling time continues to extend, the strength of the ice itself and the bond strength between it and the rut board decrease.

In addition, for the mixture with 0% rubber particle content, with the continuous increase in rubber particle content, the BPN change value of the specimen increases greatly. When the rolling time is 30 min, the BPN change value of the polyurethane gel mixture with 5%, 10% and 15% rubber particle content increases by 71.4%, 109.5% and 133.3%, respectively, which indicates that the introduction of rubber particles has a significant improvement effect on the ice-breaking performance of the mixture.

2.4.3. The Influence of Ice Thickness on Ice-Breaking Effect

In order to analyze the effect of different ice thicknesses on the ice-breaking efficiency of RPGM, two indexes of weighted average recovery and recovery rate of pendulum value (as shown in Formulas (3) and (4)) were introduced. The rutting plate specimens were formed with 10% polyurethane gel content and 15% rubber particle content. The ice thickness was set to 3 mm, and the test temperature was set to −2 °C and 2 °C, respectively. The weighted average recovery and recovery rate of pendulum value at 20 min were used to characterize the de-icing effect of the mixture. The results of specimens with different ice thicknesses are shown in Figures 16 and 17.

$$\overline{F} = \frac{\Sigma(N, \Delta D)}{\Sigma N} \tag{3}$$

$$\overline{\rho} = \frac{\Sigma[(N, \Delta D/D0)]}{\Sigma N} \tag{4}$$

where $\overline{\mathrm{F}}$ is the weighted average rise of the pendulum value, $\overline{\rho}$ is the swing value recovery rate, N is the number of rolling, ΔD is the variation of the pendulum value and D_0 is the initial pendulum value.

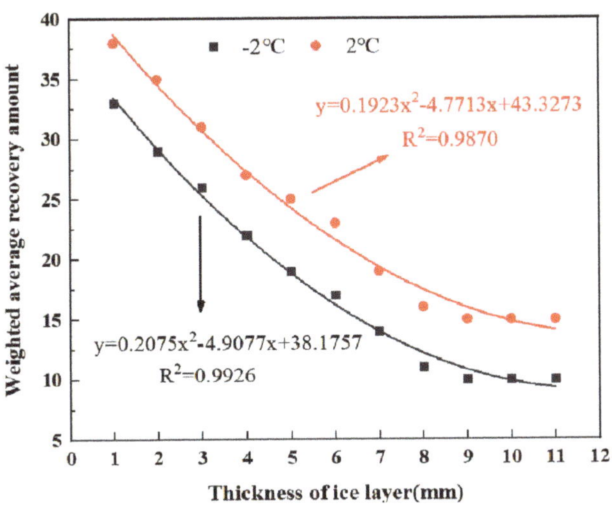

Figure 16. The change in pendulum weighted average recovery of specimens with different ice thicknesses.

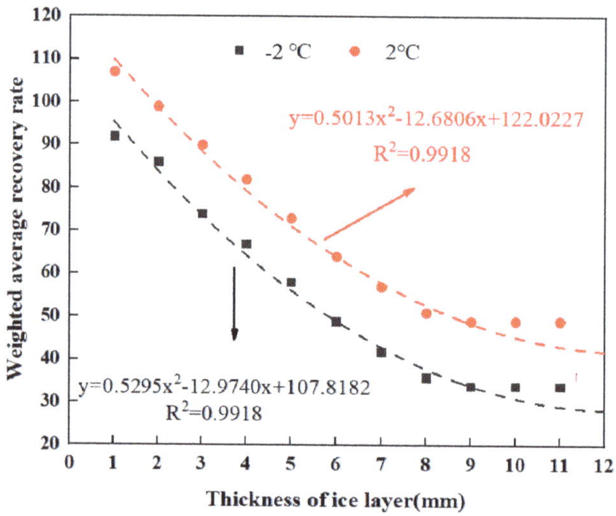

Figure 17. The change in swing value recovery rate of specimens with different ice thicknesses.

The results show that when the test temperature is set to −2 °C and 2 °C, the average weighted recovery of the pendulum value measured in the ice-breaking test and the corresponding recovery rate show a very consistent change trend. The correlation coefficient R^2 obtained after fitting is more than 98%, which fully shows that there is a very significant correlation between the influence of ice thickness on the average weighted recovery amount and the recovery rate of pendulum value. From Figure 16 to Figure 17, it can be found that with the increase in ice thickness, the weighted average recovery and the average weighted recovery rate of pendulum value both show a downward trend. This downward trend is particularly significant when the ice thickness is thinner (1–6 mm). At −2 °C, the average weighted recovery changes by 12.1%, 10.3%, 13.6% and 10.5%, respectively, with the increase in ice thickness. However, with the further increase in ice thickness, the decline rate gradually slows down. When the ice thickness reaches 9 mm, the weighted average recovery amount and the pendulum average weighted recovery rate basically tend to be stable, indicating that the ice-breaking ability of RPGM has been significantly weakened, almost losing the ice-breaking function.

2.4.4. Analysis of Ice-Breaking Mechanism

Ice is a dense crystal structure formed by water molecules at low temperatures. It has the characteristics of high hardness and strong adhesion, and it is not easy to break. The elastic modulus of ice varies with temperature, typically decreasing significantly with increasing temperature. Compared with snow, ice has a higher density and a closer structure, and an extremely thin quasi-liquid water film will be formed on the surface near the melting point. This layer of water film further reduces the adhesion between ice and the road surface but also makes it more difficult to remove the ice layer by conventional mechanical methods. As a new type of pavement ice-breaking material, the ice-breaking mechanism of RPGM mainly plays a role through the triple mechanism of thermal effect, stress effect and interface failure (Figure 18).

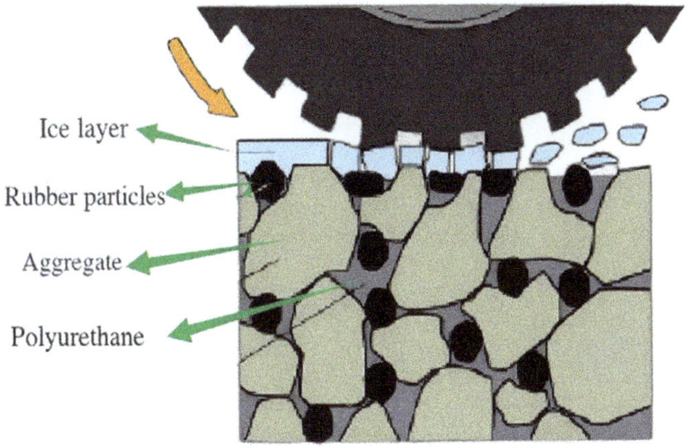

Figure 18. Ice-breaking mechanism of RPGM.

As a polymer elastomer, rubber particles will generate internal friction heat during the repeated compression and rebound process of driving load. Due to the poor thermal conductivity of rubber, the heat does not dissipate quickly, resulting in a gradual increase in the surface temperature of the particles. When the temperature is close to the melting point of ice, the local micro-area of the contact surface between ice and the mixture will melt, forming a layer of lubricating water film and weakening the bonding strength between ice and pavement. The adhesion between ice and the pavement interface is greatly reduced, and the ice layer falls off the pavement. At the same time, the RPGM has good elasticity and flexibility, which can effectively improve the deformation capacity of the road surface and change the mechanical response characteristics of the ice layer on the road surface. When the vehicle load is applied to the road surface, a large displacement will be generated, thereby changing the stress distribution of the ice layer on the road surface. Through the stress action, the bonding force between the ice layer and the road surface is destroyed. When the stress or strain of the ice layer reaches the extreme value of the damage, the ice layer reaches rupture. In addition, the rough surface of the rubber particles in the mixture forms a non-uniform contact with the ice layer, and the local stress concentration will promote the brittle fracture of the ice body. The microporous structure after polyurethane gel curing can absorb part of the ice-melting water and reduce the risk of secondary icing. It can be seen that the RPGM, by virtue of its material properties, makes the ice layer gradually loosen, break and eventually separate from the road surface, so as to achieve active de-icing. This process does not need to rely on salting or manual removal, which significantly improves the safety and traffic efficiency of winter roads while reducing maintenance costs, and it has significant environmental and economic value.

From the perspective of mechanical response characteristics, the ice layer is mainly compressed and sheared in the rectangular area below the tire, and the maximum shear stress concentration appears at the edge of the contact area, while there is a significant tensile stress concentration in the area near the rim of the double-wheel gap. Therefore, it is considered that the failure of the ice layer here is mainly caused by the instability and expansion of the composite crack (the combination of type I crack and type II crack in fracture mechanics). For the mixed fracture failure of brittle materials, the strain energy density factor theory is a widely used fracture mechanics material failure criterion. Therefore, this criterion is used to analyze the mixed fracture failure of the rubber polyurethane gel pavement ice layer.

According to the strain energy density factor criterion formula, when the polar coordinate $\theta = \theta_0$ (θ_0 is the cracking angle), the minimum strain energy density factor is $S_{min} = Sc$. The equivalent discriminant function is

$$f(K_I, K_{II}) = \frac{S_{min}}{Sc} - 1 \quad (5)$$

where S_C is the critical value of strain energy density factor, mm, K_I, K_{II} are the Mode and Mode Critical Stress Intensity Factors of Mixed Mode Crack Instability Propagation and S_C can be determined by the fracture strength test of ice material.

$$Sc = \frac{1-2v}{4\pi\mu} K_{IC}^2 \quad (6)$$

where v is the Poisson ratio, μ is the ice shear modulus and K_{IC} is the mode I fracture toughness of ice material.

$$\frac{\partial S}{\partial \theta} = 0, \ \frac{\partial^2 S}{\partial \theta^2} \quad (7)$$

$$\theta 0 = \arccos(\frac{1-2v}{3}) \quad (8)$$

When v is 0.3, θ_0 is about $-83°$. Thus, the specific expression of the discriminant function is

$$f(K_I, K_{II}) = \frac{S_{min}}{Sc} - 1 = \left(\frac{K_I}{K_{IC}}\right)^2 + 0.06617\left(\frac{K_I}{K_{IC}}\right)\left(\frac{K_{II}}{K_{IC}}\right) + 1.0917\left(\frac{K_{II}}{K_{IC}}\right)^2 - 1 \quad (9)$$

According to the strain energy density factor theory, when the discriminant function $f(K_I, K_{II}) < 0$, that is, $Smin < SC$, the mixed mode I and II cracks will not expand; when the discriminant function $f(K_I, K_{II}) = 0$, that is, $Smin = SC$, the mixed mode I and II cracks begin to destabilize. When the discriminant function $f(K_I, K_{II}) > 0$, that is, $S_{min} > S_C$, the mixed mode I and II cracks have become unstable. Therefore, according to the relationship between the discriminant function $f(K_I, K_{II})$ and 0, it can be judged whether the pavement ice layer will break. The fracture toughness K_{IC} of the mode I (open) fracture mode is about 80 kPa·$m^{1/2}$. When the temperature is 0 °C and the thickness of the ice layer is 3 mm, the elastic modulus of ice is about 3000 MPa. Assuming that the elastic modulus of RPGM is 1000 MPa, it can be calculated that

$$K_I/K_{IC} = 0.1956671387, \ K_{II}/K_{IC} = 0.8887343329 \quad (10)$$

It can be seen that K_{II} is much larger than K_I, and the fracture mode is mainly type II (hear-induced). By substituting the above values into the discriminant function, $f(K_I, K_{II}) = 0.015630523 > 0$, it can be judged that the mixed mode I and II cracks in the ice layer were unstable and expanded. In the area adjacent to the rim of the double wheel gap, the ice layer mainly shows the characteristics of crack radiation expansion dominated by shear. In this region, due to the existence of multiple initial defect cracks with random distribution of location and orientation, the composite crack forms a typical radial crack morphology during the unstable propagation process, which is consistent with the observation phenomenon of the indoor ice-breaking test. Under the repeated action of cyclic traffic load, when the crack propagation length reaches the critical size or the crack distribution density reaches the saturation degree, the interaction between the cracks will cause the stress concentration effect, which will eventually lead to local brittle fracture and the interfacial debonding of the ice layer. This mechanical process is the key mechanism for the rubber polyurethane gel pavement to realize an active ice-breaking function.

3. Conclusions

(1) The contact angle of rubber particles treated with NaOH, NaClO and KH550 decreased by 22.5%, 30.2% and 36.7%, respectively. NaOH solution improves the adhesive strength of rubber particles and polyurethane gels by eliminating zinc stearate on the rubber surface and forming a rough porous surface. The NaClO solution promoted the penetration of the adhesive molecules by removing the residual solvent on the surface of the rubber particles and forming a pore structure, thereby enhancing the bonding strength. The KH550 solution further improves the roughness of the surface of the rubber particles and the number of corrosion pores; enhances the air-entraining effect, fluidity and interfacial bonding strength; and significantly improves the working performance of the rubber particle mixture. After surface modification by three methods, the element types of rubber particles were significantly reduced, among which the element types of rubber particles treated by the KH550 solution decreased the most, indicating that the removal effect of surface impurities was the most significant.

(2) The freeze–thaw splitting strength of the mixture with four kinds of rubber particles increased greatly when the amount of polyurethane gel reached 10%. Under the condition of fixed rubber particle content, the growth trend of freeze–thaw splitting strength of the specimen increases first and then slows down with the increase in polyurethane gel content. When the content of rubber particles is 10%, the splitting strength ratio increases by 1.1%, 1.4%, 0.5% and 0.3%, respectively, when the content of polyurethane gels increases from 9–11%. When the content of polyurethane gels is 10%, its water damage resistance can meet the requirements of use, and the optimum polyurethane gel content of the mixture is determined to be 10%.

(3) With an increase in rubber particle content, the dynamic stability of the polyurethane gel mixture shows a trend of gradual increase, which is 6.2%, 18.2% and 23.5% higher than that of undoped rubber particles, respectively, and much higher than that of asphalt mixture, indicating that its anti-rutting performance is significantly enhanced. Compared with the mixture without rubber particles, the maximum bending strain increased by 11.8%, 25.1% and 31.7%, respectively, showing excellent deformation ability. The residual stability increased first and then decreased with the increase in rubber particle content, and the residual stability increased by 1.4%, 3.3% and 0.5%, respectively. The anti-scattering performance increased with the increase in rubber content, and an excessive amount would lead to an increase in scattering loss rate, but it could still be maintained below 5%, indicating that it still had good water stability under immersion conditions. Compared with the AC-13 asphalt mixture, the fatigue life of four kinds of rubber particle content mixtures increased by 2.9 times, 3.8 times, 4.3 times and 4.0 times, respectively. The fatigue performance of the polyurethane gel mixture decreased with an increase in rubber particle content. Compared with the ordinary asphalt mixture, the friction coefficient of four kinds of rubber particle content increased by 14.7%, 16.1%, 19.1% and 22.3%, respectively, which further verified its excellent skid resistance.

(4) Compared with the traditional asphalt mixture, RPGM shows superior de-icing performance, and with an increase in rubber particle content, its ice-breaking effect is significantly improved. Compared with the AC-13 asphalt mixture, the BPN change values of polyurethane gel mixtures with different rubber particle contents increased by 0.6 times, 1.8 times, 2.4 times and 2.8 times, respectively, under the rolling time of 30 min. The BPN change values of 5%, 10% and 15% RPGMs increased by 71.4%, 109.5% and 133.3%, respectively, compared with those of polyurethane gel mixtures without rubber particles. The average weighted recovery of the ice thickness to the pendulum value and the average weighted recovery rate of the pendulum value decrease with an increase in ice thickness, especially when the ice thickness is

1–6 mm. When the ice thickness reaches 9 mm, the two tend to be stable, indicating that the ice-breaking ability of the RPGM is significantly weakened. Under the action of traffic load, the RPGM can make the ice layer gradually fall off through stress, thermal effect and interface damage, indicating that RPGM exhibits strong potential for field application, subject to further long-term durability verification in real-world conditions. The ice layer damage is characterized by a mixed fracture mode dominated by a type II fracture.

4. Materials and Methods

4.1. Rubber Particles

In this paper, the cube-shaped rubber particles provided by Lingshou County Tairun Mineral Products Co., Ltd. (Shijiazhuang City, Hebei Province, China) are selected, which are concave and convex, with no obvious agglomeration on the surface and burr phenomenon. The specific technical indicators are shown in Table 5, all of which meet the technical requirements of existing road rubber particles.

Table 5. Technical index of rubber particles.

Technology Index	Moisture Content/%	Apparent Density/g/cm^3	Shore Hardness/%	Elastic Modulus/MPA	Slender Flat Particle Content/%	Carbon Black Content/%
technical requirement	<1	1.10–1.30	55–80	≥5	≤10	25–38
test result	0.22	1.153	69	10	3.9	32

4.2. Polyurethane Gels

In this study, a two-component polyurethane gel provided by Jiangxi Zhanbang Technology Co., Ltd. (Fuzhou City, Jiangxi Province, China) was composed of polyols (component A) and isocyanates (component B). Referring to the relevant technical specifications [32–34], the performance of the selected two-component polyurethane gels were tested. The test results are shown in Table 6.

Table 6. Properties of polyurethane gel binder.

Testing Item	Technical Requirement	Test Result
density	actual measurement	1.4 g/cm^3
viscosity	≥1	3.5 mPa·s
tensile strength	≥2	7.0 MPa
breaking elongation	≥150	298%
surface dry time	-	2 h
hard drying time	-	10 h

4.3. Modifier

(1) NaOH modifier

In this study, NaOH solution provided by Zibo Linnuo Chemical Co., Ltd. (Zibo City, Shandong Province, China) was used. NaOH solution shows a very broad application prospect in the engineering practice of rubber particle surface modification due to its simple modification process and low cost. In this study, NaOH was used as a granular solid, and the effective component content was 96%.

(2) NaClO modifier

In this study, sodium hypochlorite provided by Tianjin Tongxin Chemical Co., Ltd. (Tianjin, China) was used. The modification process of sodium hypochlorite is relatively simple. It is a common modification method to modify the surface of rubber particles by sodium hypochlorite. The index of NaClO solution used in this study is shown in Table 7.

Table 7. Technical index of sodium hypochlorite solution.

Project	Purity	Active Chlorine	Free Alkali (in NaOH)	Fe	As	Heavy Metals (in Pb)
index	analytically pure	≥5.5%	0.1–1.0%	≤0.003%	≤0.0005%	≤0.002%

(3) KH550 modifier

In this study, KH550 silane coupling modifier provided by Guangzhou Yinuo Chemical Technology Co., Ltd. (Guangzhou City, Guangdong Province, China) was used. Silane coupling agent is widely used in the field of surface modification of rubber particles. In this study, the analytically pure KH550 silane coupling modifier was used, and the main physical properties are shown in Table 8.

Table 8. Main physical properties of KH550.

Physical Property	Appearance	Boiling Point/°C	Specific Gravity	Solubility
Numerical and Description	Colorless Liquid	208	0.947	Soluble in water and organic solvents

4.4. Natural Aggregate

The natural aggregates used in the test are provided by Zhengzhou Zhengfa Municipal Construction Co., Ltd., Zhengzhou, China, and the technical indicators of the materials used are shown in Table 9.

Table 9. Technical indexes of natural aggregate.

NO.	Type	Materials	Technical Indexes
1	Coarse aggregate	Basalt	Apparent specific gravity (13.2 mm~16 mm) 2.745 Apparent specific gravity (9.5 mm~13.2 mm) 2.736 Apparent specific gravity (4.75 mm~9.5 mm) 2.724 Apparent specific gravity (2.36 mm~4.75 mm) 2.753 Water absorption (13.2 mm~16 mm) 1.1% Water absorption (9.5 mm~13.2 mm) 0.9% Water absorption (4.75 mm~9.5 mm) 0.7% Water absorption (2.36 mm~4.75 mm) 1.2% Crush value 18.2%
2	Fine aggregate	Limestone	Apparent specific gravity (1.18 mm~2.36 mm) 2.776 Apparent specific gravity (0.6 mm~1.18 mm) 2.792 Sand equivalent (1.18 mm~2.36 mm) 75% Sand equivalent (0.6 mm~1.18 mm) 77%
3	Mineral fines	Limestone	Apparent specific gravity 2.654 No agglomeration Hydrophilicity 0.72

4.5. Rubber Particle Performance Test

(1) Contact angle test

The German LAUDA Scientific (Lauda-Königshofen. Germany) contact angle measuring instrument LSA100 was used to microscopically analyze the surface of rubber particles with different treatment methods. The morphological characteristics of the gas–solid–liquid three-phase interface were captured by a high-resolution microscopic imaging system. The water contact angle of rubber particles after different modification treatments can accurately evaluate the improvement effect of surface wettability and provide a theoretical basis for optimizing the interface compatibility between rubber particles and cementitious material matrix.

(2) SEM test

Scanning electron microscopy (SEM) (provided by Shenyang Huayi Times Technology Co., Ltd. in Shenyang, Liaoning Province, China) can scan the surface morphology of the sample in a vacuum environment through a high-focusing electron beam and image it in combination with the principle of electron optics. It has the advantages of high resolution, continuous magnification and simple sample preparation. In this paper, the SEM test was used to observe the microstructure of the rubber particles, and the changes in the surface morphology of the steel slag before and after the optimization treatment were analyzed. The field emission scanning electron microscope with the model Quanta 450 was selected.

(3) EDS test

Energy-Dispersive Spectroscopy (EDS) is a micro-area composition analysis technology based on scanning electron microscopy. By detecting the energy distribution of these characteristic X-rays, the elemental composition and relative content of the sample surface can be qualitatively or quantitatively analyzed. Combined with the morphological changes from the scanning electron microscope, the changes in the surface elements of the original rubber particles and different modified rubber particles can be explored.

4.6. Gradation Design

With reference to the gradation design method of asphalt mixture, in order to take into account the structural strength and deformation performance of the mixture, this paper takes the AC-13 asphalt mixture gradation as the benchmark and uses the gradation median as the design gradation. The gradation curve is shown in Figure 19.

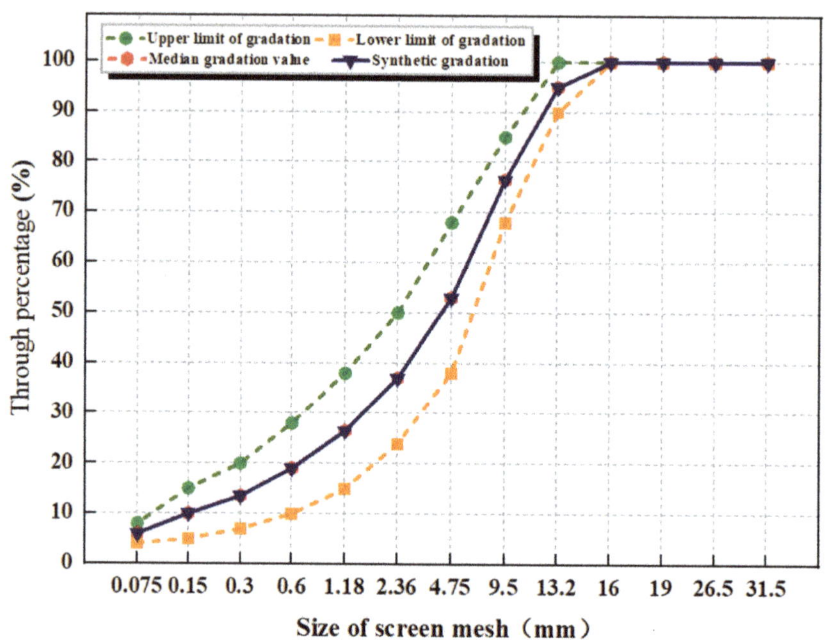

Figure 19. Synthetic grading curve.

4.7. Determination of Polyurethane Gel Dosage

In order to determine the optimal amount of polyurethane gels, this paper selects the freeze–thaw splitting strength ratio as the evaluation index. The ratio of the splitting strength after freeze–thaw to the splitting strength before freeze–thaw is the splitting strength ratio. The freeze–thaw splitting strength of four kinds of rubber particles under different polyurethane gel dosages is measured. The splitting strength of the specimen is calculated according to Formulas (11) and (12).

$$R_{T1} = 0.006287 \times P_{T1}/h_1 \tag{11}$$

$$R_{T2} = 0.006287 \times P_{T2}/h_2 \tag{12}$$

where R_{T1} is the splitting tensile strength of the first group of single specimens without freeze–thaw cycles, MPa; R_{T2} is the splitting tensile strength of the second group of single specimens subjected to freeze–thaw cycles, MPa; P_{T1} is the test load value of the first group of single specimens, N; P_{T2} is the test load value of the second group of single specimens, N; h_1 is the height of the first group of single specimens, mm; and h_2 is the height of the second group of single specimens, mm.

4.8. Road Performance Test of Mixture

4.8.1. High-Temperature Performance

The rutting test was used to evaluate the high-temperature stability of RPGM. The rutting tester model is HYCZ-5C, the test temperature is 60 °C, the load wheel pressure is 0.7 MPa, the deformation of the test time is 45 min and 60 min and the dynamic stability is calculated according to Formula (13).

$$DS = \frac{(t_2 - t_1) \times N}{d_2 - d_1} \times C_1 \times C_2 \tag{13}$$

where DS is the dynamic stability of mixture, time/mm; d_1 and d_2 are the deformations at t_1 (45min) and t_2 (60min), mm; C_1 is the type correction coefficient of the testing machine, and the value is 1.0; C_2 is the coefficient of the specimen, and the value is 1.0; and N is the rolling speed of the test wheel, which is 42 times/min.

4.8.2. Low-Temperature Performance

The low-temperature bending test was used to evaluate the low-temperature crack resistance of RPGM. The test temperature was −10 °C, and the constant rate of 50 mm/min was loaded until the specimen was destroyed. The failure strain was calculated according to Equation (14).

$$\varepsilon_B = \frac{6 \times h \times d}{L^2} \tag{14}$$

where ε_B is the maximum bending strain, $\mu\varepsilon$; h is the height of the specimen, mm; L is the span of the specimen, mm; and d is the mid-span deflection when the specimen is destroyed, mm.

4.8.3. Water Stability

The water damage resistance of RPGM was evaluated by the immersion Marshall test and the immersion dispersion test. Two groups of standard Marshall specimens were prepared, with 4 in each group. One group was soaked in a 60 °C water bath for 30 min, and the stability was tested. The other group was soaked for 48 h, and the stability was tested. The stability of the two groups was tested, and the residual stability was calculated according to Formula (15).

$$MS = \frac{MS_1}{MS_0} \times 100 \tag{15}$$

where MS is the immersion residual stability of the specimen,%; MS_1 is the stability of the specimen after soaking for 48 h, kN; and MS_0 is the stability of the specimen after soaking for 30 min, kN.

The specimens after curing were divided into two groups: one group to carry out the standard dispersion test, and the other group was immersed in a water bath at a constant temperature of 60 °C for 48 h. After the immersion, the specimens were taken out and allowed to stand at room temperature for 24 h. Then, the scattering test was carried out on the specimens, and the mass loss of the specimens before and after immersion was measured. The scattering loss of the mixture was calculated according to Formula (16).

$$\Delta S = \frac{m0 - m1}{m0} \times 100 \tag{16}$$

where ΔS is the scattering loss of asphalt mixture, %; m_0 is the mass of the specimen before the test, g; and m_1 is the residual mass of the specimen after the test, g.

4.8.4. Fatigue Property

The fatigue performance of RPGM was verified by the trabecular three-point bending test. The rutting plate specimen after curing is divided into a 30 mm × 35 mm × 250 mm small beam specimen, and the force is applied to the position of the specimen at the two ends of the distance. The fatigue test is carried out under three stress ratios of 0.3, 0.4 and 0.5. The loading frequency is 10 Hz and the test temperature is 15 °C.

4.8.5. Slip Resistance

According to the method of JTG 3450-2019 in 'Highway Subgrade and Pavement Field Test Procedures' [31], the pendulum friction coefficient tester is used to measure and record the test temperature and the measured pendulum value BPN.

$$\mathrm{BPN}_{20} = \mathrm{BPN}_T + \Delta\mathrm{BPN} \tag{17}$$

where BPN_{20} is converted to the pendulum value at standard temperature 20 °C, BPN_T is the pendulum value of road surface temperature T, and ΔBPN is the temperature correction value.

4.9. Indoor Ice-Breaking Test

By simulating the actual traffic load mechanism, the rutting test can simulate the service environment of different working conditions by regulating multiple parameters, such as load, test temperature and geometric size. In view of these characteristics, the simulation method can be applied to the evaluation of pavement de-icing performance. In order to quantitatively characterize the ice-breaking effect of the road surface, this study uses the pendulum value test method, controls the ice thickness through the modified rutting plate mold and sets the rolling time to 50 min. We analyzed the pendulum value change value under different wheel rolling times and quantitatively evaluated the ice-breaking ability of the RPGM (as shown in Figures 20 and 21).

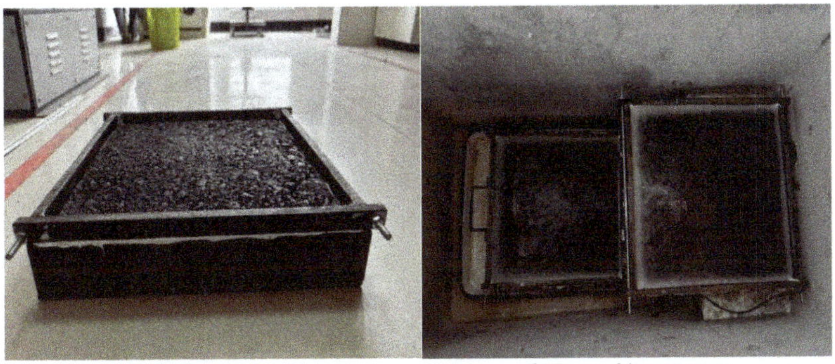

(a) Optimized rut wrench mold (b) Ice-making process

Figure 20. Ice-breaking test.

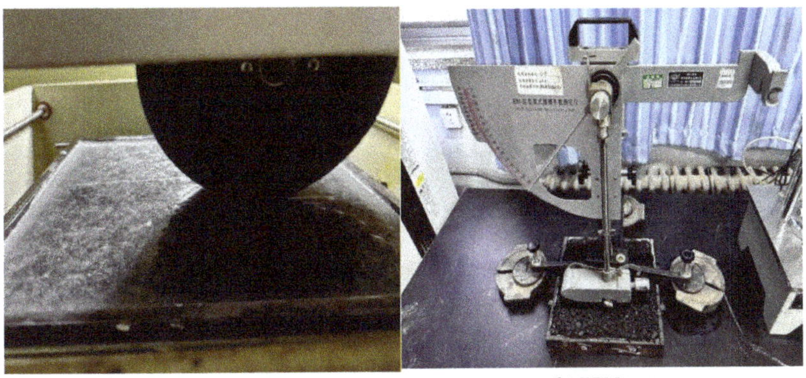

(a) Wheel tracking test (b) BPN test

Figure 21. Ice-breaking test.

Author Contributions: Y.C.: Conceptualization, project administration, supervision, funding acquisition, writing—review and editing. Z.L.: Data curation, writing—review and editing. T.G.: Methodology. C.F.: Writing—review and editing. J.Y. and P.G.: Investigation. C.W. and B.B.: Validation, investigation. W.Z.: Visualization. D.T.: Writing—original draft, writing—review and editing. J.F.: Writing—review and editing, data curation, validation, investigation. All authors have read and agreed to the published version of the manuscript.

Funding: This work was supported by a planned project supported by the science and technology innovation team of universities and colleges in Henan province (24IRTSTHN011); the Central Plains Science and Technology Innovation Leader Project (244200510031); Key scientific and technological projects in Henan province (252102240031; 252102230050); and the Special Plan for Key Scientific Research Projects of Higher Education Institutions in Henan Province to Serve Industry Development (25CY022).

Institutional Review Board Statement: Not applicable.

Informed Consent Statement: Not applicable.

Data Availability Statement: Some or all of the data, models, or code that support the findings of this study are available from the corresponding author upon reasonable request.

Conflicts of Interest: The authors declare no conflicts of interest.

References

1. Liu, T.; Guo, N.; Tan, Y.; You, Z.; Jin, X. Research status and development trend of phase change materials for road use. *Mater. Introd.* **2020**, *34*, 23179–23189.
2. Das, B.P.; Das, S.; Siddagangaiah, A.K. Probabilistic modeling of fatigue damage in asphalt mixture. *Constr. Build. Mater.* **2021**, *269*, 121300. [CrossRef]
3. Tan, Y.; Li, J.; Xu, H. Perception and early warning of snow and ice conditions on cold roads. *Basic Sci. China* **2020**, *22*, 9–15+34.
4. Dong, Q.; Du, Y.C.; Guo, M. Review of Academic Research on Pavement Engineering in China. *Chin. J. Highw.* **2024**, *37*, 1–81.
5. Liu, Z.; Sha, A.; Jiang, W. Salt asphalt pavement research progress: Salt material, mixture and its performance and evaluation. *Chin. J. Highw.* **2019**, *32*, 18–31+72.
6. Sajid, H.U.; Kiran, R.; Qi, X.; Bajwa, D.S.; Battocchi, D. Employing corn derived products to reduce the corrosivity of pavement deicing materials. *Constr. Build. Mater.* **2020**, *263*, 120662. [CrossRef]
7. Chen, Y.; Tan, Y.; She, H.; Zhang, M.; Jiang, X.; Guo, P.; Li, Y.; Zhang, Y. Characteristics of slow-release ice and snow melting micro-surfacing materials. *Int. J. Pavement Eng.* **2023**, *24*, 2120986. [CrossRef]
8. Chen, Y.; Li, Z.; Zhao, C.; Guo, T.; Wang, Z.; Li, J.; Gao, D. Study on environmentally friendly slow-release active melting ice and snow coating materials. *Chin. J. Highw.* **2020**, *33*, 155–167.
9. Li, Z.; Guo, T.; Chen, Y.; Yu, L.; Niu, X.; Yang, X.; Jin, L. Study on road performance and electrothermal performance of poured conductive asphalt concrete. *Adv. Mater. Sci. Eng.* **2022**, *2022*, 1–15. [CrossRef]
10. Wang, C.; Han, X.; Chen, J.; Hou, R.; Zheng, S. Conductive heat effect of guss conductive asphalt concrete. *Mater. Introd.* **2018**, *32*, 3891–3899.
11. Hasan, R.; Ali, A.; Decarlo, C.; Elshaer, M.; Mehta, Y. Laboratory evaluation of electrically conductive asphalt mixtures for snow and ice removal applications. *Transp. Res. Rec.* **2021**, *2675*, 48–62. [CrossRef]
12. Tan, Y.; Zhang, C.; Xu, H.; Tian, D. Summarization of research on snow melting and ice melting characteristics and road performance of active de-icing pavement. *Chin. J. Highw.* **2019**, *4*, 1–17.
13. Chen, Y.; Li, Z. Deicing mechanism of crumb rubber asphalt pavement. *J. Cent. South Univ. (Nat. Sci. Ed.)* **2013**, *44*, 2073–2081.
14. Liang, C.; Zhang, H.; Gu, Z.; Xu, X.; Hao, J. Study on Mechanical and Viscoelastic Properties of Asphalt Mixture Modified by Diatomite and Crumb Rubber Particles. *Appl. Sci.* **2020**, *10*, 8748. [CrossRef]
15. Li, S.; Ke, Y.; Xie, L.; Zhao, Z.; Huang, X.; Wang, Y.; Wang, Z. Study on the aging of three typical rubber materials under high-and low-temperature cyclic environment. *e-Polymers* **2023**, *23*, 20228089. [CrossRef]
16. Ma, Z.; Wei, H.; Wei, D.; Jiang, B.; Wang, X. Study on snow melting performance evaluation and optimization design of conductive rubber electric heating pavement. *Constr. Build. Mater.* **2025**, *470*, 140556. [CrossRef]
17. Shan, W.; Zhang, S. Study on the road performance of terminal carboxylated nitrile rubber-modified epoxy asphalt permeable concrete. *Materials* **2025**, *18*, 1691. [CrossRef]
18. Sun, M.; Hou, D.; Geng, L.; Yan, Z.; Bi, Y.; Huang, Z.; Ren, S.; Wang, B. Study on road performance and mechanical properties of multi-gravel polyurethane concrete. *Silic. Bull.* **2024**, *43*, 746–756.
19. Cao, Z.; Hao, Q.; Xu, S.; Han, X.; Yi, J.; Sun, G. Preparation and performance evaluation of bio-based polyurethane modified asphalt binders: Towards greener and more sustainable asphalt modifier. *Constr. Build. Mater.* **2025**, *476*, 141209. [CrossRef]
20. Hesami, S.; Sadeghi, V.; Azizi, A. Investigation of modified bitumen's rheological properties with synthesized polyurethane by MDI-PPG reactive prepolymers. *J. Thermoplast. Compos. Mater.* **2019**, *143*, 741–749. [CrossRef]
21. Torzs, T.; Lu, G.; Monteiro, A.O. Hydraulic properties of polyurethane-bound permeable pavement materials considering unsaturated flow. *Constr. Build. Mater.* **2019**, *212*, 422–430. [CrossRef]
22. Zheng, Y.; Han, S.; Zheng, H. Design, fabrication, and laboratory performance evaluation of polyurethane poroelastic road surfaces (PERS) mixtures. *Constr. Build. Mater.* **2025**, *473*, 141030. [CrossRef]
23. Gao, J.; Chen, J.; Meng, X.; Wang, H.; Xu, N. Research on the selection of polyurethane adhesive and direct tensile properties of polyurethane rubber particle mixture. *Case Stud. Constr. Mater.* **2023**, *18*, e01728. [CrossRef]
24. Chen, J.; Xie, M.; Hao, W.; Xie, P.; Huang, W. Experimental study on anti-icing and deicing performance of polyurethane concrete as road surface layer. *Constr. Build. Mater.* **2018**, *161*, 598–605. [CrossRef]
25. Chen, J.; Yin, X.; Wang, H.; Ding, Y. Evaluation of durability and functional performance of porous polyurethane mixture in porous pavement. *J. Clean. Prod.* **2018**, *188*, 12–19. [CrossRef]
26. Zou, B.; Yin, J.; Cao, C.; Long, X. Mechanical performance analysis of rubber elastic polymer-polyurethane reinforced cement-based composite grouting materials. *J. Polym. Mat.* **2025**, *42*, 255–275. [CrossRef]
27. Agaavriloaie, L.; Oprea, S.; Barbuta, M.; Florentina, L. Characterisation of polymer concrete with epoxy polyurethane gel acryl matrix. *Constr. Build. Mater.* **2012**, *37*, 190–196. [CrossRef]
28. Min, S.; Bi, Y.; Zheng, M.; Chen, S.; Li, J. Evaluation of a cold-mixed high-performance polyurethane mixture. *Adv. Mater. Sci. Eng.* **2019**, *2019*, 1–12. [CrossRef]

29. Li, G.; Tian, X.; Gao, K.; Wu, Q.; Huang, S.; Xie, Z. Study on the performance and microscopic mechanism of activated crumb rubber synergistic polyurethane composite modified asphalt. *Constr. Build. Mater.* **2024**, *450*, 138739. [CrossRef]
30. Wang, D.; Liu, P.; Leng, Z.; Leng, C.; Lu, G.; Buch, M.; Oeser, M. Suitability of PoroElastic Road Surface (PERS) for urban roads in cold regions: Mechanical and functional performance assessment. *J. Clean. Prod.* **2017**, *165*, 1340–1350. [CrossRef]
31. *JTG 3450-2019*; Specification for Field Test of Highway Subgrade and Pavement. Ministry of Transport: Beijing, China, 2019.
32. *GB/T 16777-2008*; Test Method for Architectural Waterproofing Coatings. Quality Inspection Press: Beijing, China, 2008.
33. *GB/T 4472-2011*; Determination of Relative Density of Chemical Products. Standard Press: Beijing, China, 2011.
34. *JTG E20-2011*; Test code for asphalt and asphalt mixture of highway engineering. People' s Traffic Press: Beijing, China, 2011.

gels

MDPI

Article

A Study on the Performance of Gel-Based Polyurethane Prepolymer/Ceramic Fiber Composite-Modified Asphalt

Tengteng Guo [1,2,3,4], Xu Guo [1], Yuanzhao Chen [1,2,3,4,*], Chenze Fang [1,2,3,4], Jingyu Yang [1,2,3,4], Zhenxia Li [1,2,3,4], Jiajie Feng [1], Hao Huang [1], Zhi Li [1], Haijun Chen [1,2,3,4] and Jiachen Wang [5]

1 School of Civil Engineering and Transportation, North China University of Water Resources and Electric Power, Zhengzhou 450045, China; guotth@ncwu.edu.cn (T.G.); 17538255803@163.com (X.G.); fangchenze@ncwu.edu.cn (C.F.); yangjingyu@ncwu.edu.cn (J.Y.); zhenxiali2009@ncwu.edu.cn (Z.L.); 18027459877@163.com (J.F.); 15951287427@163.com (H.H.); 15076861657@163.com (Z.L.); chenhaijun@ncwu.edu.cn (H.C.)

2 Technology Innovation Center of Henan Transport Industry of Utilization of Solid Waste Resources in Trafffc Engineering, North China University of Water Resources and Electric Power, Zhengzhou 450045, China

3 Henan Province University-Enterprise Research and Development Center for Green, Low-Carbon and High-Performance Road Materials, Zhengzhou 450045, China

4 Henan Province Engineering Technology Research Center of Environment Friendly and High-Performance Pavement Materials, Zhengzhou 450045, China

5 Department of Electrical Engineering, College of Science and Technology, University of Nottingham Ningbo China, Ningbo 315100, China; ssyjw19@nottingham.edu.cn

* Correspondence: cyz740513@ncwu.edu.cn

Abstract: In order to solve various problems in traditional roads and extend their service life, new road materials have become a research hotspot. Polyurethane prepolymers (PUPs) and ceramic fibers (CFs), as materials with unique properties, were chosen due to their synergistic effect: PUPs provide elasticity and gel-like behavior, while CFs contribute to structural stability and high-temperature resistance, making them ideal for enhancing asphalt performance. PUPs, a thermoplastic and elastic polyurethane gel material, not only enhance the flexibility and adhesion properties of asphalt but also significantly improve the structural stability of composite materials when synergistically combined with CF. Using response surface methodology, an optimized preparation scheme for PUP/CF composite-modified asphalt was investigated. Through aging tests, dynamic shear rate (DSR) testing, bending rate (BBR) testing, microstructure scanning (MSCR), scanning electron microscopy (SEM), atomic force microscopy (AFM), and infrared spectroscopy (IR), the aging performance, rheological properties, permanent deformation resistance, microstructure, and modification mechanism of PUP/CF composite-modified asphalt were investigated. The results indicate that the optimal preparation scheme is a PUP content of 7.4%, a CF content of 2.1%, and a shear time of 40 min. The addition of the PUP and CF significantly enhances the asphalt's aging resistance, and compared with single-CF-modified asphalt and base asphalt, the PUP/CF composite-modified asphalt exhibits superior high- and low-temperature rheological properties, demonstrating stronger strain recovery capability. The PUP forms a gel network structure in the material, effectively filling the gaps between CF and asphalt, enhancing interfacial bonding strength, and making the overall performance more stable. AFM microscopic morphology shows that PUP/CF composite-modified asphalt has more "honeycomb structures" than matrix asphalt and CF-modified asphalt, forming more structural asphalt and enhancing overall structural stability. This study indicates that the synergistic effect of PUP gel and CF significantly improves the macro and micro properties of asphalt. The PUP forms a three-dimensional elastic gel network in asphalt, improving adhesion and deformation resistance. Using response surface methodology, the optimal formulation (7.4% PUP, 2.1% CF) improves penetration (↓41.5%), softening point

https://doi.org/10.3390/gels11070558

(↑6.7 °C), and ductility (↑9%), demonstrating the relevance of gel-based composites for asphalt modification.

Keywords: gel material; polyurethane prepolymer; ceramic fiber; rheological properties

1. Introduction

Traditional asphalt pavement is prone to typical problems such as rutting, cracking, and potholes in high-temperature environments, especially due to heavy-duty vehicles and frequent traffic loads [1–5]. The accelerated degradation of pavement structural performance will not only lead to a substantial decrease in the service life of roadways but will also result in a significant rise in maintenance and repair costs. In order to address this issue, researchers have conducted experiments to assess the combinations and proportions of various modifiers, aiming to evaluate their effects on asphalt performance. This study seeks to develop tailored modified asphalt solutions that cater to specific engineering requirements. Some scholars have found that adding fiber to asphalt mixture can significantly enhance the mechanical properties of the mixture and effectively improve its performance under high- and low-temperature conditions. This method also enhances the mixture's water stability and fatigue resistance, thereby extending the service life of asphalt pavement and reducing maintenance costs [6–12].

Polyurethane, an organic polymer composed of hard segments (isocyanates) and soft segments (polyols), where the former enhances rigidity and the latter imparts good toughness, and gel materials—colloidal or polymeric systems with solid-like behavior due to three-dimensional network structures whose ability to encapsulate particles and adjust mechanical behavior makes them critical in asphalt design, particularly for enhancing elasticity and durability—are both key components in this context. [13–19]. PUP contains reactive -NCO groups that, during mixing, react with hydroxyls in asphalt to form a urethane network. This crosslinked gel structure enhances elasticity, fills voids, and bridges weak interfacial regions between fibers and asphalt, improving deformation resistance [20–22]. As a crucial intermediate in the synthesis of polyurethane materials, polyurethane prepolymer (PUP) is synthesized through the reaction of R-N=C=O groups with active hydrogen-containing compounds. During the reaction, the N=C double bond in the isocyanate group is broken, and active hydrogen is transferred to the N atom, ultimately forming a urethane structure (R-NHCOO) [23–29]. Akimov, Liu et al. [30,31] added polyurethane prepolymer into matrix asphalt at 140 °C through high-speed shearing to prepare polyurethane-modified asphalt. Experimental analyses showed that the anti-aging performance of the modified asphalt was improved, and its stability was good. Infrared spectroscopy confirmed that the isocyanate groups in polyurethane react with the hydroxyl groups in asphalt to form new chemical bonds through group bonding. Fang Ying et al. [32] determined the optimal parameters for preparing polyurethane prepolymer-modified asphalt, finding that its performance is best at high temperature but its temperature sensitivity is strongest at 52–82 °C. Cuadri et al. [33] prepared polyurethane-modified asphalt by using castor oil instead of polyols to react with diisocyanates, and the results showed that the rheological properties and rutting resistance of castor oil-based polyurethane-modified asphalt were both improved. Vural Kök et al. [34] synthesized polyurethane derivatives by polymerizing 4,4′-diphenylmethane diisocyanate with novel modified palm oil-based polyols to modify asphalt. The study showed that when the curing condition was 24 h at 85 °C (compared with 1 h), the rutting factor of the asphalt increased by 256%, and the optimal modification process parameters were determined by optimizing the curing time, temperature, NCO/OH molar ratio, and PUP content. Rabindra K Padhan et al. [35] found that in situ polymerization enables better dispersion of polymers in asphalt, and a new type of polyurethane-modified asphalt synthesized in situ with terephthalamide and MDI in asphalt improved the low-temperature, high-temperature, and fatigue properties of the asphalt.

Ceramic fiber, a fibrous material made of ceramic materials, is characterized by its light weight, high strength, high temperature resistance, low thermal conductivity, good chemical stability, and excellent thermal insulation performance [36,37]. It has gradually attracted attention in the asphalt field: its low thermal conductivity can reduce heat accumulation in asphalt pavements, delay asphalt softening, and reduce the risk of high-temperature rutting; its chemical stability can slow down asphalt aging and extend pavement service life. WAN Jiuming et al. [38] used DSR to confirm that ceramic fibers can significantly enhance the high-temperature performance of asphalt, and scanning electron microscopy (SEM) and atomic force microscopy (AFM) observations showed that ceramic fibers have good dispersibility in asphalt. Arabani M, Shabani A et al. [39,40] found that adding ceramic fibers to asphalt can improve its high-temperature performance, but its low-temperature performance decreases slightly; additionally, ceramic fibers can enhance the permanent deformation resistance and fatigue life of asphalt mixtures, with a recommended dosage of 3%. Zhou Haicheng et al. [41,42] found that the addition of ceramic fibers significantly enhances the high-temperature performance of asphalt mixtures but also causes a slight reduction in low-temperature performance. Xiao Ziwei [43] found that nano-AAT/ceramic fiber composite-modified asphalt, although with slightly weakened low-temperature performance, has excellent high-temperature deformation resistance and shows significant advantages in pavement performance, including high-temperature stability, low-temperature crack resistance, and water stability.

In summary, it is evident that different fibers can significantly enhance specific properties of asphalt and asphalt mixtures. Ceramic fibers, known for their exceptional high-temperature and corrosion resistance, can markedly improve the high-temperature stability, mechanical strength, and fatigue resistance of asphalt, thereby effectively extending the service life of pavements. However, their improvement effect on asphalt's low-temperature performance is limited, and when the fiber dosage exceeds a certain amount, it may instead reduce the low-temperature crack resistance of asphalt. A common problem with fiber-modified asphalt is the poor dispersibility of fibers in asphalt, which makes it prone to agglomeration during mixing and affects the modification effect. Ceramic fibers have highly inert surfaces and weak compatibility with asphalt, making them prone to segregation during storage and possibly causing shedding during long-term use. Surface modification methods, such as NaOH alkali treatment and silane coupling agents (KH-550), have been proposed and used in this study to improve fiber dispersion and chemical compatibility with asphalt.

2. Results and Discussion

2.1. The Best Preparation Scheme of PUP/CF Composite-Modified Asphalt

2.1.1. Analysis of Response Surface Method Test Results

According to the level of influencing factors, 17 sets of test schemes corresponding to the response indicators were designed and generated. As shown in Table 1, in order to ensure the reliability and stability of the model and reduce the model error, five repeated tests were carried out at the center point of the parameter design.

Table 1. Design-Expert-optimized experimental design.

Serial Number	Polyurethane Prepolymer Content%	Ceramic Fiber Content%	Shear Time Min	Penetration	Softening Point	Ductility
1	4	1	30	42.7	52.1	18.5
2	8	1	30	40.5	53.3	20.2
3	4	3	30	38.1	55.6	17.6
4	8	3	30	36.5	56.5	19.6
5	4	2	20	40.6	54.6	18.9
6	8	2	20	38.7	55.7	20.8
7	4	2	40	40.0	55.1	19.5
8	8	2	40	37.8	56.0	21.0
9	6	1	20	42.2	52.7	19.5
10	6	3	20	38.8	56.2	18.7
11	6	1	40	41.2	53.0	20.1
12	6	3	40	37.3	56.4	19.8
13	6	2	30	38.2	55.4	20.9
14	6	2	30	38.5	55.5	20.8
15	6	2	30	39.1	55.7	20.9
16	6	2	30	38.7	55.6	21.2
17	6	2	30	38.5	55.5	20.9

According to the data in Table 1, multiple regression analysis was carried out, and A (polyurethane prepolymer content), B (ceramic fiber), and C (shear time) were used as response surface variables. The response surface models of penetration, softening point, and ductility were established by using the software Design-Expert 13 and were expressed as (1)~(3), respectively. The response surface diagrams of the influencing factors affecting the response value are shown in Figures 1–4.

$$X = 38.6 - 0.9875A - 1.99B - 0.5C + 0.15AB - 0.075AC - 0.125BC + 0.125A^2 + 0.725B^2 + 0.55C^2 \quad (1)$$

$$X = 55.54 + 0.5125A + 1.7B + 0.1625C - 0.075AB - 0.05AC - 0.025BC - 0.0195A^2 - 0.97B^2 + 0.005C^2 \quad (2)$$

$$X = 20.94 + 0.8875A - 0.325B + 0.3125C + 0.075AB - 0.1AC + 0.125BC - 0.72A^2 - 1.25B^2 - 0.17C^2 \quad (3)$$

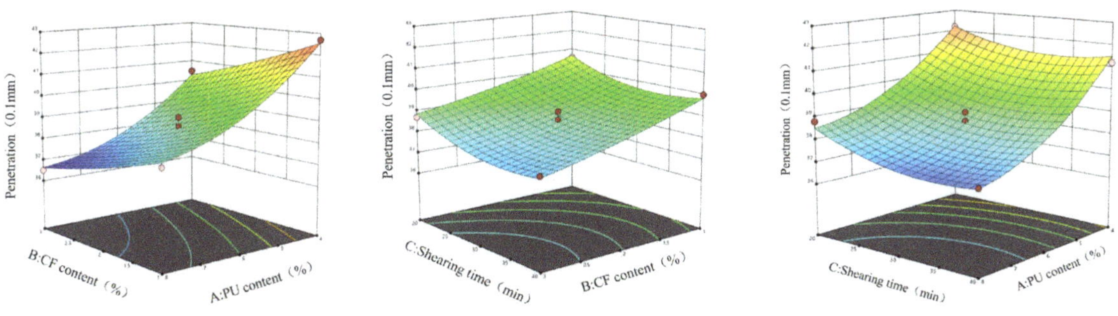

(**a**) A-B (**b**) A-C (**c**) B-C

Figure 1. Response surface of three factors to penetration.

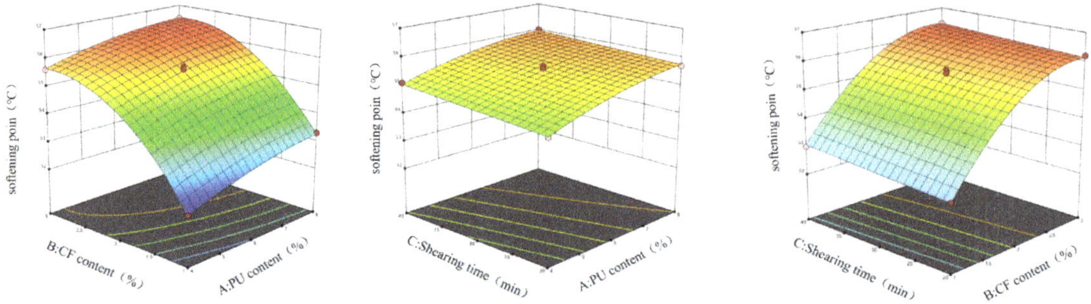

(**a**) A-B (**b**) A-C (**c**) B-C

Figure 2. Response surface of three factors to softening point.

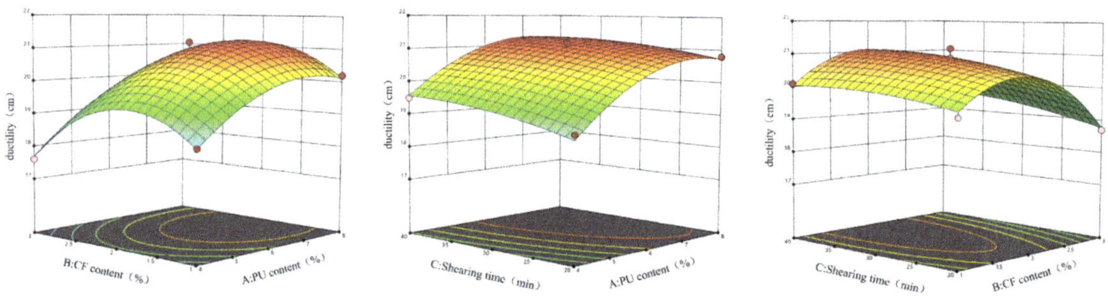

(**a**) A-B (**b**) A-C (**c**) B-C

Figure 3. Response surface of three factors to ductility.

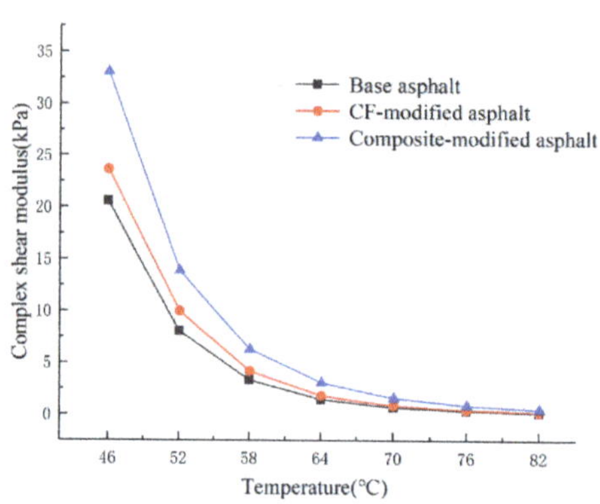

Figure 4. Complex modulus test results.

It can be seen from Figure 1 that when the shear time is constant, an increase in polyurethane prepolymer content and ceramic fiber content will make the penetration decrease, but an increase of just the polyurethane prepolymer content will make the slope of the response surface steeper, which indicates that the increase in the polyurethane prepolymer has a significant effect on the penetration of asphalt. When the content of ceramic fiber is constant, the increase in polyurethane prepolymer content and shear time will make the penetration decrease. However, when A is 4%, with the increase in shear time, the penetration shows a trend of decreasing first and then increasing. The response surface in Figure 1c is approximately flat, which indicates that the comprehensive influence of ceramic fiber content and shear time on asphalt penetration is relatively stable.

It can be seen from the response surface in Figure 2a that with the increase in A, the softening point gradually increases, but the increase is small. When B is 1%, with the increase in A, the softening point increases from 52 °C to 53.2 °C. This shows that the addition of the polyurethane prepolymer can improve the softening point of asphalt, but the effect is relatively mild. It can be seen from Figure 2b that the response surface is approximately flat, which indicates that the combined effect of the polyurethane prepolymer content and shear time on the softening point of asphalt is relatively stable, and there may be no strong interaction between the two. From Figure 2c, it can be seen that with the increase in B, the response curve is steeper, and when the shear time changes, the softening point changes less, indicating that the influence of B on the softening point is more significant.

Based on the steepness of the surface in Figure 3a, the influence of factor B on the change in asphalt ductility is more significant than that of factor A, which indicates that the change in ceramic fiber content is more sensitive to the change in ductility. As can been seen by the similar trend of the two factors in relation to ductility change, it is speculated that there is a certain interaction between factor A and factor B. It can be seen from Figure 3b that the change in factor A has a more significant effect on the steepness of the surface, indicating that the polyurethane prepolymer content has a greater influence on the ductility of the asphalt. With the increase in the PUP content, the ductility of the asphalt increases first and then decreases. It can be seen from Figure 3c that there is an interaction effect of ceramic fiber content and shear time on the ductility of the response value. With the change in B, the surface is more steep, indicating that the influence of ceramic fiber content on asphalt ductility is more significant than that of shear time. When the shear time is constant, with the increase in ceramic fiber content, the ductility increases first and then decreases.

2.1.2. Response Surface Optimization

According to the requirements of the relevant specifications of road asphalt, combined with the test purpose, a response surface optimization analysis was carried out. The lower the penetration of asphalt, the better the high-temperature stability, so the minimum penetration was used; the higher the softening point of asphalt, the stronger its high-temperature stability, so the maximum softening point was used. The greater the ductility of the asphalt, the stronger its low-temperature cracking resistance, so the maximum value of ductility was used. According to the performance requirements, the response surface method was used to optimize the performance, and the optimization results of the response value preparation parameters were obtained, as shown in Table 2.

Table 2. Optimization value of preparation parameters.

Preparation Parameters	PUP (%)	CF (%)	Shearing Time (min)
optimal value	7.4	2.1	40

The performance of asphalt preparation was optimized by the comprehensive response surface results, and the optimum preparation conditions of modified asphalt were determined as follows: the content of polyurethane prepolymer was 7.4%, the content of ceramic fiber was 2.1%, and the shear time was 40 min. These values were determined via RSM optimization and validated through experimental tests. The error between the predicted and actual values was less than 3%, confirming the statistical reliability of the model.

2.1.3. Validation of the Best Dosage of Composite Modification

According to the optimized preparation parameters, the preparation of PUP/CF composite-modified asphalt was carried out, and the three indicators were tested. The test results were compared with the predicted values, as shown in Table 3.

Table 3. Properties of the composite modified asphalt with the optimal dosage.

Indicators	Needle Penetration (0.1 mm)	Softening Point (°C)	Ductility (cm)
Predicted value	38.6	55.54	20.94
Measured value	38.2	56.2	20.4

It can be seen that the error between the measured value and the predicted value is small, not exceeding 3%. This shows that the model can well describe the relationship between variables and also reflects that the selection of factors and the setting of levels are more reasonable.

2.2. *Aging Performance Analysis*

After testing the matrix asphalt, 2% CF-modified asphalt and PUP/CF composite-modified asphalt were subjected to 85 min RTFOT; the changes in the three indexes of penetration, softening point, and ductility before and after aging were measured as shown in Table 4.

Table 4. Asphalt RTFOT indicators before and after aging.

Performance Index	Matrix Asphalt		CF-Modified Asphalt		PUP/CF Composite-Modified Asphalt	
	Before Aging	After Aging	Before Aging	After Aging	Before Aging	After Aging
Mass (g)	35.140	35.018	35.312	35.258	35.374	35.344
Penetration at 25 °C (0.1 mm)	66.1	53.7	55.9	40.5	40.6	34.7
Softening Point (°C)	50.8	53.7	53.3	56.4	57.5	60.2
Mass Loss (%)	0.348		0.152		0.086	
Penetration Ratio (%)	69.6		72.5		85.4	
Softening Point Increase (°C)	2.9		2.1		1.7	

It can be seen from Table 4 that after aging, the penetration of the three kinds of asphalt showed a significant downward trend. Compared with the matrix asphalt, the residual penetration ratio of CF-modified asphalt increased by 2.9%, indicating that CF improved the anti-aging performance of asphalt. The residual penetration of PUP/CF composite-modified asphalt was 12.9% higher than that of CF-modified asphalt, indicating that the addition of PUP further improved the anti-aging performance. The softening point of the three kinds of asphalt increased after aging. The minimum increase in PUP/CF composite-modified asphalt was 1.7 °C, and the maximum increase in softening point of matrix asphalt was 2.9 °C. The addition of modifiers made the softening point increment decrease gradually, indicating that CF and PUP composite modification can improve the anti-aging performance of asphalt. The mass loss of matrix asphalt, CF-modified asphalt, and PUP/CF composite-modified asphalt was 0.348%, 0.152%, and 0.086%, respectively. The mass loss of PUP/CF composite-modified asphalt and CF-modified asphalt was reduced by 0.196%

and 0.262%, respectively, compared with that of matrix asphalt, indicating that CF can effectively improve the anti-aging ability of asphalt and reduce the mass loss. The addition of PUP can effectively inhibit mass loss of asphalt and improve the anti-aging performance of asphalt.

2.3. *Analysis of Dynamic Shear Rheological Test*

2.3.1. Temperature Scanning Analysis

The temperature scanning test results of PUP/CF composite-modified asphalt are shown in Figures 4 and 5.

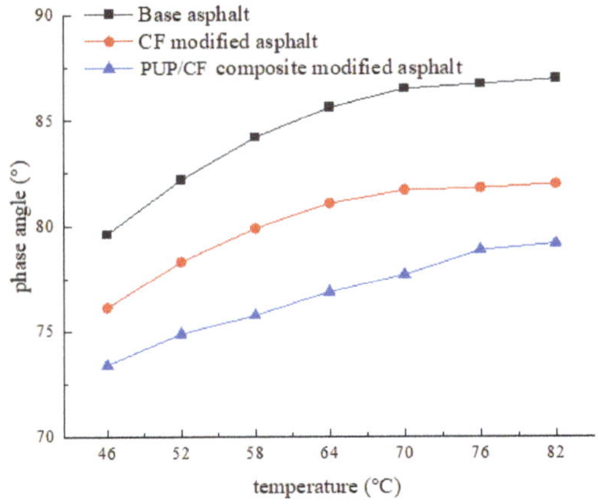

Figure 5. Phase angle test results.

It can be seen from Figure 4 that the complex shear modulus of the three kinds of asphalt decreases with the increase in temperature. Under different temperature conditions, the complex shear modulus of PUP/CF composite-modified asphalt is the largest. On the whole, the complex shear modulus of the PUP/CF composite-modified asphalt is significantly higher than that of both the matrix asphalt and the CF-modified asphalt at low temperatures. However, as the temperature increases, the complex shear modulus gradually decreases and approaches the level of the matrix asphalt, although it remains consistently higher than that of the matrix asphalt. It can be seen from Figure 5 that the phase angle of the three kinds of asphalt increases with the increase in temperature. The δ of matrix asphalt increased from 79.62° to 86.99°, that of CF-modified asphalt increased from 76.13° to 82.0°, and that of PUP/CF-modified asphalt increased from 73.40° to 79.19°. The higher the temperature, the greater the viscosity of the asphalt, resulting in an increase in δ. The phase angle of PUP/CF-modified asphalt is the smallest at the same temperature.

It can be seen from Figure 6 that the rutting factor decreases significantly with the increase of temperature, and the rutting factor of PUP/CF composite modified asphalt is the largest, followed by CF modified asphalt, and the matrix asphalt is the smallest. However, as the temperature rises to a certain extent, the gap between the three rutting factors gradually narrows. This is due to the transition of asphalt from an elastic state to a viscous state at high temperature. The viscous component increases, the elastic component decreases, and the asphalt is more likely to deform, so the rutting factor will decrease. At 46 °C, the maximum rutting factor of PUP/CF composite-modified asphalt is 34.50 kPa, which is 10.17 kPa larger than that of CF-modified asphalt and 13.57 kPa larger than that of matrix asphalt, indicating that CF plays a role of filling and supporting asphalt to prevent excessive deformation at high temperature. PUP can fill the gap between fibers, and its internal structure is more stable; so, the resistance to deformation of asphalt is improved, and the rutting factor increases.

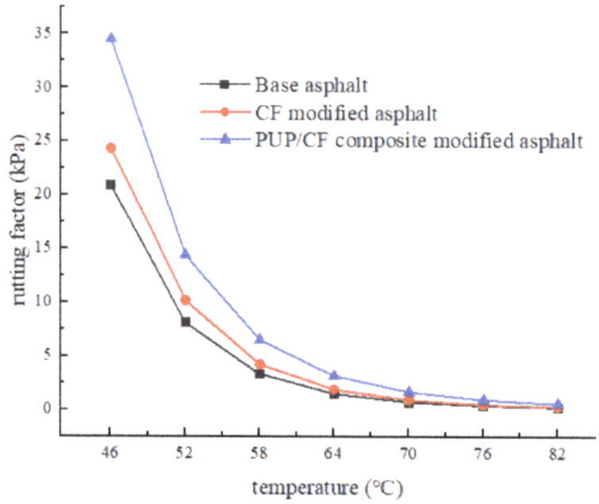

Figure 6. Rutting factor–temperature curve.

2.3.2. Frequency Scanning Analysis

(1) G* analysis of Different Asphalt Complex Moduli

The variation in the complex modulus of asphalt with loading frequency at different temperatures was explored in detail. According to the test results, the logarithm was taken and the complex modulus (lgG*)–angular frequency (lgω) curve was drawn, as shown in Figure 7.

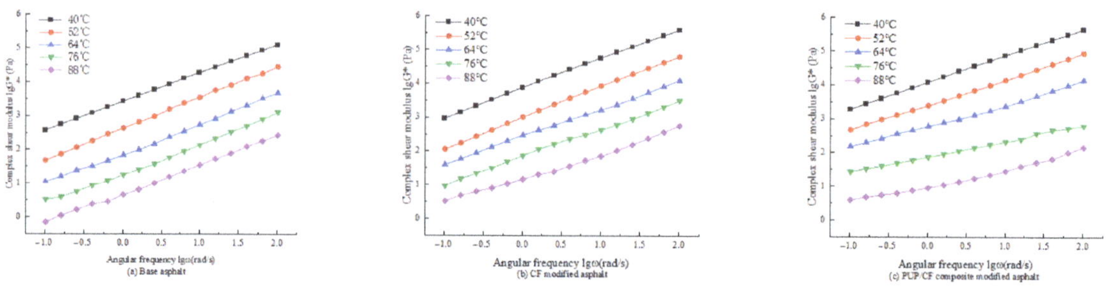

Figure 7. Asphalt lgG^*-$lg\omega$ relationship diagram.

It can be seen from Figure 7 that the complex shear modulus of different asphalts increases with the increase in angular frequency at the same temperature, and the two show an approximate linear correlation. This is because when the angular frequency increases, the load action time is shortened, the elastic characteristics of the asphalt are highlighted, and the elastic deformation increases, making the complex shear modulus increase. The higher angular frequency corresponds to the high speed of the vehicle, and the complex shear modulus is the ability of the asphalt to resist deformation. Under the same temperature and the same frequency, the complex shear modulus of PUP/CF composite-modified asphalt is the largest, and the matrix asphalt is the smallest. This shows that the addition of PUP increases the elastic properties of asphalt, and CF increases the stiffness of asphalt. The combination of the two makes the asphalt show better anti-deformation ability.

(2) Time–temperature equivalent master curve construction and analysis

By comparing the mechanical properties at different temperatures with those at the reference temperature, the shift factor of each temperature relative to the reference temperature was determined. According to the displacement factor, displacement was carried out, and the main curve of lgG^*-lgω was obtained. Based on the displacement factor at the test temperature of 40 °C, the master curve of the composite modulus at the reference temperature of 40 °C was drawn, as shown in Figure 8.

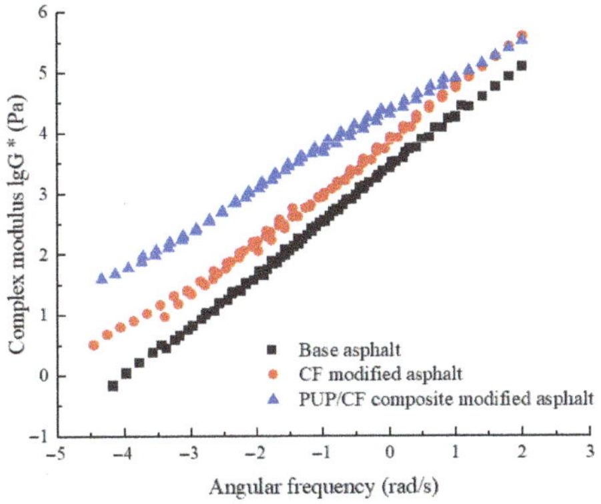

Figure 8. The main curves of lgG^*-lgω of asphalt.

According to the analysis of Figure 8, it can be concluded that under the condition of high temperature and low frequency, the complex shear modulus of matrix asphalt is the lowest, indicating that its high-temperature deformation resistance is weak; the complex shear modulus of CF-modified asphalt is slightly higher than that of matrix asphalt, and CF has good thermal stability. The complex modulus of PUP/CF composite-modified asphalt is significantly higher than that of CF-modified asphalt and matrix asphalt, indicating that the synergistic effect of PUP and CF can effectively enhance the high-temperature performance of asphalt. At low temperature and high frequency, as the angular frequency increases, the complex shear modulus of the three asphalts gradually increases. Among them, CF-modified asphalt gradually tends to PUP/CF composite-modified asphalt. PUP/CF composite-modified asphalt is the largest, because PUP has excellent flexibility and low-temperature performance and can improve the flexibility of asphalt in low-temperature environments. CF plays a role in enhancing the skeleton in asphalt, which greatly improves the overall strength and stiffness of asphalt. When PUP and CF are used to modify asphalt, PUP can fill the tiny voids that may exist between the CF and asphalt, enhance the bonding force between the fiber and asphalt, and make the synergy between them closer. They complement each other's advantages, significantly improving the elastic properties of asphalt and enhancing its ability to resist deformation. Therefore, the addition of PUP and CF significantly improves the deformation resistance of asphalt.

2.4. Multi-Stress Creep Recovery Test

The test results are shown in Figure 9. Under a creep cycle of 0.1 and 3.2 kPa stress levels, the strain is gradually increasing. It can be seen from Figure 9a,b that the strain level of the matrix asphalt in a cycle period shows almost no recovery ability, indicating that the matrix asphalt has relatively weak resistance to deformation when subjected to stress. It can be seen from Figure 9a,b that under the same stress level, the cumulative strain of PUP/CF composite-modified asphalt is lower than that of CF-modified asphalt. At 0.1 kPa, both asphalts have good recovery ability, but at 3.2 kPa, the recovery strain ability of the two modified asphalts becomes weaker; compared with the matrix asphalt, the cumulative strain is greatly reduced, indicating that PUP and CF can give asphalt better resistance to deformation and effectively inhibit strain accumulation under stress. All tests were performed in triplicate, and the results are reported as the mean ± standard deviation. One-way ANOVA ($\alpha = 0.05$) was used to assess the significance of differences between modified and unmodified asphalt.

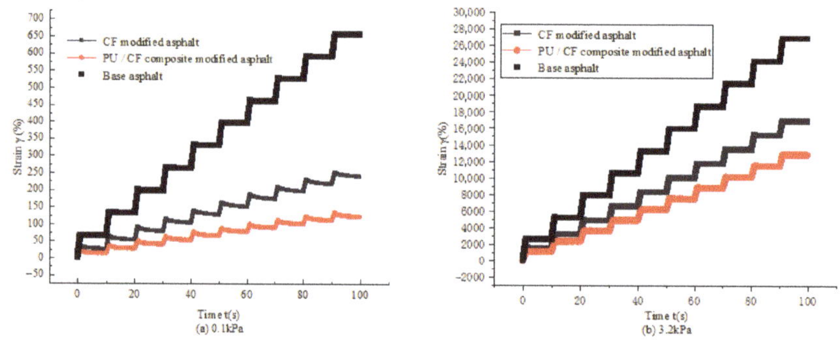

Figure 9. Strain variation with time under different stress levels.

The data obtained from the test were used to calculate R and Jnr under different stresses, and the results are shown in Figure 10.

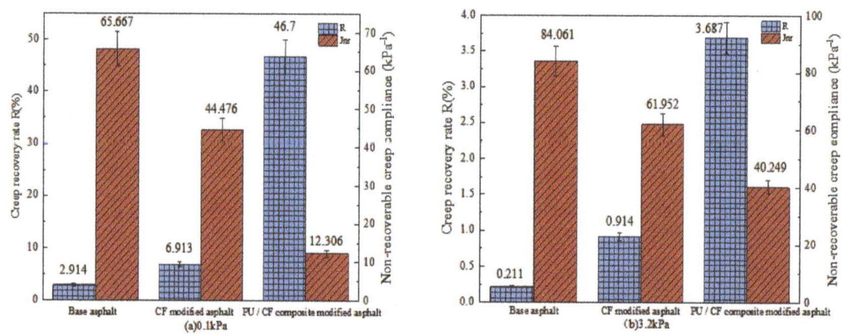

Figure 10. R and Jnr of three kinds of asphalt under different stress.

It can be seen from Figure 10 that under the stress of 0.1 kPa, the R value of matrix asphalt is the smallest, and the R value of CF-modified asphalt is not significantly higher than that of matrix asphalt, which is only increased by 3.999%. The R value of PUP/CF composite-modified asphalt is the largest, which is 43.786% higher than that of matrix asphalt. It shows that the addition of CF has no obvious effect on the strain recovery of asphalt. The chemical structure and physical properties of PUP enhance the elastic composition of CF-modified asphalt, improve the flexibility and elasticity of composite modified asphalt, and enhance the resistance to deformation of asphalt. It can be seen from (b) that compared with the stress of 0.1 kPa, the R of the three asphalts at the stress level of 3.2 kPa is greatly reduced. Under the action of large stress, their recovery deformation ability is weakened, but PUP/CF composite-modified asphalt have a relatively higher performance than CF-modified asphalt and matrix asphalt. The performance is the best, indicating that the addition of PUP and CF improves the creep recovery ability of asphalt, but under large stress, the improvement effect is weakened.

2.5. Bending Creep Stiffness Test Analysis

The results of the bending creep stiffness test are shown in Figure 11a. It can be seen that the stiffness modulus of matrix asphalt, CF-modified asphalt, and PUP/CF composite-modified asphalt increases with the decrease in temperature. At −6 °C, −12 °C, and −18 °C, CF-modified asphalt has a bending creep stiffness 11.8%, 13%, and 41.7% lower than that of matrix asphalt, and PUP/CF composite-modified asphalt has a bending creep stiffness 35.1%, 49.1%, and 118.4% lower than that of matrix asphalt. This shows that in a low-temperature environment, the effect of CF on the anti-deformation ability of asphalt is relatively limited. At low temperature, the brittleness of asphalt itself increases, and the reinforcement effect of CF struggles to offset the adverse effect of low temperature on asphalt performance, while the addition of PUP enhances the low-temperature performance of CF-modified asphalt. It can be seen from Figure 11b that the creep rate decreases with the decrease in temperature. At the three temperatures of −6 °C, −12 °C, and −18 °C, the creep rate of PUP/CF composite-modified asphalt is the largest, and that of matrix asphalt is the smallest. The creep rate of CF-modified asphalt increases by 0.03, 0.023, and 0.028, respectively, at the three temperatures, and the creep rate of PUP/CF-modified asphalt increases by 0.097, 0.085, and 0.093, respectively, compared with matrix asphalt. CF mainly relies on physical hindrance to reduce the creep rate, and the improvement in low-temperature creep performance of asphalt is limited. For PUP in PUP/CF composite-modified asphalt, its activity at low temperature is relatively strong, and the elastic effect of PUP still makes the creep rate of asphalt relatively high, so the low-temperature rheological properties of PUP/CF composite-modified asphalt are the best.

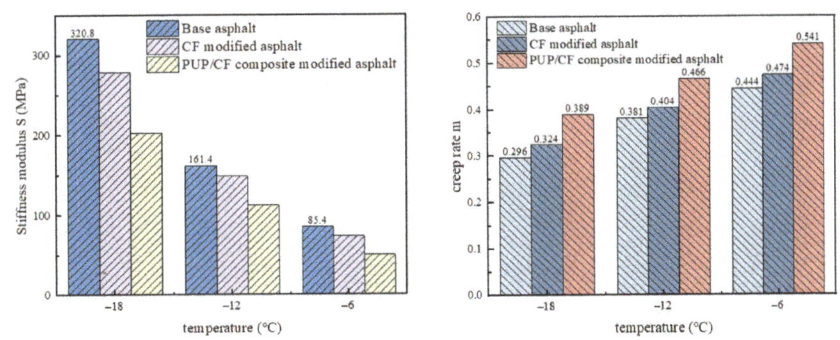

(**a**) Change in modulus of elasticity S (**b**) Change in creep rate m

Figure 11. The variation in stiffness modulus and creep rate with temperature.

Compared with base asphalt, the PUP/CF composite modification significantly improves tensile strength (by ~25%), fatigue life (by ~30%), and high-temperature rutting resistance (by ~20%), while also enhancing interfacial bonding and microstructural uniformity.

2.6. Scanning Electron Microscope Test Analysis

The scanning electron microscope morphology of matrix asphalt, CF-modified asphalt, and PUP/CF composite-modified asphalt was studied, as shown in Figures 12–14.

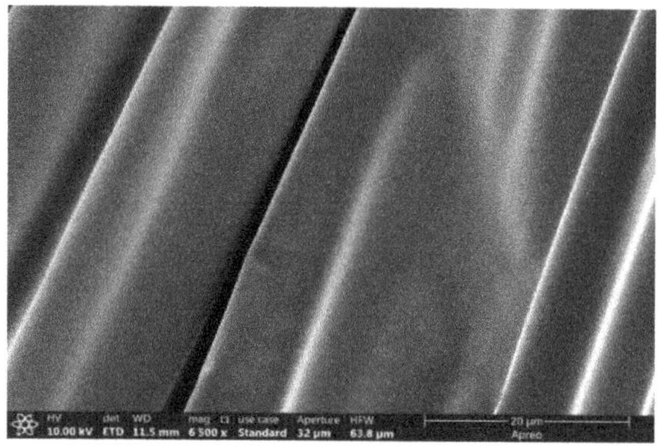

Figure 12. Microstructure of matrix asphalt.

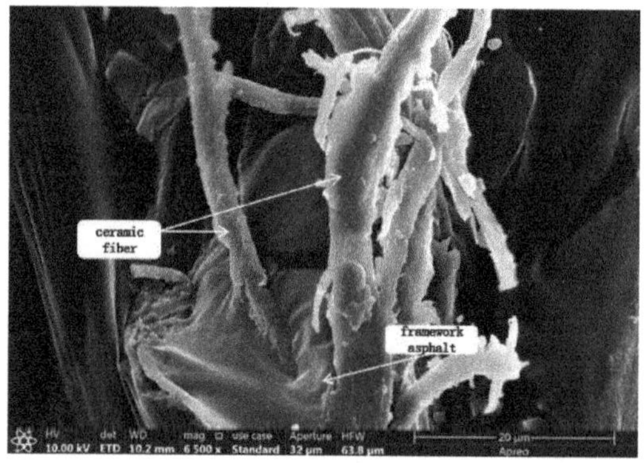

Figure 13. Microstructure of CF-modified asphalt.

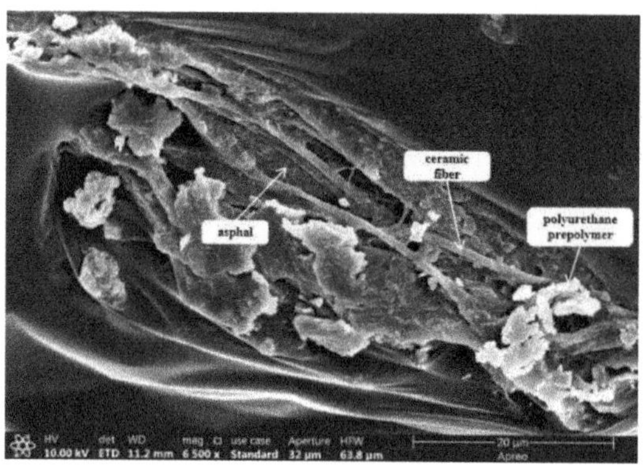

Figure 14. Microstructure of PUP/CF composite-modified asphalt.

The analysis of Figures 12–14 shows that the surface of the matrix asphalt is relatively smooth, the micro-morphology is evenly distributed, the surface is flat, and there is no obvious fluctuation and fracture. There are no impurities, holes, or cracks on the surface, indicating that the internal structure is dense and evenly distributed. In CF-modified asphalt, a large amount of asphalt is attached around CF, and an asphalt film is formed on the surface of the fiber, which can transform free asphalt into structural asphalt. When stressed, the force can be transferred from asphalt to CF, which enhances the mechanical properties of the whole material and makes asphalt more stable. CF shows a certain distribution state in asphalt, and the fibers are intertwined to form a three-dimensional network structure. Under the action of PUP, CF is closely combined with asphalt, and there is no obvious agglomeration phenomenon, indicating that CF and PUP have good dispersion in asphalt. The surface of CF is wrapped by PUP and asphalt, which enhances the interfacial bonding between CF and asphalt.

2.7. Atomic Force Microscope Test Analysis

The results of atomic force microscopy of matrix asphalt, CF-modified asphalt, and PUP/CF composite-modified asphalt are shown in Figures 15–17.

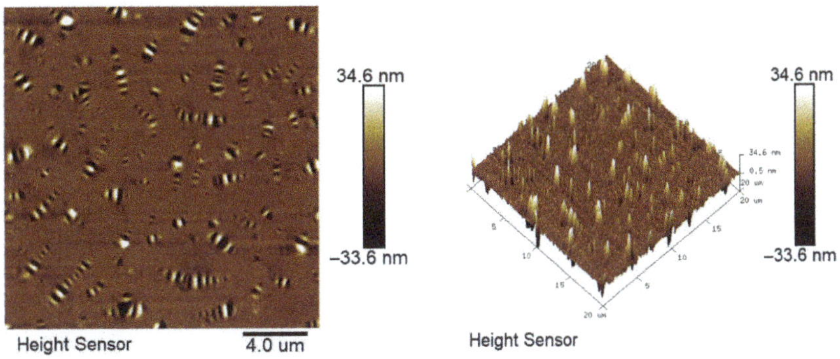

Figure 15. Microscopic morphology of matrix asphalt.

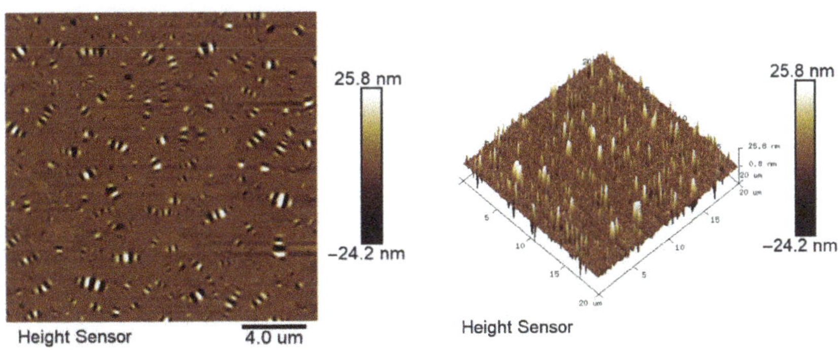

Figure 16. Micro-morphology of CF-modified asphalt.

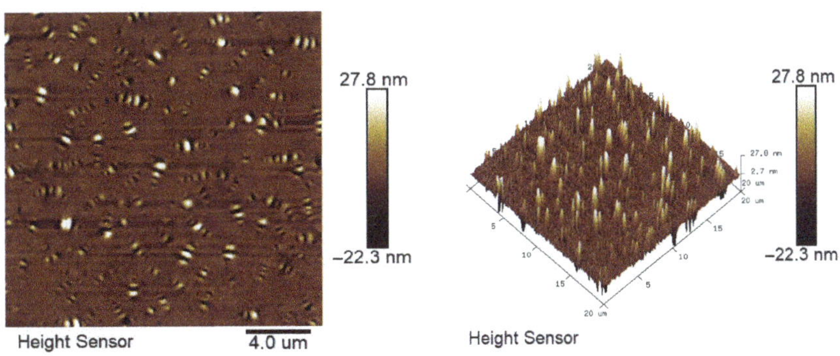

Figure 17. Microscopic morphology of PUP/CF-modified asphalt.

The sol–gel process is a key chemical method for synthesizing high-purity ceramic materials at lower temperatures than in conventional solid-phase reactions. The method facilitates precise control of composition, microstructure, and morphology, and sol–gel-derived ceramic fibers and matrices are critical in high-performance composites.

The hydrolysis sol–gel process involves a continuous reaction, with hydrolysis being the reaction of metal alcohol salts with water and polycondensation being the formation of M-O-M bonds from the hydrolyzed monomers via dehydration or dehydrogenation. The resulting colloidal suspension (sol) is transformed into a porous three-dimensional network (gel) suitable for oxide ceramics (SiO_2, TiO_2, Al_2O_3) and homogeneous doping and preparation of organic–inorganic hybrid materials. The non-hydrolyzed sol–gel process comprises direct condensation using the reaction between halides and oxygen donors or alcohol salts. An aluminosilicate (Al_2O_3-SiO_2) fiber-reinforced polyurethane matrix can be prepared by using the sol–gel method. The selected polyurethane prepolymer is a partial reaction product of isocyanate and polyol, retaining the active -NCO group. With performance advantages, the three-dimensional network polyurethane structure is generated by a temperature-controlled curing reaction under the action of a chain-expanding crosslinking agent. The nanoscale uniformity of the aluminosilicate fibers optimizes the fiber/matrix interfacial bonding, the low defect rate of the sol–gel fibers significantly improves the fracture toughness of the composites, and the flexible network of the polyurethane matrix mitigates the interfacial failure caused by thermal stress.

From Figures 15–17, it can be seen that the microscopic morphology of asphalt shows 'bee-like structures' with different depths and alternating black and white. These 'bee-like structures' are the aggregates formed by asphaltenes in asphalt through van der Waals forces and π-π stacking to form a rigid skeleton. The resin and saturates/aromatics are filled as dispersion medium to form a soft-phase region. The structure is shown as a convex light-colored area in the phase diagram, and the color of the surrounding depression is darker, reflecting the viscoelastic differences in different regions. CF modified asphalt has more small-sized 'bee-like structures' compared to matrix asphalt, and the dispersion is more uniform. This is because the addition of CF changes the rheological properties of asphalt, increases its viscosity and elasticity, decreases the mobility of asphalt molecules, and enhances the interaction between molecules. Asphaltenes that may have formed large-sized 'bee-like structures' can now only form smaller 'bee-like structures'. CF forms a three-dimensional network structure in asphalt, which limits the free movement of asphaltene molecules and forces them to arrange in a smaller space to form a more uniform 'bee-like structure'. Compared with CF-modified asphalt and matrix asphalt, PUP/CF composite-modified asphalt has more 'bee-like structures', which is because the unique molecular structure and properties of polyurethane prepolymer interact with asphalt molecules and change the asphalt, indicating that the gel-like polyurethane network is uniformly distributed within the asphalt matrix, contributing to a more stable structural asphalt phase.

2.8. Infrared Spectrum Test Analysis

The test results of matrix asphalt, CF-modified asphalt, and PUP/CF composite-modified asphalt are shown in Figure 18.

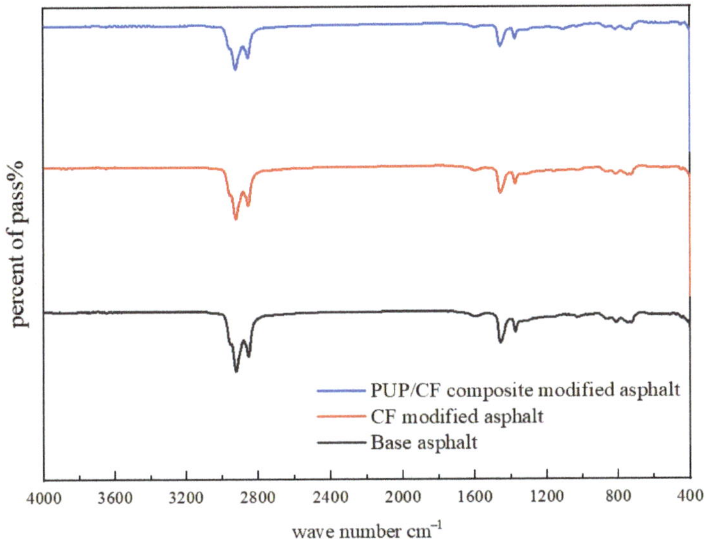

Figure 18. Infrared spectra of asphalt.

The infrared spectrum of matrix asphalt in Figure 18 shows that there are two significant characteristic absorption peaks at 2919 cm^{-1} and 2851 cm^{-1}, which are related to the stretching vibration of methyl (-CH) and methylene ($-CH_2-$). A characteristic peak with low intensity appears at 1601 cm^{-1}, which is usually related to the C=C stretching vibration of aromatic hydrocarbons. Medium-intensity stretching vibration peaks appear at 1455 cm^{-1} and 1372 cm^{-1}, which are related to the bending vibration of methylene ($-CH_2-$) and the symmetrical bending vibration of methyl ($-CH_3-$). From 867 cm^{-1} to 721 cm^{-1}, there are multiple absorption peaks related to the out-of-plane bending vibration of the C-H group of aromatic compounds. The infrared spectrum of CF-modified asphalt is basically the same as that of matrix asphalt, indicating that there is no chemical reaction between CF and asphalt. The peak intensity of PUP/CF composite-modified asphalt increases at 1595 cm^{-1}. Because the benzene ring structure in polyurethane prepolymer enters the asphalt system through chemical bonding or physical blending, the peak intensity is enhanced. The PUP molecule has an isocyanate (-NCO) active group, and no absorption peak is found at 2270 cm^{-1}, because it is related to the carboxyl group (-COOH) and hydroxyl group (-OH) in the asphalt.

3. Conclusions

(1) The three-factor and three-level optimization test was designed using the response surface method, and 17 groups of modified asphalt preparation schemes were created. The penetration, softening point, and ductility were used as response values. The influence of each factor on the response values and the interactions between each influencing factor were analyzed. The preparation scheme was optimized, and the optimal preparation scheme for composite-modified asphalt was determined. The polyurethane prepolymer content was 7.4%, the ceramic fiber content was 2.1%, and the shear time was 40 min.

(2) PUP/CF composite-modified asphalt exhibits the largest residual penetration ratio before and after aging, along with the smallest mass loss and softening point increment, indicating that PUP and CF enhance asphalt's aging resistance, leading to superior aging performance. Its rutting factor is higher than that of CF-modified

asphalt and matrix asphalt, showing better anti-rutting ability. Based on the time–temperature equivalence principle, the fitted complex shear modulus–frequency curve and viscoelastic master curve (using displacement factors) reveal that it has better high-temperature performance under low-temperature and high-frequency or high-temperature and low-frequency conditions.

(3) PUP/CF composite-modified asphalt has the best recovery strain capacity under low stress. At high stress levels, the recovery strain capacity of PUP/CF composite-modified asphalt is weakened, but the cumulative strain is significantly lower than that of matrix asphalt. Unlike previous studies focusing on single modifiers, this work combines gel-forming PUP with ceramic fibers (CFs) to form a hybrid microstructure, which not only results in significantly enhanced rheological and aging properties but also improves the flexibility and elasticity of composite-modified asphalt while enhancing its resistance to deformation.

(4) The stiffness modulus of PUP/CF composite-modified asphalt was significantly lower than that of matrix asphalt, which decreased by 35.1%, 49.1%, and 118.4% at −6 °C, −12 °C, and −18 °C, respectively. Compared with CF-modified asphalt, it is reduced by 11.8%, 13%, and 41.7%. The creep rate of PUP/CF composite-modified asphalt is large at three temperatures, indicating that PUP and CF have a good effect on the low-temperature rheological properties of asphalt.

(5) SEM observations show that carbon fiber (CF) is encapsulated by asphalt with minor voids which are filled by polyurethane prepolymer (PUP), strengthening CF–asphalt interfacial bonding via co-encapsulation for more stable performance. AFM micrographs reveal that PUP/CF composite-modified asphalt has more and larger 'honeycomb-like structures', indicating greater structural stability. Infrared analysis shows that PUP engages in hydrogen bonding and weak chemical reactions with asphalt, achieving modification through a synergistic combination of physical (predominant) and chemical means. This leverages PUP and ceramic fiber advantages: PUP physically encapsulates CF to reduce voids and enhance load transfer, and acts as a precursor to form a 3D elastic gel network that bridges CF–asphalt interfaces, boosting durability, mechanical resilience, and thermal stability under stress.

(6) In contrast to existing studies that investigate CF or PUP in isolation, this work focuses on the synergistic effects of gel-forming polyurethane prepolymers and ceramic fibers to enhance asphalt's durability, stability, and resistance to deformation. The purpose is to develop a composite-modified asphalt suitable for extreme temperature conditions. Compared with base asphalt, the PUP/CF composite modification significantly improves tensile strength (by ~25%), fatigue life (by ~30%), and high-temperature rutting resistance (by ~20%) while also enhancing interfacial bonding and microstructural uniformity.

4. Materials and Methods

4.1. Matrix Asphalt

In this study, 70# road petroleum asphalt provided by Zhengfa Municipality of Zhengzhou City was selected as the base asphalt, and the basic properties of the base asphalt were tested according to the relevant regulations [44]. The test results are shown in Table 5.

Table 5. Basic performance index of asphalt.

Performance Index		Test Results	Unit	Technical Requirements
Penetration (25 °C)		66.1	0.1 mm	60~80
Softening point		50.8	°C	≥46
Ductility (5 cm/min, 10 °C)		30.2	cm	≥20
Flash point		270	°C	≥260
Density (15 °C)		1.136	g/cm^3	measured value
After aging	Quality change	−0.122	%	≤±0.8
	Softening point increment	2.9	°C	≤8 °C
	Penetration ratio	69.6	%	≥61

4.2. Polyurethane Prepolymer

Polyurethane prepolymer is an intermediate product in the process of polyurethane synthesis which is formed by the partial reaction of isocyanate and polyol. It contains unreacted -NCO groups and can react with chain extenders to form polyurethane under certain temperature conditions. Under specific conditions, this polyurethane prepolymer reacts with asphalt components to form a three-dimensional crosslinked structure, exhibiting typical gel behavior. In this paper, the polyether polyurethane prepolymer produced by Jining Liduo Chemical Industry was selected, and its performance was determined according to the relevant specifications [45], as shown in Table 6.

Table 6. Basic properties of polyurethane prepolymers.

Performance Index	Unit	Test Results
NCO content	(%)	5.1 ± 0.2
State	/	Colorless transparent liquid
Viscosity	(85 °C/MPa.s)	350
Hardness	Shore A	90 ± 2
Tensile strength	(MPa)	30
Elongation at break	(%)	420
Rebound	(%)	32

4.3. Ceramic Fiber

The ceramic fiber (aluminum silicate) used in this study was purchased from Zhengzhou Xinyang Refractory Co., Ltd., with main components of Al_2O_3 (38–40%), ZrO_2 (15–17%), and Fe_2O_3 (0.2%). The fibers were fabricated via melt-spinning. Its characteristics include high-temperature resistance, excellent chemical stability, and environmental protection. Its basic performance indicators are shown in Table 7.

Table 7. Basic performance indicators of ceramic fiber.

Performance Index		Ceramic Fiber (Aluminum Silicate Fiber)
Classification Temperature (°C)		1400
Diameter (m)		3–5
Slag ball content (%)		≤15
Chemical composition (%)	Al_2O_3	38–40
	Fe_2O_3	0.2
	ZrO_2	15–17

4.4. Surface Modification of Ceramic Fiber

During the production, processing, or use of ceramic fibers, fiber particles may stick together or aggregate, forming larger clumps or agglomerates. This agglomeration phenomenon can adversely affect the performance of ceramic fibers, such as thermal conductivity, insulation, and mechanical strength. Therefore, surface modification treatment is performed on ceramic fibers to enhance their dispersibility and minimize agglomeration, thereby ensuring their stability and reliability. This paper used NaOH solution and a silane coupling agent (KH-550) to modify the surface of ceramic fibers cut into 6 mm lengths. The dispersion properties of the treated fibers were evaluated and analyzed. NaOH solution was selected because its strong alkalinity can remove impurities from the surface of ceramic fibers, roughen the surface, and introduce polar groups to improve wettability. Silane coupling agents were selected because their molecules can react with the hydroxyl groups on the surface of ceramic fibers and organic matrices at both ends, enhancing the compatibility between fibers and media through chemical bonding, thereby improving dispersibility and reducing agglomeration.

4.4.1. Ceramic Fiber Modified by NaOH Solution

We prepared sodium hydroxide solutions with mass fractions of 3%, 4%, and 5%. We added ceramic fibers to sodium hydroxide solutions of different concentrations, placed them on a magnetic stirrer, heated them to 60 °C, and maintained a constant temperature for 0.5 h. As shown in Figure 19a–c.

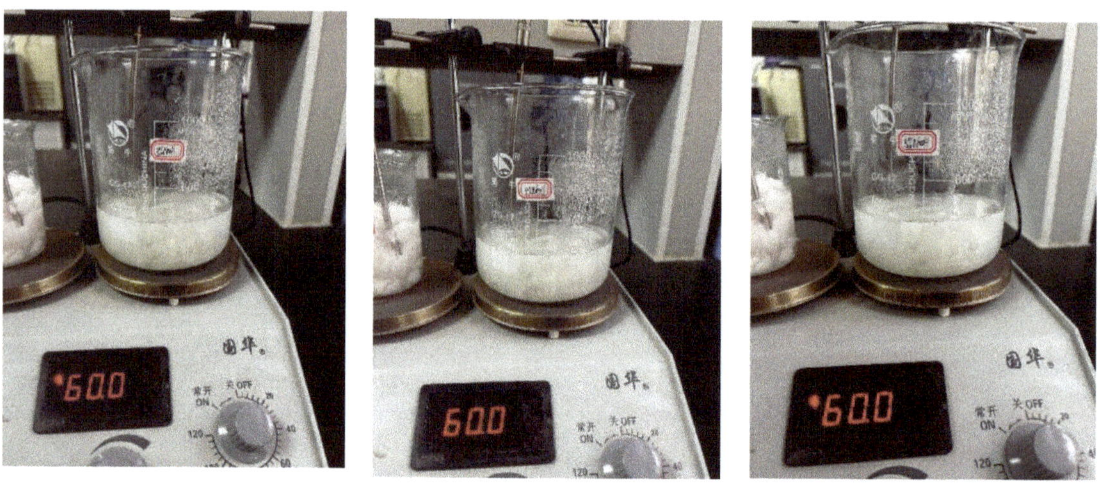

(**a**) 3%NaOH (**b**) 4%NaOH (**c**) 5%NaOH

Figure 19. Modification with different concentrations of NaOH.

4.4.2. KH-550 Solution-Modified Ceramic Fibers

As shown in Figure 20, we mixed anhydrous ethanol and deionized water in a 2:8 ratio by weight to prepare the dissolving solution. We added 4%, 6%, and 8% coupling agents to the solution, stirred it evenly, and let it sit for 30 min to allow the silane coupling agent to hydrolyze fully. We put the ceramic fibers into different concentrations of KH-550 solution, heated them to 40 °C, and kept them at that temperature for 0.5 h.

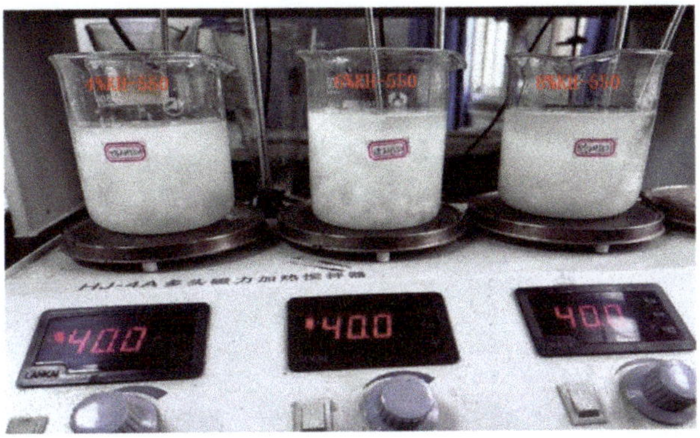

Figure 20. KH-55-modified ceramic fibers in different concentrations.

4.5. MOCA

In this paper, 3,3-dichloro-4,4-diaminodiphenylmethane (MOCA) was selected. The chain-extending crosslinking agent MOCA can react with the isocyanate group in the polyurethane prepolymer to extend the molecular chain and form a three-dimensional network structure, thereby improving the mechanical, heat resistance, and chemical resistance of the polyurethane gel material. Its performance is shown in Table 8.

Table 8. Basic performance of MOCA.

Performance Index	Appearance	Molecular Weight	Melting Point (°C)	Structural Formula
Test results	Yellow particles	267.16	105	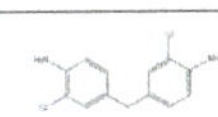

4.6. Test Scheme

4.6.1. The Optimum Preparation of PUP/CF Composite-Modified Asphalt Based on Response Surface Methodology

According to the Box–Behnken design method in the response surface method, the experimental design of PUP/CF composite-modified asphalt was carried out by using the analysis software Design-Expert 13. The polyurethane prepolymer content (4~8%), ceramic fiber content (1~3%), and shear time (20~40 min) in the preparation process of modifying asphalt were selected as response variables. A three-factor and three-level optimization test was designed to study the effects of polyurethane prepolymer content, ceramic fiber content, and shear time on penetration (0.1 mm), softening point (°C), and 10 °C ductility (cm). A mathematical regression model between influencing factors and response values was established, and the optimal preparation scheme of composite-modified asphalt was determined.

4.6.2. Rotating Film Oven Aging Test

The aging test of asphalt was carried out by using the rotating thin-film oven test (RTFOT). The asphalt sample was placed in a rotating thin-film oven and heated at a certain temperature. The rotating film can make the asphalt sample uniformly heated, ensuring that it is fully in contact with the air, and simulate the aging process in the actual environment. The thermal stability and volatility of asphalt can be evaluated by measuring the mass change, viscosity change, and softening point change of asphalt samples before and after heating.

4.6.3. Dynamic Shear Rheological Test

Dynamic shear test (DSR) is an important test method for evaluating the rheological properties of asphalt and its modified materials under high-temperature and low-frequency conditions. This test is mainly used to determine the viscoelastic behavior of asphalt. Temperature scanning is an important test method for evaluating the rheological properties of asphalt with temperature changes. The strain level was 10%, the temperature range was 46~82 °C, the temperature interval was 6 °C, and the angular frequency was 10 rad/s. Frequency scanning is a test method for measuring the mechanical properties of viscoelastic materials such as asphalt at different frequencies. The test temperature was set at 40~88 °C, the temperature interval was 12 °C, the frequency range was 0.1~100 rad/s, and the strain level was controlled at 1%.

4.6.4. MSCR Test

The MSCR test is based on the creep theory. During the test, a constant axial stress was applied to the asphalt and maintained for a certain time to cause creep deformation of the specimen. Then, the stress was unloaded, and the asphalt was allowed to recover for a certain period of time. The deformation of the specimen in each loading-recovery cycle was observed and recorded, including recoverable strain and unrecoverable strain. Repeated loading–recovery cycles were performed at two common stress levels of 0.1 kPa and 3.2 kPa. The loading time was 1 s, the unloading time was 9 s, and the number of cycles was 10 times.

4.6.5. Bending Creep Stiffness Test

BBR evaluates the low-temperature rheological properties of asphalt by measuring the bending deformation of the beam sample at a certain temperature. The basic principle is that the asphalt sample is prepared into a long strip, and then a constant load is applied in the test. The low-temperature performance of the asphalt is judged by measuring the deformation of the beam in a certain period of time. In the test, PUP/CF composite-modified asphalt was tested at −6 °C, −12 °C, and −18 °C, and the stiffness modulus S and creep rate m were measured.

4.6.6. Scanning Electron Microscopy Test

This study used a scanning electron microscope model JSM-7500F manufactured by Shanghai Bahe Instrument Technology Co., Ltd. (Shanghai, China). The test employed electron optics principles to emit a low-energy electron beam onto the asphalt surface. The electron beam interacts with the asphalt atom, and the generated signal is processed to generate an observation image. Different from ordinary microscopy, scanning electron microscopy can enlarge the material to nanometer scale and obtain detailed observations of the microstructure and distribution of the material. In the study of composite-modified asphalt, by adjusting different magnifications, the bonding state and distribution of the admixture and asphalt can be clearly observed, and the differences in the microstructure of the two can be distinguished so as to further analyze the modification mechanism of the modifier on asphalt.

4.6.7. Atomic Force Microscope Test

Using the JSM-7610FPlus atomic force microscope provided by Jieouluo Trading Co., Ltd., it is possible to observe the nanoscale structure of the asphalt surface with a resolution of up to 0.1 nanometers. The microstructure of asphalt can be understood more deeply, and the modification mechanism can be analyzed. The scanning frequency of this test was 1

Hz, the scanning pixel size was 512 × 512, the image scanning area was 20 μm × 20 μm, the resolution was 10 nm, and the experimental temperature was 25 °C.

4.6.8. Infrared Spectroscopy Test

A TENSOR 37 Fourier transform infrared spectrometer from Bruker Spectrometer Instruments was used. The scanning range as 4000~500 cm^{-1}. By comparing the infrared spectra of asphalt before and after modification, the change in absorption peak can be observed. If a new absorption peak appears in the modified spectrum, it indicates that the modifier reacts with the asphalt to form a new functional group. If the position or intensity of some original absorption peaks change, it may mean that the chemical structure of the asphalt has been altered due to modification.

Author Contributions: Writing original draft preparation, T.G., X.G. and Y.C.; writing—review and editing, T.G., Z.L. (Zhenxia Li), X.G., Y.C. and C.F.; investigation, J.Y., H.C. and J.F., validation, J.W., H.H. and Z.L. (Zhi Li). All authors have read and agreed to the published version of the manuscript.

Funding: This work was supported by a planned project supported by the science and technology innovation team of universities and colleges in Henan province (24IRTSTHN011); the Central Plains Science and Technology Innovation Leader Project (244200510031); the Key scientific and technological projects in Henan province (252102240031; 252102230050); and the Special Plan for Key Scientific Research Projects of Higher Education Institutions in Henan Province to Serve Industry Development (25CY022).

Institutional Review Board Statement: Not applicable.

Informed Consent Statement: Not applicable.

Data Availability Statement: Some or all of the data, models, or code that support the findings of this study are available from the corresponding author upon reasonable request.

Conflicts of Interest: The authors do not have any conflicts of interest with other entities or researchers.

References

1. Rao, Z.; Wang, Y.; Cui, S.; Li, M. Interpretation of the key points of highway construction in the 14th Five-Year Plan. *China Highw.* **2022**, *623*, 28–32.
2. Bai, X.; Jia, Q. Disease analysis and treatment maintenance of asphalt pavement of expressway. *Road Constr. Mach. Constr. Mech.* **2016**, *33*, 76–79.
3. Chen, Q.; Ge, T.; Li, X.; Wang, C. Road area pollution cleaning technology for asphalt pavement: Literature review and research propositions. *J. Clean. Prod.* **2025**, *493*, 144975. [CrossRef]
4. Wang, C.; Lan, X.; Cong, Y.; Peng, S.; Huang, S.; Chen, Q. Evaluation of skid resistance of pavement maintenance energy-absorbing seal based on surface texture characteristics. *Measurement* **2025**, *245*, 116588. [CrossRef]
5. Chen, Q.; Lan, X.; Li, A.; Sun, X.; Wang, C. The novel rapid curing pavement maintenance seal with a low environmental impact: Preparation and performance evaluation. *Wear* **2025**, *566–567*, 205919. [CrossRef]
6. Huang, S.; Liu, G.; Wu, Y.; Zhao, Y.; Zhai, J.; Xiong, R. Study on crack resistance of fiber modified asphalt under medium temperature. *Highway* **2025**, *70*, 328–335.
7. Mrema, A.H.; Noh, S.-H.; Kwon, O.-S.; Lee, J.-J. Performance of Glass Wool Fibers in Asphalt Concrete Mixtures. *Materials* **2020**, *13*, 4699. [CrossRef]
8. Zhang, T.; Wang, L.; Liu, L. Experimental study on road performance of mixed fiber asphalt mixture. *Highway* **2018**, *63*, 5.
9. Tang, G. *Study on the Properties of Bamboo Fiber Asphalt Mortar and Its Mixture Performance*; Xi'an University of Science and Technology: Xi'an, China, 2021.
10. Fan, Z.; Wang, C.; Wang, Z.; Li, Y.; Feng, L.; Tan, S. Fog seal with polymer composite modified emulsified asphalt: Road performance and environmental adaptability. *Wear* **2025**, *562–563*, 205672. [CrossRef]
11. Feng, G.; Jiang, W.; Liu, J.; Zhang, Q. A novel green nonaqueous sol-gel process for preparation of partially stabilized zirconia nanopowder. *Process. Appl. Ceram.* **2017**, *11*, 220–224. [CrossRef]
12. Zhang, Q.; Jiang, W.H.; Liu, J.M.; Guo, F. Low temperature synthesis of ultrafine Al_2TiO_5 powders by hydrolytic sol-gel method. *Mater. Sci. Forum* **2016**, *848*, 324–327.

13. Zhang, X.; Wang, G.; Liu, Z.; Su, J.; Hu, M.; Zhao, Y. Study on the properties and modification mechanism of polyether TPUP modified asphalt. *Highway* **2024**, *69*, 63–71.
14. Zhou, L.; Zhang, H. Research on rheological properties and road performance of polyurethane modified asphalt. *J. Chongqing Univ. Technol. Nat. Sci.* **2022**, *36*, 142–147.
15. Wei, B.; Gong, X.; Jiang, W.; Qin, L.; Fan, Y. Study on the properties of magnetorheological gel based on polyurethane. *J. Appl. Polym. Sci.* **2010**, *118*, 2765–2771. [CrossRef]
16. Jiang, W.H.; Hu, Z.; Liu, J.M. Study on low-tanperature synthesis of iron-stabilized aluminium titanate via non-hydrolytic sol-gel method. *J. Syn. Cryst.* **2011**, *40*, 465–469.
17. Feng, G.; Jiang, F.; Jiang, W.; Liu, J.; Zhang, Q.; Wu, Q.; Hu, Q.; Miao, L.; Liang, J. Low-temperature preparation of novel stabilized aluminum titanate ceramic fibers via nonhydrolytic sol-gel method through linear self-assembly of precursors. *Ceram. Int.* **2019**, *45*, 18704–18709. [CrossRef]
18. Bao, Y.; Jiang, W.H.; Feng, G.; Liu, J.; Wu, Q. Low Temperature Preparation of Aluminum Titanate Film via Sol-Gel Method. *Adv. Mater. Res.* **2014**, *936*, 238–242. [CrossRef]
19. Fu, K.L.; Jiang, W.H.; Liu, J.M.; Feng, G.; Pan, M. Study on mullite whiskers preparation via non-hydrolytic sol-gel process combined with molten salt method. *Mater. Sci. Forum* **2016**, *848*, 295–300. [CrossRef]
20. Wei, H.Y.; Jiang, W.H.; Lin, J. Comparative research on the synthesis of aluminum titanate powders by nonhydrolytic and hydrolytic sol-gel method. *J. Inorg. Mater.* **2009**, *24*, 199–203. [CrossRef]
21. Jiang, W.; Wei, H.; Feng, G.; Zhou, Y.; Yu, Y. Effect of oxygen donor alcohols on low temperature nonhydrolytic sol-gel synthesis of aluminum titanate. *J. Chin. Ceram. Soc.* **2008**, *36*, 11.
22. Jiang, W.H.; Yang, Y.H.; Zhu, Q.X.; Liu, J.M. Iron-zircon pigments prepared by non-hydrolytic sol-gel method at low temperature. *Adv. Mater. Res.* **2012**, *412*, 223–226. [CrossRef]
23. Zhang, Z.; Huang, T.; Zhu, Y.; Lv, W.; Sun, J. The effect of PUP soft segment structure type on the performance of PUP modified asphalt. *J. Chang'an Univ. Nat. Sci. Ed.* **2021**, *41*, 1–9.
24. Yu, C.; Wang, J.; Li, J.; Sun, Y. Application progress of polyurethane prepolymer modified asphalt. *Polym. Mater. Sci. Eng.* **2024**, *40*, 156–168.
25. Guo, G.; Cong, L.; Yang, F.; Tan, L. Progress in the application of polyurethane materials in pavement engineering. *Road Traffic Sci. Technol.* **2020**, *37*, 1–10.
26. Lv, W.; Liu, H.; Chang, P.; Huang, T.; Zhang, Z. Research progress on the application of polyurethane modified asphalt in pavement engineering. *New Chem. Mater.* **2022**, *50*, 227–230.
27. Park, D.; Wu, W.; Wang, Y. A functionalizable reverse thermal gel based on a polyurethane/PEG block copolymer. *Biomaterials* **2011**, *32*, 777–786. [CrossRef]
28. Baillif, P.Y.; Tabellout, M.; Emery, J.R. Ultrasonic investigation of polyurethane gel forming systems. *Macromolecules* **1999**, *32*, 3432–3437. [CrossRef]
29. Liu, X.; Yu, K.; Sun, J.; Guo, W.; Qian, K. Effect of shear thickening gel on structure and properties of flexible polyurethane foam. *Smart Mater. Struct.* **2021**, *30*, 125008. [CrossRef]
30. Akimov, A.E.; Valentina, V.Y.; Mikhail, S.L.; Vasilij, P.D.; Sergei, S.I.; Aleksandr, S.I.; Andrey, V.K.; Anton, S.P. Development of an energy-efficient method of obtaining polymer-modified bitumen with high operational characteristics via polymer–bitumen concentrate application. *J. Compos. Sci.* **2024**, *8*, 337. [CrossRef]
31. Liu, M.; Han, S.; Shang, W.; Qi, X. New polyurethane modified coating for maintenance of asphalt pavement potholes in winter-rainy condition. *Prog. Org. Coat.* **2019**, *133*, 368–375. [CrossRef]
32. Fang, Y.; Xie, W.; Yang, J. Preparation and rheological behavior of polyurethane prepolymer modified asphalt. *Funct. Mater.* **2019**, *50*, 6197–6205.
33. Cuadri, A.A.; García-Morales, M.; Navarro, F.J.; Partal, P. Processing of bitumens modified by a bio-oil-derived polyurethane. *Fuel* **2014**, *118*, 83–90. [CrossRef]
34. Baha, V.K.; Ercan, A.; Mehmet, Y.; Mustafa, A. Investigation on the properties of new palm-oil-based polyurethane modified bitumen. *Constr. Build. Mater.* **2021**, *289*, 123152.
35. Padhan, R.K.; Gupta, A.A. Preparation and evaluation of waste PET derived polyurethane polymer modified bitumen through in situ polymerization reaction. *Constr. Build. Mater.* **2018**, *158*, 337–345. [CrossRef]
36. Xu, L.; Zhang, Z.; Li, B.; Ru, Y. Research Progress of Artificial Ceramic Fibers. *Synth. Fiber Ind.* **2021**, *44*, 76–80.
37. Wang, Q.; Zhao, B.; Han, X. Properties and Preparation of Ceramic Fibers. *China Ceram.* **2019**, *55*, 10–18, 26.
38. Wan, J.; Wu, S.; Xiao, Y.; Liu, Q.; Schlangen, E. Characteristics of Ceramic Fiber Modified Asphalt Mortar. *Materials* **2016**, *9*, 788. [CrossRef]
39. Mahyar, A.; Amir, S.; Hossein, H.G. Evaluation of the ceramic fiber modified asphalt binder. *Constr. Build. Mater.* **2019**, *205*, 377–386. [CrossRef]

40. Arabani, M.; Shabani, A.; Hamedi, G.H. Experimental Investigation of Effect of Ceramic Fibers on Mechanical Properties of Asphalt Mixtures. *J. Mater. Civ. Eng.* **2019**, *31*, 04019203.1–04019203.12. [CrossRef]
41. Zhou, H.; Pan, Q. Study on the effect of ceramic fiber addition on the rheological properties of asphalt. *Highw. Eng.* **2022**, *47*, 166–171.
42. Wang, X.; Zhou, H.; Zhang, X.; Fan, T. Analysis of road performance and modification mechanism of ceramic fiber asphalt mixture. *J. Chongqing Jiaotong Univ. (Nat. Sci. Ed.)* **2022**, *41*, 100–106.
43. Xiao, Z. *Study on Properties of Nano AAT/Ceramic Fiber Composite Modified Asphalt and Mixture*; Chongqing Jiaotong University: Chongqing, China, 2023.
44. *JTG E20-2011*; Test Procedures for Asphalt and Asphalt Mixtures for Highway Engineering. People's Transportation Publishing House: Beijing, China, 2011.
45. *GB/T 16777-2008*; Test Methods for Building Waterproofing Coatings. China Quality Inspection Press: Beijing, China, 2008.

gels

Article

Study on the Adaptability of FBG Sensors Encapsulated in CNT-Modified Gel Material for Asphalt Pavement

Tengteng Guo [1,2,3,4], Xu Guo [1], Yuanzhao Chen [1,2,3,4,*], Chenze Fang [1,2,3,4], Jingyu Yang [1,2,3,4], Zhenxia Li [1,2,3,4], Jiajie Feng [1], Jiahua Kong [1], Haijun Chen [1,2,3,4], Chaohui Wang [5], Qian Chen [5] and Jiachen Wang [6]

1 School of Civil Engineering and Transportation, North China University of Water Resources and Electric Power, Zhengzhou 450045, China; guotth@ncwu.edu.cn (T.G.); 17538255803@163.com (X.G.); fangchenze@ncwu.edu.cn (C.F.); yangjingyu@ncwu.edu.cn (J.Y.); zhenxiali2009@ncwu.edu.cn (Z.L.); 18027459877@163.com (J.F.); 18539291281@163.com (J.K.); chenhaijun@ncwu.edu.cn (H.C.)

2 Henan Province Engineering Technology Research Center of Environment Friendly and High-Performance Pavement Materials, Zhengzhou 450045, China

3 Technology Innovation Center of Henan Transport Industry of Utilization of Solid Waste Resources in Traffic Engineering, North China University of Water Resources and Electric Power, Zhengzhou 450045, China

4 Henan Province University-Enterprise Research and Development Center for Green, Low-Carbon and High-Performance Road Materials, Zhengzhou 450045, China

5 School of Highway, Chang'an University, Xi'an 710064, China; wchh0205@chd.edu.cn (C.W.); chenqian@chd.edu.cn (Q.C.)

6 Department of Electrical Engineering, College of Science and Technology, University of Nottingham Ningbo China, Ningbo 315100, China; ssyjw19@nottingham.edu.cn

* Correspondence: cyz740513@ncwu.edu.cn; Tel.: +86-13608696351; Fax: +86-0371-69127209

Abstract: To prolong the service life of asphalt pavement and reduce its maintenance cost, a fiber Bragg grating (FBG) sensor encapsulated in carboxylated carbon nanotube (CNT-COOH)-modified gel material suitable for strain monitoring of asphalt pavement was developed. Through tensile and bending tests, the effects of carboxylated carbon nanotubes on the mechanical properties of gel materials under different dosages were evaluated and the optimal dosage of carbon nanotubes was determined. Infrared spectrometer and scanning electron microscopy were used to compare and analyze the infrared spectra and microstructure of carbon nanotubes before and after carboxyl functionalization and modified gel materials. The results show that the incorporation of CNTs-COOH increased the tensile strength, elongation at break, and tensile modulus of the gel material by 36.2%, 47%, and 17.2%, respectively, and increased the flexural strength, flexural modulus, and flexural strain by 89.7%, 7.5%, and 63.8%, respectively. Through infrared spectrum analysis, it was determined that carboxyl (COOH) and hydroxyl (OH) were successfully introduced on the surface of carbon nanotubes. By analyzing the microstructure, it can be seen that the carboxyl functionalization of CNTs improved the agglomeration of carbon nanotubes. The tensile section of the modified gel material is rougher than that of the pure epoxy resin, showing obvious plastic deformation, and the toughness is improved. According to the data from the calibration experiment, the strain and temperature sensitivity coefficients of the packaged sensor are 1.9864 pm/μm and 0.0383 nm/°C, respectively, which are 1.63 times and 3.61 times higher than those of the bare fiber grating. The results of an applicability study show that the internal structure strain of asphalt rutting specimen changed linearly with the external static load, and the fitting sensitivity is 0.0286 με/N. Combined with ANSYS finite element analysis, it is verified that the simulation analysis results are close to the measured data, which verifies the effectiveness and monitoring accuracy of the sensor. The dynamic load test results reflect the internal strain change trend of asphalt mixture under external rutting load, confirming that the encapsulated FBG sensor is suitable for the long-term monitoring of asphalt pavement strain.

https://doi.org/10.3390/gels11080590

Keywords: asphalt pavement; CNT-modified gel material; fiber grating sensor; calibration test; performance study

1. Introduction

Asphalt pavement is the main structure type of domestic expressways. Because of its unique engineering advantages, it is very important in expressway construction [1]. Compared with other forms of roads, asphalt pavement has the advantages of convenient maintenance, shock absorption and noise reduction, rapid construction, and recycling. However, due to the influence of various unfavorable factors in the use of asphalt pavement, rutting, subsidence, cracks, and other diseases often occur [2]. Traditional pavement monitoring methods have problems such as low accuracy, low frequency, and strong destructiveness. It is difficult to achieve long-term and continuous monitoring [3], which makes it difficult to detect and deal with pavement diseases in time. Fiber grating sensors show great potential in the monitoring of asphalt pavement due to their advantages of anti-electromagnetic interference, corrosion resistance, and high sensitivity [4], which can provide accurate data support for pavement health assessment. However, in the actual use process, fiber Bragg grating (FBG) sensors have problems such as large differences in modulus from the pavement structure and weak shear resistance, which can easily cause measurement errors or sensor damage. Therefore, it is of great significance to use appropriate packaging materials to protect FBG sensors [5].

FBG sensors have shown superior performance in the field of structural monitoring, so they have been widely used in the field of civil engineering. Meng S et al. [6] proposed an implantable cantilever sensing beam based on FBG to monitor the permanent deformation of subgrade in seasonally frozen areas under vehicle load and freeze–thaw cycles, and verified its feasibility through three years of field tests. Liu et al. [7] tested the strain response of four kinds of base asphalt pavement under a 100 kN dynamic load based on FBG sensors and revealed the compression–tension–compression cycle in the surface layer and the tensile strain characteristics of the base layer. They found that reducing the stiffness of the cement stabilized the base layer and maintaining modulus continuity can optimize the strain distribution and improve the bearing capacity of pavement. Liao et al. [8,9] established a moving load identification model of asphalt pavement by combining the measured data of FBG sensors and a BP neural network, and verified the accuracy of this method for vehicle load identification by finite element simulation. Li Jianxin et al. [10] established a monitoring method for concrete crack propagation through FBG sensors and a plastic damage model, verified the quantitative relationship between damage factor and crack width, and provided an effective means for structural damage assessment. In summary, FBG sensors have been successfully applied to measure and monitor many factors, such as pavement strain, temperature, deformation, and damage, achieving significant results. However, there are still challenges in the embedding process, survival rate, accuracy, data demodulation technology, and other aspects of FBG sensors.

In order to ensure that the sensor is not damaged during the normal use of asphalt pavement, there are higher requirements for the strength, corrosion resistance, high temperature resistance, and wear resistance of the packaging material. Shi Q.Q. et al. [11–13] prepared highly oriented CNT/EP composites by a continuous impregnation stretching and step pressing process. The tensile strength and toughness of the CNT/EP composites were 3.5 GPa and 80.2 J cm^{-3}, respectively, which are better than those of traditional CNT and carbon fiber-reinforced composites. Song X. et al. [14] modified carbon nanotubes (CNTs) on electrospun PCL nanofibers by ultrasonic assistance to construct a flexible interwoven structure of CF/EP laminates. After curing, PCL phase separation caused the CNTs to disperse uniformly while maintaining the glass transition temperature of the epoxy resin. Chen et al. [15] used amino-modified multi-walled carbon nanotubes and a low concentration of polyetherimide to synergistically toughen epoxy resin. After testing, the fracture toughness, impact strength, and bending strength of epoxy resin were significantly improved under the synergistic effect. Xin et al. [16–18] prepared epoxy resin composites using aligned multi-walled carbon nanotubes. The effects of different carbon nanotube contents on the mechanical, electrical, morphological, and fatigue properties of CNT/EP composites were studied, and the excellent mechanical durability of this composite was verified. Epoxy resin (EP) has excellent properties, such as high adhesion, temperature resistance, corrosion resistance, and processability after curing [19], but there are high brittleness defects. Carbon nanotubes (CNTs) are ideal reinforcement materials due to their unique hollow structure and high aspect ratio, high strength and high modulus [20]. In this paper, CNT-reinforced EP composites were selected as the packaging substrate for fiber Bragg grating (FBG) sensors. Zhong et al. [21] used three kinds of pressure-sensitive packaging materials, including polycarbonate, polyethylene, and epoxy resin. The pressure sensitivity is about 200 times higher than that of bare fiber grating, and the mechanical strength is high. Huang et al. [22] manufactured all-silicon sensors, using silicon glass for the substrate and packaging materials. The sensing principle and performance test of the tilt sensor are described in detail. The test results show that the packaged FBG has good packaging quality and sensing performance. Luo et al. [23] used epoxy resin as the adhesive material for sensor packaging and found that the smaller the thermal expansion coefficient of the packaging adhesive material, the smaller the influence on the output performance of the sensor in high-temperature environments.

In summary, FBG sensors provide a new technical means for asphalt pavement health monitoring by virtue of their anti-electromagnetic interference, corrosion resistance, high sensitivity, and other characteristics. However, they still face problems, such as mismatch with structural modulus and weak shear resistance in pavement applications, which can easily lead to measurement errors or sensor damage. EP has become a potential choice for FBG packaging materials due to its excellent adhesion, high temperature resistance, and chemical corrosion resistance, but its inherent brittleness limits its application in complex environments. CNTs can effectively enhance the mechanical properties of EP due to their high stiffness, high strength, and high aspect ratio. Therefore, the use of CNT/EP composites to encapsulate FBG sensors can not only effectively alleviate the stress concentration problem caused by the difference in modulus between the sensor and the pavement but can also enhance its shear resistance, fatigue resistance, and environmental adaptability, thereby improving the survival rate and monitoring reliability of the sensor in the high-temperature, high-load, and complex mechanical environments of asphalt pavement.

2. Results and Discussion

2.1. Analysis of Mechanical Properties

2.1.1. Tensile Properties Analysis

Figure 1a–c present the results of the tensile property tests of the composites.

It can be seen in the figure that under the condition of the same amount of epoxy resin, curing agent, and accelerator, the tensile strength, tensile modulus, and elongation at break of carboxylated carbon nanotubes/epoxy resin composites were improved by adding different amounts of carboxylated carbon nanotubes to the epoxy resin matrix. When the content of carboxylated carbon nanotubes was 0.3 wt%, the tensile strength and elongation at break of the composites reached 31.54 MPa and 3.87%, which were 36.2%

and 47% higher than those of the pure epoxy resin, respectively. The tensile modulus of carboxylated carbon nanotubes/epoxy resin composites reached a maximum of 2794.5 MPa when the content of carbon nanotubes was 0.5 wt%, which was 17.2% higher than that without carbon nanotubes. It can be seen that with the change in the amount of carbon nanotubes added, the tensile strength, tensile modulus, and elongation at break of the composites show a trend of increasing first and then decreasing.

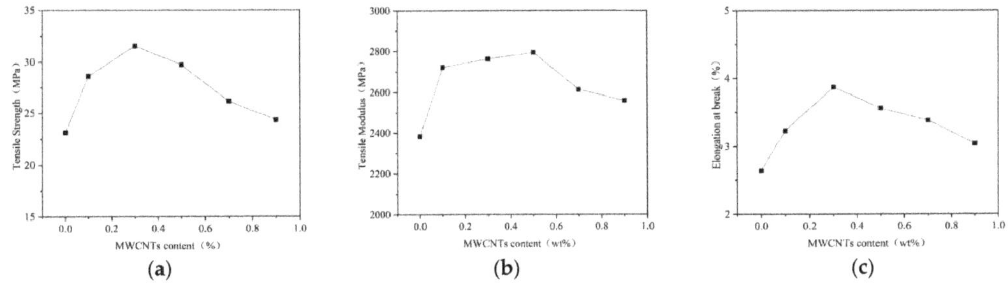

Figure 1. Tensile properties test results of composite materials. (**a**) Tensile strength of composite materials. (**b**) Tensile modulus of composites. (**c**) Fracture elongation of composite materials.

This phenomenon shows that when an appropriate amount of carbon nanotubes is added to epoxy resin, they can be uniformly dispersed throughout the material system. However, as the carbon nanotube content further increases beyond the critical value, the carbon nanotubes cannot continue to maintain a good dispersion state, resulting in uneven internal structure of the composite material, making it more prone to damage.

2.1.2. Bending Performance Analysis

Figure 2a–c show the results of composite materials in bending tests.

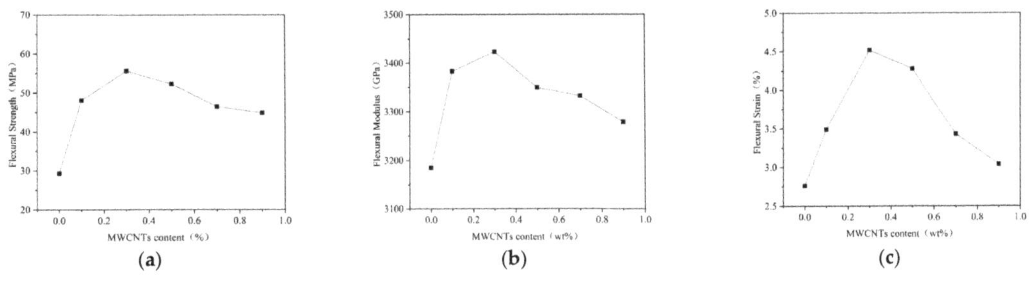

Figure 2. Bending test results of composite materials. (**a**) Bending strength of composite materials. (**b**) Bending modulus of composite materials. (**c**) Bending strain of composite materials.

It can be seen that the addition of carbon nanotubes (CNTs) to epoxy resin matrix can significantly improve the flexural properties of composites. When the CNT content was 0.3 wt%, the flexural strength (55.61 MPa), flexural modulus (3423.6 MPa), and flexural strain (4.52%) of the carboxylated CNT/epoxy resin composites reached the maximum values, which were 89.7%, 7.5%, and 63.8% higher than those of pure epoxy resin, respectively. The improvement in the flexural strength and flexural strain was particularly significant. When the CNT content exceeded 0.3 wt%, the flexural properties of the composites began to decrease, indicating that the CNTs agglomerated, affecting the properties.

Tensile and flexural properties tests showed that the addition of 0.3 wt% CNT optimized the mechanical properties of epoxy resin composites. Further increases in CNT content will lead to a decrease in performance. It is confirmed that 0.3 wt% is the best addition ratio, which can not only give full play to the enhancement effect of CNTs but can also avoid the problem of agglomeration and uneven dispersion caused by excessive addition.

2.2. Infrared Spectrum Analysis of Carboxylated Carbon Nanotubes

The multi-walled carbon nanotubes and carboxylated multi-walled carbon nanotubes were studied by a wavenumber–transmittance test. The data obtained from the test were summarized into the infrared spectrum, and then the characteristic peaks were compared and analyzed. The test results are shown in Figure 3.

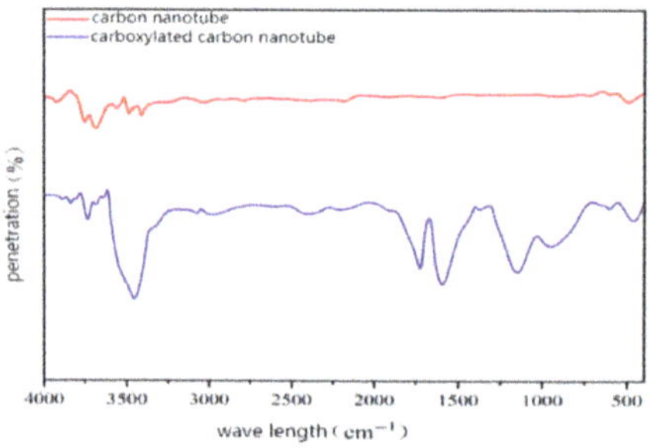

Figure 3. Infrared spectra of carbon nanotubes before and after modification.

It can be seen in Figure 3 that the infrared spectrum of pure carbon nanotubes shows a stretching vibration peak of the O-H bond in the range of 3500 cm^{-1} to 3700 cm^{-1}. This may be due to the fact that the surface of untreated carbon nanotubes contains trace impurities containing O-H groups or has adsorbed water from the air. Comparing the infrared spectra of carbon nanotubes before and after carboxylation, new absorption peaks were observed near 1200 cm^{-1}, 1600 cm^{-1}, and 1700 cm^{-1}. These characteristic peaks correspond to the stretching vibration of the C-O bond, the bending vibration of the O-H bond, and the stretching vibration of the C=O bond in the carboxyl group, respectively, which indicates that the carboxyl (COOH) group is formed on the surface of the carbon nanotubes after carboxylation treatment. In addition, an obvious absorption peak was observed at about 3450 cm^{-1}, where the absorption peak is related to the stretching vibration of the O-H bond, indicating the presence of hydroxyl (OH) or water molecules on the surface. These new chemical groups change the surface properties of carbon nanotubes, enabling them to form stronger chemical bonding or physical adsorption with epoxy resin, thereby improving the interfacial bonding strength between carbon nanotubes and epoxy resin.

2.3. SEM Micro-Morphology Characterization Analysis

2.3.1. Morphology Characterization Analysis of Carbon Nanotubes Before and After Modification

Figures 4 and 5 present SEM photos of the untreated multi-walled carbon nanotubes and carboxylated multi-walled carbon nanotubes, magnified 200,000 times.

Scanning electron microscopy (SEM) observations showed that the surface of the unmodified carbon nanotubes was smooth and the tube wall structure was complete and tightly entangled into a network structure. The surface of the carboxylated carbon nanotubes was fuzzy and rough, the entanglement was reduced, and the arrangement was loose. This was due to the surface defects induced by mixed acid treatment, which provided grafting sites for -COOH/-OH groups. The introduction of surface groups enhances the polarity of carbon nanotubes and effectively weakens the interactions between the tubes through electrostatic repulsion and hydrogen bonding, thereby reducing entanglement. This indicates that carboxylation treatment can significantly reduce the agglomeration tendency of carbon nanotubes, improve their dispersion, and provide higher surface activity.

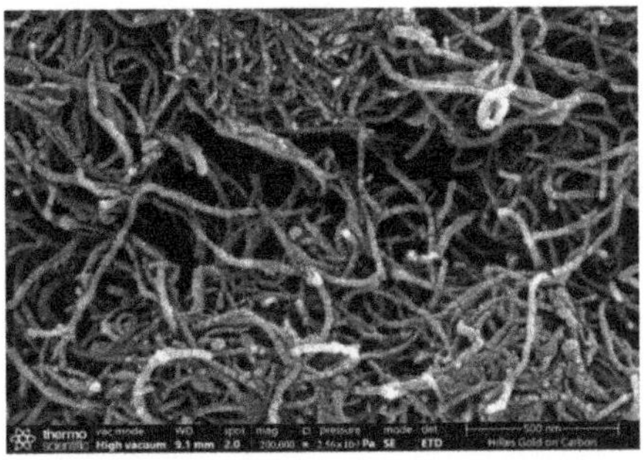

Figure 4. Unprocessed carbon nanotubes, magnified 200,000 times.

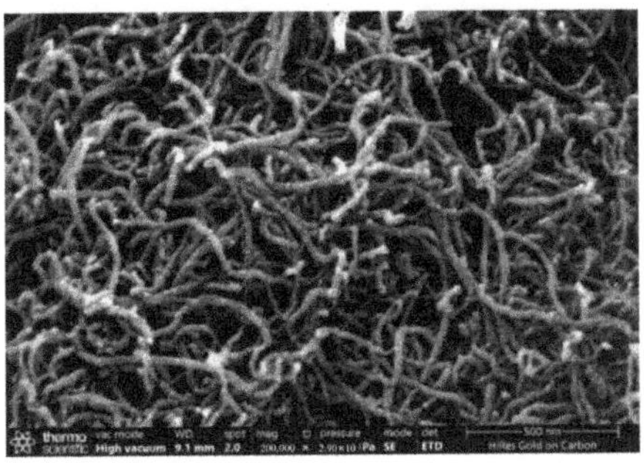

Figure 5. Carboxylated carbon nanotubes, magnified 200,000 times.

2.3.2. Analysis of Tensile Fracture Surface Morphology of Composites

Figures 6 and 7 present SEM diagrams of the tensile fracture surfaces of pure epoxy resin and carboxylated carbon nanotube/epoxy resin composites at the optimum content.

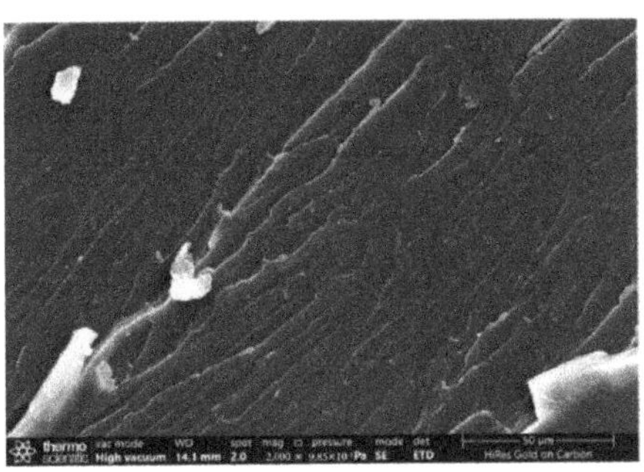

Figure 6. Tensile fracture surface of pure epoxy resin.

According to the observation results of scanning electron microscopy shown in Figure 6, at magnification of 2000 times, the tensile fracture surface of the pure epoxy resin shows a typical brittle fracture morphology. The fracture surface is relatively smooth and flat, the crack propagation path shows an obvious linear arrangement, and there are fewer crack branches. This morphological feature shows that under the tensile load, the microcracks inside the pure epoxy resin expand rapidly and connect with each other, and sudden fracture occurs almost without an obvious plastic deformation stage.

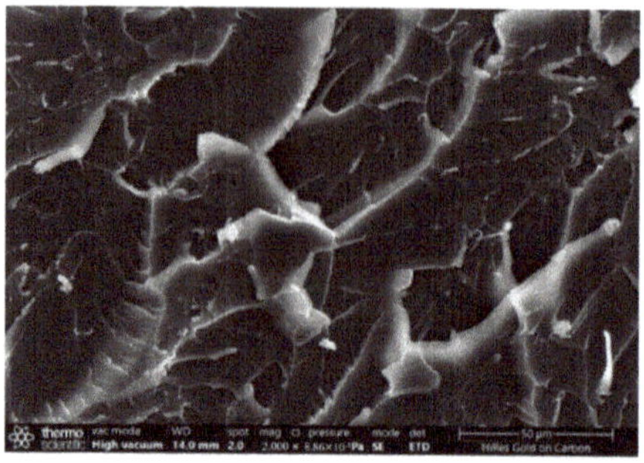

Figure 7. Tensile fracture surface of composite materials.

In contrast, as shown in Figure 7, at the same magnification, the tensile fracture surface of the composite material is rougher, and there are a large number of uneven tearing and plastic deformation traces. At the same time, the crack propagation path is tortuous and complex, and there are secondary cracks with radial distribution. These phenomena indicate that the composite material undergoes an obvious plastic deformation stage before fracture. This change is likely due to the introduction of carbon nanotubes, which leads to the effective transmission and dispersion of external stress. When the epoxy resin matrix initially cracks under the action of external force, CNTs, as a nano-scale reinforcing material, can hinder the direct propagation of cracks, forcing cracks to deflect or bifurcate, thereby extending the crack propagation path. This indicates that the addition of carbon nanotubes can not only effectively bear the external applied force but can also absorb the energy in the fracture process, thus significantly improving the tensile properties and toughness of the composites.

2.4. Calibration Test Analysis

2.4.1. Analysis of Strain Calibration Test

Since the measured experimental data are discrete, the least squares fitting method was used to fit the data. The fitting curves are shown in Figure 8a–c, including the relationship between load and micro-strain, the relationship between load and central wavelength, and the relationship between micro-strain and wavelength change.

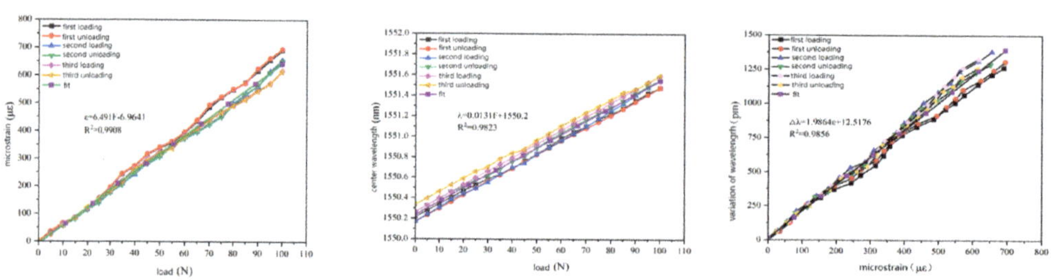

(a) (b) (c)

Figure 8. Strain calibration test results. (**a**) The relationship between load and micro-strain. (**b**) The relationship between load and center wavelength. (**c**) The relationship between micro-strain and wavelength change.

It can be seen in Figure 8 that the fitted relationships between load and micro-strain, load and center wavelength, micro-strain and wavelength change are 6.494 μm/N, 0.0131 nm/N, and 1.9864 pm/μm, respectively. The correlation coefficient exceeds 0.98. This indicates that the packaging material exhibits good elastic behavior, good stability, and repeatability during loading and unloading. By analyzing the three loading and unloading processes, it can be concluded that during the initial loading and unloading process, the change in the micro-strain of the packaging material is not completely linear, and there may be some residual strains. However, as the number of loading and unloading steps increases, the behavior of the packaging material becomes gradually stable.

As presented in Section 2.3, the theoretical value of the axial strain sensitivity coefficient of the bare fiber is 1.22 pm/μm. The strain sensitivity coefficient of the packaged FBG sensor reaches 1.9864 pm/μm. This means that the strain sensitivity of the encapsulated sensor is about 1.63 times higher than that of the bare fiber, significantly enhancing the sensitivity of strain monitoring.

2.4.2. Temperature Calibration Test Analysis

The least square method was used to fit the calibration test data of three heating and cooling cycles, and the fitting curve of the center wavelength of the sensor with the change of temperature was obtained, as shown in Figure 9.

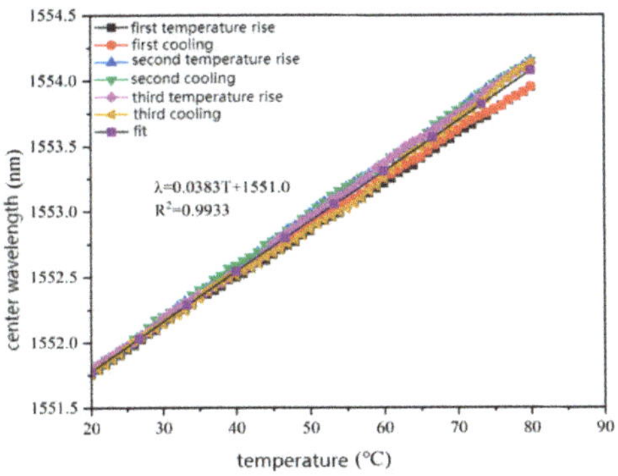

Figure 9. The relationship between temperature and central wavelength.

It can be seen in Figure 9 that the encapsulation of fiber grating by carboxylated carbon nanotube/epoxy resin composite material will not destroy the temperature sensing characteristics of the sensor. The encapsulated sensor shows good thermal stability and repeatability after multiple heating and cooling cycles. This is suitable for the application scenario of asphalt pavement, which requires long-term temperature monitoring. After multiple temperature cycles, the fitted correlation coefficient exceeded 0.99, indicating that the sensor has good linearity. The temperature sensitivity of the sensor was 0.0383 nm/°C, which is 3.61 times higher than the theoretical temperature sensitivity coefficient of bare fiber of 10.6 pm/°C, calculated in the second chapter. In the temperature cycle test of 20 °C → 80 °C → 20 °C, the change in the center wavelength of the sensor was strictly linear with the temperature (R2 > 0.99). The temperature sensitivity was 0.0383 nm/°C, and the three cycle data overlapped, with no thermal hysteresis phenomenon and stable performance in a high-temperature environment.

2.5. Applicability Analysis of the Sensor

2.5.1. Static Load Test Analysis

In the static load test of the rutting specimen, according to the change in the central wavelength, the strain change in the corresponding load at the sensor embedding position was calculated by the fitting curve formula shown in Figure 10. The relationship curve between the external load and the calculated strain was obtained by the least square fitting of the three loading and unloading cycle data, as shown in Figure 10.

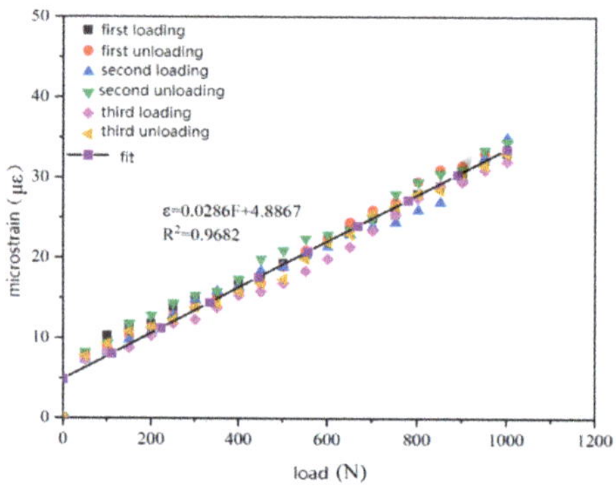

Figure 10. Relationship between load and strain in static load test.

According to the fitting results in the Figure 10, it can be seen that there is a linear relationship between the strain change in the internal structure of the asphalt concrete rut specimen detected by the FBG sensor and the change in the external static load. With the adjustment of the applied static load, the internal strain monitored by the sensor shows a linear change trend accordingly. The load/shear force direction indirectly changes the sensitivity of the sensor by affecting the stress distribution of the packaging material, the interface bonding state, and the enhancement efficiency of CNTs. The static load test verified that the strain transfer efficiency was high under vertical load. The horizontal shear load may lead to a decrease in sensitivity due to interface defects.

Based on the results of the static load test, it can be seen that the linear fitting sensitivity of the applied external static load and the internal structural strain of the rutting specimen monitored by the fiber Bragg grating demodulator was 0.0286 με/N, and the correlation coefficient was R2 = 0.9682, indicating that the linear relationship is good. With the increase in external load, the strain of the sensor buried position also increased, which can well reflect the strain change inside the asphalt mixture rutting specimen.

2.5.2. ANSYS Finite Element Analysis

(1) Build models and set attributes

A model was established according to the actual size of the specimen. The size of the rutting specimen model was 300 mm × 300 mm × 50 mm, and the size of the sensor model was 10 mm × 10 mm × 100 mm. Because only the analysis and calculation of strain were carried out, only the elastic modulus and Poisson's ratio of the material were defined. According to the specification requirements, the elastic modulus of AC-13 asphalt mixture material is 1400 MPa, and the Poisson's ratio is 0.25; the elastic modulus of carbon nanotube/epoxy resin composites is 2800 MPa, and the Poisson's ratio is 0.35.

(2) Meshing and adding load

The rut specimen model was meshed by SOLID186 ten-node tetrahedron, and the unit size was set to 5 mm. The sensor model was meshed by SOLID186 twenty-node hexahedron. In order to make the calculation result more accurate, the sensor model mesh was encrypted, and the unit size was 1 mm. The finite element model is shown in Figures 11 and 12. Fixed loads were added to the four sides of the model and the bottom surface. The static load was arranged at the center of the upper surface of the model as a circular uniform load with a diameter of 150 mm.

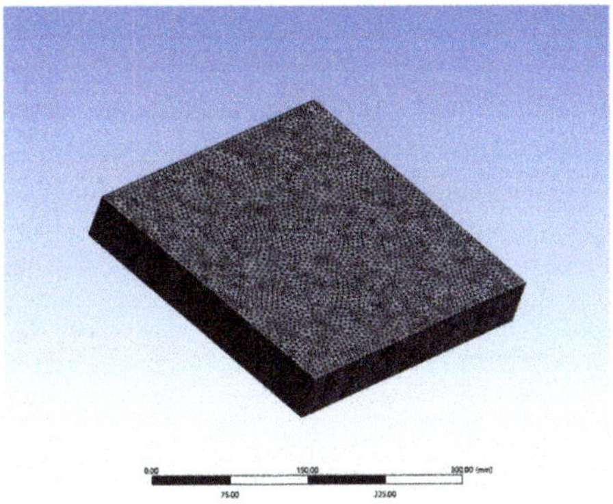

Figure 11. Rutting specimen model.

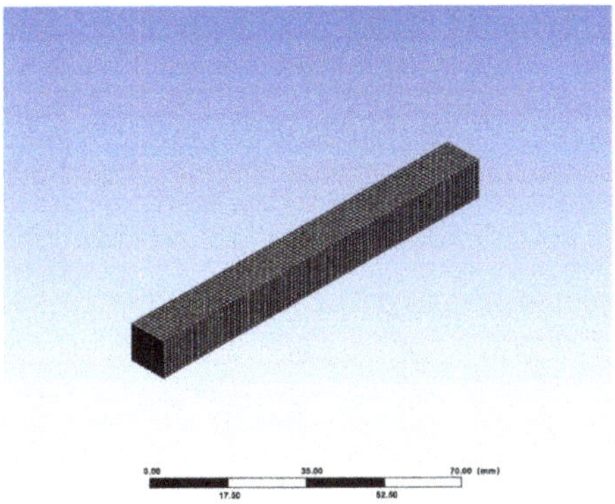

Figure 12. Sensor model.

(3) Solution analysis

The circular uniform load was added to the upper surface of the asphalt mixture rutting test piece, the load of each stage was set to 49.98 N, and the load was applied cumulatively over 20 cycles. A strain cloud diagram was obtained after the finite element calculation, as shown in Figure 13.

Origin 2021 software was used to draw a scatter plot of the obtained data, and the data were fitted by the least squares method to obtain the fitting curve of the load and strain in ANSYS finite element simulation analysis, as shown in Figure 14.

It can be seen in Figure 14 that the slope between the strain and load of the asphalt mixture rutting specimen simulated by finite element analysis was 0.0336 $\mu\varepsilon/N$ under static load, and the correlation coefficient exceeded 0.99. However, compared with the slope of the fitting curve of 0.0286 $\mu\varepsilon/N$ in the static load test, there is a certain deviation. Therefore, the strain sensing coefficient θ was introduced, and $\theta = 0.85$ was obtained by comparing the measured value with the theoretical value. This deviation may be caused by many factors. Firstly, during the fabrication of the sensor, the surface of the fiber grating may not have been completely clean, resulting in insufficient curing and bonding with the epoxy resin matrix, leading to slight slip between the two. Secondly, the epoxy resin and curing agent inevitably produced bubbles during the heating and curing process. Although the defoamer can inhibit the formation of bubbles, there is still a small amount of residue. In addition, in the ANSYS finite element simulation, it was assumed that the sensor and the asphalt mixture were completely bonded, and there may have been a small gap between the two in the actual situation. These factors may have led to errors in the monitoring process of the sensor, which in turn affected the sensitivity of the sensor. Under the action of external load, the stress distribution of the high-aspect-ratio device is more uniform along the length direction, which can reduce the end effect and improve the strain transfer efficiency. The low-aspect-ratio device has relatively stronger compressive and shear resistance, and is more suitable for high-stress areas.

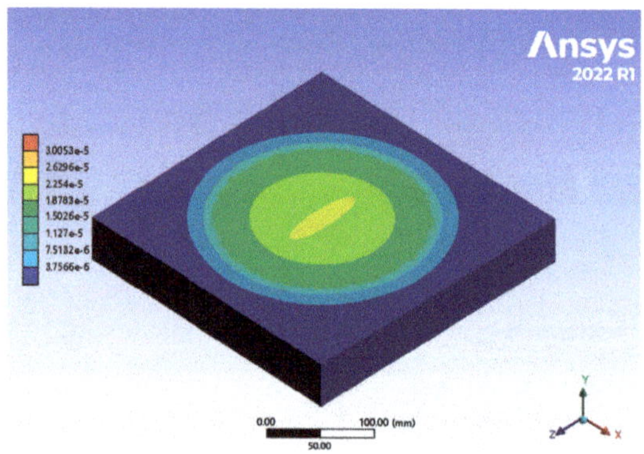

Figure 13. Strain distribution cloud map.

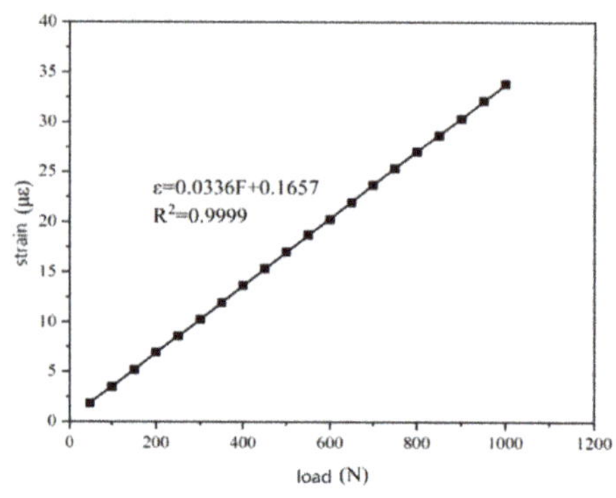

Figure 14. The relationship between load and strain.

Although there was a certain error between the finite element simulation and the actual test, the response trends of the two were basically the same, which verifies the effectiveness of the sensor and the accuracy of the monitoring process. In general, the actual test results can better reflect the strain response law of asphalt mixture under static load, and the finite element simulation further verifies the reliability of sensor detection. Although there were problems such as fiber grating surface cleanliness, bubble residue during epoxy resin curing, and imperfect interface bonding between the sensor and the asphalt mixture, these factors did not significantly affect the overall performance of the sensor.

2.5.3. Dynamic Load Test Analysis

A dynamic load rutting test was used to simulate the dynamic load of asphalt pavement with driving vehicles, and the performance of the sensor under dynamic load was evaluated. The rutting test was carried out for 1 h, and the internal strain of the specimen under the action of dynamic load changed. According to the collected data, the waveform is shown in Figure 15.

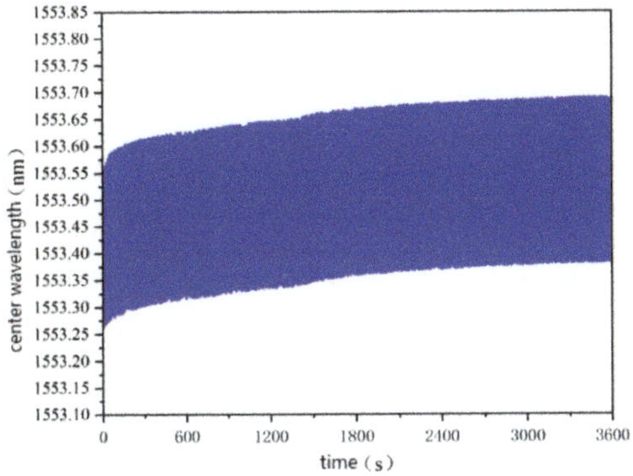

Figure 15. Diagram of the sensor wavelength changes in the rutting test.

In the image, it can be seen that after the 1h rutting dynamic load test, the central wavelength change range of the sensor was about 430 pm. The internal strain of the corresponding asphalt concrete structure was calculated by the fitting curve formula in Figure 14. It was about 210 με.

Because of the large amount of data, it is difficult to see the change trend, so the difference between the peak value and the initial wavelength was used for plotting, and the relationship curve between the difference and the time change is shown in Figure 11.

It can be seen in Figure 16 that the relationship between the change in the center wavelength of the sensor and the time in the rutting test follows a cubic polynomial change rule. It can be observed that the coefficient of the monomial is positive, which indicates that the wavelength variation λ shows an increasing trend with the increase in the test time t in the initial stage, and there is an obvious growth period. However, due to the negative coefficient of the quadratic term, the growth rate of the wavelength variation gradually slows down over time, eventually leveling off. The coefficient of the cubic term is very small, and the impact on the overall trend can be ignored.

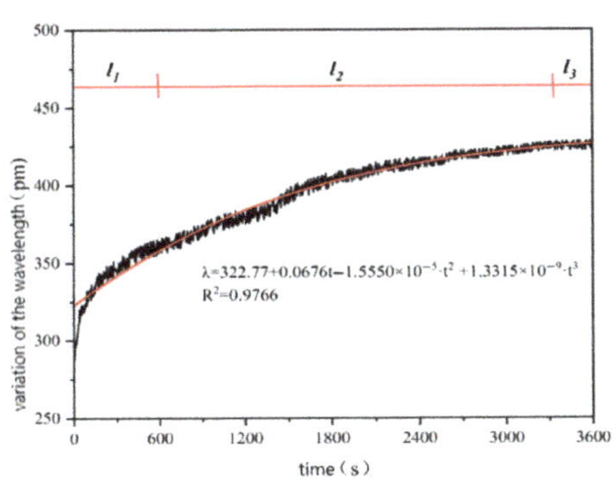

Figure 16. The relationship between wavelength change and time.

Therefore, Figure 16 is roughly divided into three stages. In the l_1 (0–600 s) stage, the central wavelength changes significantly and the increase is large. Subsequently, with the progress of the rutting test, it can be seen that the change in the center wavelength of the sensor in the l_2 (600–3300 s) stage shows a steady upward trend, and the wavelength change in the l_3 (3300–3600 s) stage gradually levels off, with a small increase, almost reaching a stable state, indicating that the wavelength change has basically stagnated and there is no obvious fluctuation. The sensor can still work stably under multi-directional complex load environment and meet the long-term monitoring requirements of asphalt pavement, but the packaging process needs to be optimized to reduce the direction dependence.

The change trend of the central wavelength of these three stages reflects the internal strain change trend of asphalt concrete under the action of external rutting load, which is of great significance for studying the internal structure response law of asphalt concrete. After an hour-long rutting test, the sensor showed good working performance and no damage, meeting the requirements of long-term monitoring of asphalt pavement strain. The results show that the strain monitored by the sensor was highly linear with the load, and the fitting sensitivity was 0.0286 με/N (R2 = 0.9682). In the dynamic load test of simulated vehicle wheel load (70 MPa of tire pressure, 42 times/min rolling) for 1 h, the center wavelength variation range was only 430 pm (corresponding to strain 210 με), and there was no abnormal fluctuation or signal interruption, indicating that the stability under load was good.

3. Conclusions

(1) When the content of carboxylated carbon nanotubes (CNTs) in epoxy resin (EP) was 0.3 wt%, the tensile and flexural properties of CNT/EP composites were optimal. When the content exceeded this amount, the performance showed a downward trend, indicating that 0.3 wt% is the best content. Infrared spectroscopy confirmed that carboxyl groups were successfully grafted on the surface of CNTs by the mixed acid reflux method, and the characteristic absorption peaks were located at 1200 cm^{-1}, 1600 cm^{-1}, 1700 cm^{-1}, and 3450 cm^{-1}, respectively. This modification significantly improved the dispersion and interfacial bonding strength of CNTs in EP.

(2) According to scanning electron microscopy analysis, after carboxylation treatment, the agglomeration of carbon nanotubes was significantly reduced, the size of the aggregates was significantly reduced, the degree of entanglement was reduced, the arrangement between carbon nanotubes was relatively loose, and the dispersion was improved. Comparative analysis of the microstructure of the tensile fracture surface of the material was carried out. The tensile fracture surface of the composite material was rougher, and there was a large number of uneven tears and plastic deformation traces. The crack propagation path was tortuous and complex, and radial secondary cracks appeared. This indicates that the addition of carbon nanotubes can effectively bear the external applied force, absorb the energy in the fracture process, and enhance the toughness of the material.

(3) Through the calibration test of the sensor, it can be concluded that the packaging material has good elastic behavior, good stability, and repeatability when subjected to external load and temperature changes. The strain sensitivity coefficient of the packaged FBG sensor reached 1.9864 pm/μm, which is about 1.63 times higher than that of the bare fiber. The temperature sensitivity of the sensor was 0.0383 nm/°C, which is an increase of 3.61-fold.

(4) According to the analysis of the applicability of the sensor, under a certain amount of static load, the internal strain of the asphalt concrete specimen monitored by the sensor showed a corresponding linear change trend. The response trends of finite

element simulation and the static load test were basically the same, verifying the effectiveness of the sensor and the accuracy of the monitoring process. Under the action of simulated wheel load, the relationship between the change in the center wavelength of the sensor and the time shows a cubic polynomial change rule, reflecting the internal strain change trend of asphalt concrete under the conditions of external wheel load.

4. Materials and Methods

4.1. Carbon Nanotubes

In this paper, carbon nanotubes were selected as multi-walled carbon nanotubes (MWCNTs) produced by Suzhou Carbonfeng Graphene Technology Co., Ltd. (Suzhou, China). The carbon nanotubes have high purity, a large aspect ratio, and a high specific surface area, and the comprehensive advantages are obvious. Multi-walled carbon nanotubes with a purity of >95 wt%, an inner diameter of 3–5 nm, an outer diameter of 8–15 nm, and a length of 3–12 μm were used.

4.2. Epoxy Resin

The gel material used in this paper was bisphenol A epoxy resin, which is a widely used high-performance thermosetting gel material. It is widely used because of its excellent mechanical properties, good adhesion, and chemical resistance. In order to achieve effective curing of epoxy resin, methyl tetrahydrophthalic anhydride (MeTHPA) was selected as the curing agent. MeTHPA is an efficient anhydride curing agent. Epoxy resin cured by anhydride curing agent usually shows high temperature resistance and mechanical properties, which is more suitable for the high-temperature environment of the asphalt pavement construction process. However, the reaction rate of MeTHPA at lower temperatures is slow, which prolongs the time required for curing and requires a higher curing temperature to complete the curing reaction. In order to solve this problem, 2,4,6-tris (dimethylaminomethyl) phenol (DMP-30) was added as an accelerator to accelerate the curing rate, allowing the curing process to occur at a relatively low temperature. In addition, defoamer, release agent, and acetone solution were also used in the experiment.

4.3. Fiber Grating

The bare fiber grating selected in this paper was produced by Jinan Dahui Photoelectric Technology Co., Ltd. (Jinan, China). It has a bare fiber grating center wavelength of 1550 ± 0.5 nm, reflectivity $\geq$90%, bandwidth $\leq$0.3 nm, and a grating area length of 10 mm.

Combined with the photosensitive characteristics of the fiber material and the sensing principle of the fiber grating, the theoretical value of the axial strain sensitivity coefficient of the quartz fiber was roughly calculated to be 1.22 pm/$\mu\varepsilon$, and the theoretical value of the temperature sensitivity coefficient was 10.6 pm/°C.

4.4. Preparation of Carboxylated Carbon Nanotubes

Due to the strong van der Waals force between carbon nanotubes, they tend to attract each other and gather together to form clusters or bundle structures, which are difficult to uniformly disperse in a polymer matrix. This agglomeration phenomenon causes the actual performance of the prepared carbon nanotube-modified gel material to fail to meet the theoretical expectations, and may even cause a small increase in strength or a decline in performance. Therefore, in this paper, the carboxyl functionalization of carbon nanotubes was carried out by the mixed acid reflux method. The modification process is shown in Figure 17. The specific steps are as follows:

(1) The mixed acid solution of concentrated sulfuric acid (H_2SO_4) and concentrated nitric acid (HNO_3) was prepared according to a volume ratio of 3:1.
(2) A certain amount of MWCNTs was placed in a clean beaker, and enough mixed acid solution was slowly added to ensure that all carbon nanotubes were completely immersed. A glass rod was used to gently stir the carbon nanotubes in the mixed acid along the wall of the beaker to initially break up the possible aggregates and ensure that the acid solution fully contacted the surface of the carbon nanotubes.
(3) The whole mixture was carefully transferred into a round-bottomed flask, and the temperature was controlled by a constant-temperature heating sleeve. The mixture was continuously heated and refluxed at 120 °C for 3 h until the carbon nanotubes were fully oxidized.
(4) After the reaction system was naturally cooled to room temperature, the reaction solution was diluted with deionized water to reduce the concentration of strong acid. The diluted solution was subjected to multiple suction filtration using a vacuum suction filtration device until a pure carboxylated carbon nanotube was obtained.
(5) In order to ensure that the residual acid was completely removed, the modified carbon nanotubes needed to be washed repeatedly with deionized water again until the carbon nanotubes were neutral. Then, the cleaned carboxylated carbon nanotubes were transferred to the preheated oven for drying treatment.

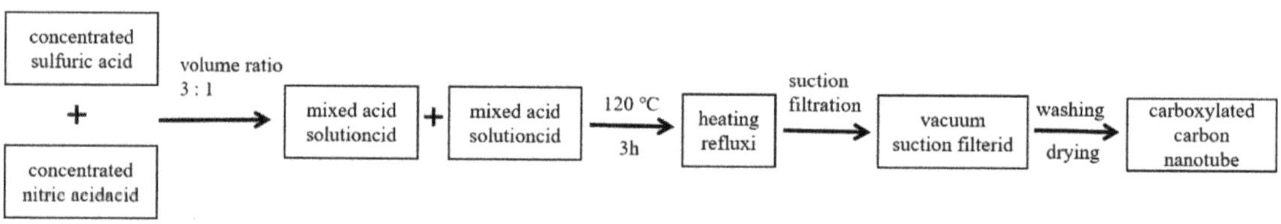

Figure 17. Flowchart of carboxylated carbon nanotubes by acid reflux.

4.5. Preparation of CNT-Modified Gel Materials

In order to achieve uniform dispersion of carbon nanotubes, the modified gel material was prepared by ultrasonic dispersion. The preparation process is shown in Figure 18.

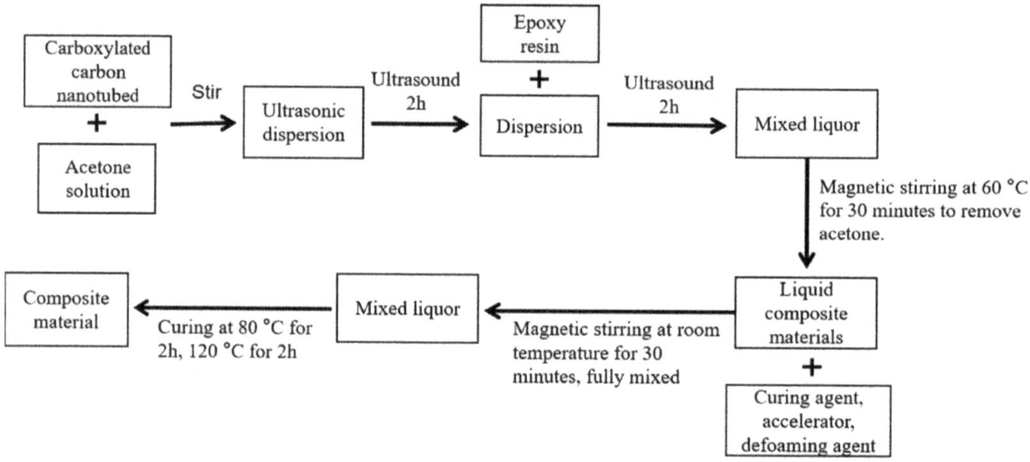

Figure 18. Preparation process of carboxylated carbon nanotubes/epoxy resin composites.

The specific steps were as follows:

(1) Carbon nanotubes with different mass percentages were added to acetone solution and treated with an ultrasonic disperser for 2 h.
(2) Epoxy resin was added to the dispersed solution according to the predetermined ratio, and ultrasonic dispersion was performed again for 2 h.
(3) The acetone solvent in the system was removed by magnetic stirring for 30 min at 60 °C. After the mixture cooled to room temperature, the anhydride curing agent was added at a mass ratio of 100:80 (epoxy resin/curing agent), and 0.5% defoaming agent and DMP-30 accelerator were added at the same time.
(4) Continuing magnetic stirring was performed for 30 min to ensure that all components were fully and evenly mixed. Then, the prepared mixed liquid was poured into the mold. According to the specific curing process, it was cured at 80 °C for 2 h, and then raised to 120 °C for 2 h to finally obtain the carboxylated carbon nanotube-reinforced epoxy resin composite sample.

4.6. Tensile and Bending Tests

In order to explore the optimal content of carboxylated multi-walled carbon nanotubes in epoxy resin, six groups of proportions were designed, and the contents of each group were 0.0%, 0.1%, 0.3%, 0.5%, 0.7%, and 0.9%, respectively. Tensile specimens and bending specimens of composite materials were prepared according to GB/T 1040.1-2018 [24] and GB/T 9341-2008 [25], respectively. The specimen is shown in Figures 19 and 20.

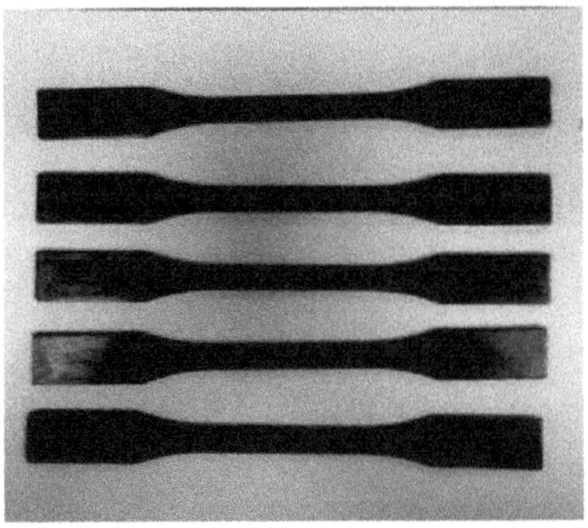

Figure 19. Carbon nanotubes/epoxy resin tensile specimens.

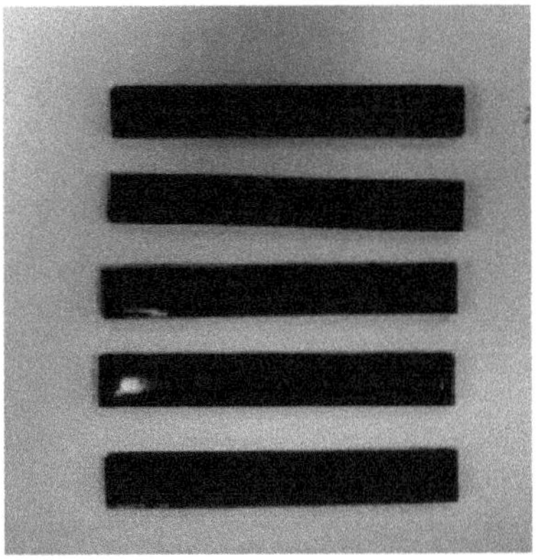

Figure 20. Carbon nanotube/epoxy resin bending specimens.

The tensile and bending properties of the prepared carboxylated carbon nanotube/epoxy resin composite specimens were tested by a microcomputer-controlled electronic universal testing machine (WDW-50C). When measuring the tensile strength, the loading rate was set to 10 mm/min, and then to 2 mm/min when measuring the elongation at break, tensile modulus, bending strength, bending modulus, and bending strain.

4.7. Fourier Transform Infrared Spectroscopy Test

In the experiment, FTIR was used to analyze the functional groups on the surface and edge of the prepared carboxylated carbon nanotubes, and the changes in the functional groups of the carbon nanotubes before and after modification were compared and observed. The instrument used a Thermo Nicolet IS5 infrared spectrometer from the Thermo Nicolet Technology Company (Waltham, MA, USA). The test range was 400 cm^{-1} to 4000 cm^{-1}, the resolution was 4 cm^{-1}, and the number of scans was 32.

4.8. Scanning Electron Microscope Test

The effect of the carboxylation process on the dispersion of carbon nanotubes was observed by comparing the original multi-walled carbon nanotubes without mixed acid treatment with the carboxylated multi-walled carbon nanotubes using the Zeiss 300 scanning electron microscope produced by German Carl's company (Wuppertal, Germany). A comparative SEM experiment was conducted on the tensile section of the tensile specimen of pure epoxy resin and the tensile specimen of the composite material with the best content of carboxylated carbon nanotubes to observe the microstructure of the fracture surface. In order to obtain a clearer image and reduce the charging effect, all samples were sprayed with gold.

4.9. Packaging of Fiber Grating Sensor

In order to improve the durability and protection of bare fiber in asphalt pavement construction, multi-level protection measures were taken for bare fiber gratings. The steps were as follows:

(1) Hytrel is a thermoplastic polyester elastomer with excellent wear resistance, chemical corrosion resistance and fatigue resistance. It can effectively protect optical fibers from the influence of the external environment and ensure that they are tightly and safely wrapped.
(2) The Hytrel loose sleeves with optical fibers are further encapsulated into armored sleeves with an inner diameter of 1.1 mm. The armored sleeves are equipped with a stainless steel protective sleeve layer, which can effectively protect the optical fiber from damage in the asphalt pavement.
(3) The FBG sensor is protected without affecting the accuracy of the sensor by encapsulating the fiber grating area with CNT/EP composites.

The sensor package structure was designed as a cuboid shape. In order to avoid the adverse effect of excessive cross-section size on the stress and strain distribution of the structure, the cross-section size was determined to be 10 mm × 10 mm × 100 mm. The sensor package structure is shown in Figure 21.

Using a special steel mold, the fiber grating with armored casing protection was inserted into the mold, and the carbon nanotube/epoxy resin composite mixture was injected. The gradient curing process (80 °C and 120 °C for 2 h each) was used to complete the curing. After demolding, the fiber grating was cured in a standard environment for 24 h. Finally, the fiber grating was fused with the jumper by a fiber splicer to prepare a complete FBG sensor. The fabricated FBG sensor is shown in Figure 22.

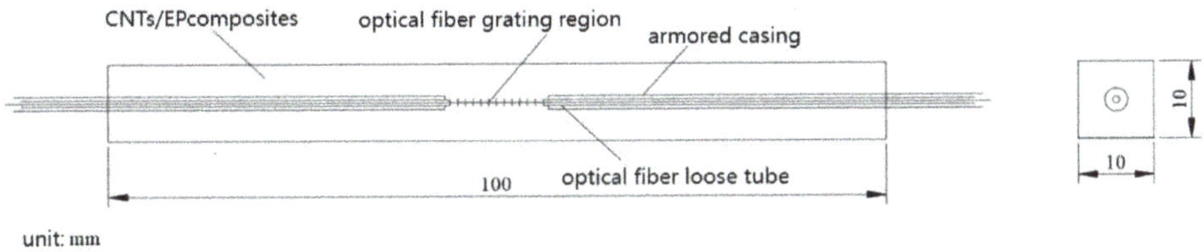

Figure 21. Package structure diagram of the FBG sensor.

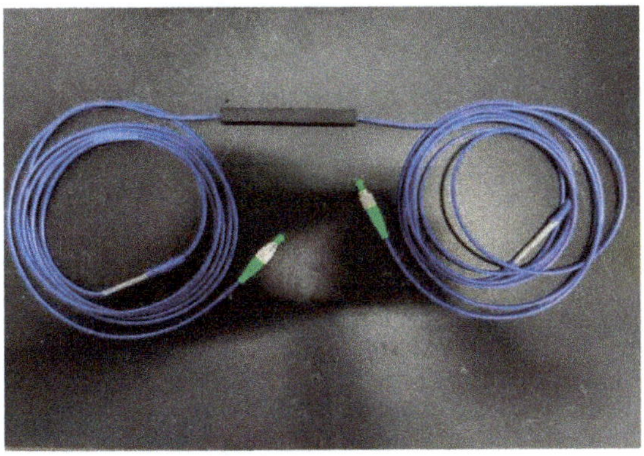

Figure 22. Physical diagram of the sensor.

4.10. Sensor Calibration Test

Although the developed package provides the necessary physical protection for the fiber grating, it changes the stress and temperature sensing characteristics of the grating, affecting its sensing performance. In order to ensure that the sensor can accurately measure strain in practical applications, it must be calibrated before use. Strain sensitivity calibration was performed at room temperature using a microcomputer-controlled electronic universal testing machine. Tensile force from 0 N to 100 N was applied to the sensor, and the center wavelength change was recorded every 5 N increase using the fiber grating demodulator. The resistance strain gauge was pasted on the surface of the sensor, and the strain change under the stress value was measured by the strain gauge. By comparing and analyzing the strain change and the center wavelength drift data of the fiber grating, the relationship curve between the center wavelength change and the strain was drawn, and the sensitivity of the sensor was finally determined to realize the strain calibration of the sensor. The temperature calibration test was carried out by the oven method. The initial temperature was 20 °C, and the final temperature was increased to 80 °C, and then the temperature was gradually decreased. During the whole process, data acquisition was carried out for every 1 °C change. In order to ensure the accuracy of the test, the strain and temperature calibration test was repeated for three cycles.

4.11. Sensor Adaptability Analysis Test

The prepared sensor was embedded in an AC-13 asphalt rutting specimen to simulate the actual embedding of the sensor in asphalt pavement. Through static load and dynamic load testing of the asphalt rutting specimen with the embedded sensor, the validity and accuracy of the sensor in the asphalt pavement were verified. The test used #70 matrix asphalt, and its performance meet the requirements of specification JTG E20-2011 [26]. The relevant performance indicators of each grade aggregate and mineral powder meet the requirements of JTG 3432-2024 [27].

The static load test adopted the method of step-by-step loading of heavy weights. In the experiment, the weight of the round cake was 5.1 kg, that is, each weight was 49.98 N. After connecting the optical fiber jumper and the optical fiber demodulator, the weights were placed in the center of the rut specimen in turn. A total of 20 weights were loaded, with a total of 999.6 N. After the loading was completed, they were unloaded one by one, and the loading and unloading cycles were performed three times.

In order to verify the accuracy of the sensor detection, ANSYS Workbench 2022 finite element software was used to simulate and analyze the static load test process, and the strain of the rut specimen under local static load was calculated. The whole process was roughly divided into the following three steps: (1) establishing the model and setting the attributes; (2) meshing and adding load; (3) performing solution analysis.

The dynamic load rutting test was carried out with reference to JTG E20-201126, and the change in the internal strain of asphalt mixture under a dynamic automobile wheel load was simulated. The test wheel was a rubber with a width of 50 mm and a tire pressure of 70 MPa $\pm$ 0.05 MPa. After 5 h of heat preservation in a 60 °C constant-temperature room, the specimens were rolled back and forth at a rolling speed of 42 times/min $\pm$ 1 times/min, and the central wavelength change during the rolling process was recorded by a fiber grating demodulator.

Author Contributions: Writing—original draft preparation, T.G., Y.C. and X.G.; writing—review and editing, Z.L., Y.C., J.Y., H.C., J.K. and J.F.; investigation, H.C., C.F., J.F., X.G., C.W., Q.C. and J.W.; data curation, C.F. All authors have read and agreed to the published version of the manuscript.

Funding: This work was supported by the Planned Project supported by the Science and Technology Innovation Team of Universities and Colleges in Henan Province (24IRTSTHN011); the Central Plains Science and Technology Innovation Leader Project (244200510031); Key Scientific and Technological Projects in Henan Province (252102240031; 252102230050); Special Plan for Key Scientific Research Projects of Higher Education Institutions in Henan Province to Serve Industry Development (25CY022).

Institutional Review Board Statement: Not applicable.

Informed Consent Statement: Not applicable.

Data Availability Statement: Data are contained within the article. Some or all of the data, models, or code that support the findings of this study are available from the corresponding author upon reasonable request.

Conflicts of Interest: The authors declare no conflicts of interest.

References

1. Lu, C.; Zhang, H.; Chen, M. Realization of high-quality development of transportation in the new era. *China J. Highw. Transp.* **2021**, *34*, 1–9.
2. Ou, J.; Zhang, J.; Duan, B.; Jiang, C.; Wang, X. Progress in research on asphalt pavement maintenance decision-making technology. *J. Beijing Univ. Technol.* **2024**, *50*, 1–12.
3. Zhou, Y.; Guo, X.; Hou, F.; Wu, J. Review of intelligent road defects detection technology. *Sustainability* **2022**, *14*, 6306. [CrossRef]
4. Ding, B.; Zhao, Q.; Chen, D.; Du, D. Technology and application progress of fiber bragg grating pressure sensing. *Study Opt. Commun.* **2024**, *50*, 75–86.
5. Feng, D.; Luo, X.; Fan, W.; Qiao, X. Strain sensing performance of material packaged fiber bragg grating in wide temperature range. *Acta Opt. Sin.* **2021**, *41*, 88–95.
6. Meng, S.; Sun, Y.; Wang, M. Fiber Bragg grating sensors for subgrade deformation monitoring in seasonally frozen regions. *Struct. Control Health Monit.* **2020**, *27*, 2472. [CrossRef]
7. Liu, H.; Ge, W.; Pan, Q.; Hu, R.; Lv, S.; Huang, T. Characteristics and analysis of dynamic strain response on typical asphalt pavement using Fiber Bragg Grating sensing technology. *Constr. Build. Mater.* **2021**, *310*, 125242. [CrossRef]

8. Liao, M.; Sheng, L.; Luo, R.; Chen, Y. The moving load identification method on asphalt roads based on the BP neural network and FBG sensor monitoring. *Constr. Build. Mater.* **2023**, *378*, 131216. [CrossRef]
9. Chen, Q.; Ge, T.; Li, X.; Li, X.; Wang, C. Road area pollution cleaning technology for asphalt pavement: Literature review and research propositions. *J. Clean. Prod.* **2025**, *493*, 144975. [CrossRef]
10. Li, J.; Zhu, W.; Ren, J.; Li, Z.; Ding, G. Research on concrete cracks damage based on FBG sensing technology. *Transducer Microsyst. Technol.* **2025**, *44*, 17–20.
11. Shi, Q.; Zhan, H.; Mo, R.; Wang, J. High-strength and toughness carbon nanotube fiber/resin composites by controllable wet-stretching and stepped pressing. *Carbon* **2022**, *189*, 1–9. [CrossRef]
12. Chen, Q.; Lan, X.; Li, A.; Sun, X.; Wang, C. The novel rapid curing pavement maintenance seal with a low environmental impact: Preparation and performance evaluation. *Wear* **2025**, *566*, 205919. [CrossRef]
13. Wang, C.; Lan, X.; Cong, Y.; Peng, S.; Huang, S.; Chen, Q. Evaluation of skid resistance of pavement maintenance energy-absorbing seal based on surface texture characteristics. *Measurement* **2025**, *245*, 116588. [CrossRef]
14. Song, X.; Gao, J.; Zheng, N.; Zhou, H.; Mai, Y.-W. Interlaminar toughening in carbon fiber/epoxy composites interleaved with CNT-decorated polycaprolactone nanofibers. *Compos. Commun.* **2021**, *24*, 100622. [CrossRef]
15. Chen, Z.; Luo, J.; Huang, Z.; Cai, C.; Tusiime, R.; Li, Z.; Wang, H.; Cheng, C.; Liu, Y.; Sun, Z.; et al. Synergistic toughen epoxy resin by incorporation of polyetherimide and amino groups grafted MWCNTs. *Compos. Commun.* **2020**, *21*, 100377. [CrossRef]
16. Xin, X.; Liang, M.; Yao, Z.; Su, L.; Zhang, J.; Li, P.; Sun, C.; Jiang, H. Self-sensing behavior and mechanical properties of carbon nanotubes/epoxy resin composite for asphalt pavement strain monitoring. *Constr. Build. Mater.* **2020**, *257*, 119404. [CrossRef]
17. Li, S.; Yao, Y. Synergistic improvement of epoxy composites with multi-walled carbon nanotubes and hyperbranched polymers. *Compos. Part B Eng.* **2019**, *165*, 293–300. [CrossRef]
18. Fan, Z.; Wang, C.; Wang, Z.; Li, Y.; Feng, L.; Tan, S. Fog seal with polymer composite modified emulsified asphalt: Road performance and environmental adaptability. *Wear* **2025**, *562*, 205672. [CrossRef]
19. Peng, L.; Fu, Q.; Li, Z.; Lin, M.; Qian, Y.; Kong, X. Research progress in environmentally friendly epoxy resin materials. *Insul. Mater.* **2024**, *57*, 1–16.
20. Zeng, L.; Li, R.; Chen, Y. Tensile test and finite element simulation of carbon nanotube/epoxy resin composites. *J. Compos.* **2024**, *41*, 2909–2922.
21. Lv, H.; Zhong, W.; Qin, L.; Zhang, K. Characteristics of polymer-encapsulated fiber grating pressure sensors. *Laser* **2020**, *41*, 63–67.
22. Huang, L.Q.; Xiong, L.; Guo, Y.X.; Hu, Z.C. All-Silicon Packaging Technology for Fiber Bragg Gratings and Its Application in Tilt Sensor. *IEEE Sens. J.* **2023**, *22*, 22627–22636. [CrossRef]
23. Luo, H.; Lei, C.; Li, R.; Zhang, S.; Zhang, J.; Xiao, C.; Wang, D. Study on the effect of packaging adhesive materials on the performance of high temperature pressure sensors. *J. Test Meas. Technol.* **2025**, *39*, 27–32+95.
24. *GB/T1040.1-2018*; Plastics—Determination of Tensile Properties—Part 1: General Principle. Standards Press of China: Beijing, China, 2018.
25. *GB/T 9341-2008*; Plastics—Determination of Flexural Properties. Standards Press of China: Beijing, China, 2018.
26. *JTG E20-2011*; Standard Test Methods of Bitumen and Bituminous Mixtures for Highway Engineering. China Communications Press: Beijing, China, 2011.
27. *JTG 3432-2024*; Test Methods of Aggregate for Highway Engineering. China Communications Press: Beijing, China, 2024.

gels

MDPI

Article

Quantum-Dot-Based Molecularly Imprinted Hydrogel for Rapid Detection of Homocysteine

Xin Zhang *, Jiarong Liang, Binglei Zheng, Pengfei Jiao and Qian Xu *

Research Center of Henan Provincial Agricultural Biomass Resource Engineering and Technology, College of Life Science, Nanyang Normal University, Nanyang 473061, China; 13620667641@163.com (J.L.); 13459281791@163.com (B.Z.); jiaopf@nynu.edu.cn (P.J.)

* Correspondence: zxnuny@nynu.edu.cn (X.Z.); xiaoqian7666@nynu.edu.cn (Q.X.)

Abstract: Elevated levels of homocysteine (Hcy) are associated with various pathological conditions including atherosclerosis, hypertension, and cardiovascular diseases. In this work, quantum-dot-based molecularly imprinted hydrogels (QD@MIHs) were developed by integrating L-cysteine-modified ZnS quantum dots (QDs)with highly selective molecular imprinting technology for rapid homocysteine detection. The QD@MIPHs were fabricated using a dual-functional monomer system (acrylamide and methacrylic acid) through surface coating of the Hcy molecularly imprinted polymer gel onto the QDs. Under optimal conditions, the response time of the QD@MIPHs for Hcy detection was 5 min. When the Hcy concentration ranged from 0.1 to 10.0 μM, the fluorescence quenching of the QD@MIHs showed a good linear relationship with Hcy concentration (R^2 = 0.9972), with a corresponding detection limit of 0.027 μM. In addition, the constructed QD@MIPHs showed no significant response to other interfering substances, demonstrating the high selectivity of the prepared material. Practical sample analysis revealed that the recovery rates of Hcy ranged from 94.34% to 104.1%, with relative standard deviations (RSD, n = 3) between 3.56% and 7.17%. This study provides a novel tool and method for rapid Hcy detection with significant potential in biomedical diagnostics and preventive-healthcare applications.

Keywords: quantum dots; molecularly imprinted hydrogel; homocysteine; fluorescence sensor

1. Introduction

Homocysteine (Hcy) is a crucial intermediate metabolite in the methionine and cysteine metabolic pathways in humans [1]. Under physiological conditions, serum homocysteine is metabolized via enzymatic reactions into glutathione and *S*-adenosylmethionine, participating in protein biosynthesis and cellular metabolism maintenance, thereby playing a pivotal role in both metabolic regulation and immune function [2–4]. However, when this metabolic process is disrupted by factors such as genetic predisposition, nutritional status, unhealthy lifestyle, aging, chronic diseases, or certain medications, Hcy and its metabolites accumulate in the blood, leading to elevated homocysteine levels (hyperhomocysteinemia) [5–8]. Studies have shown that a variety of diseases such as stroke, depression, Alzheimer's disease, cardiovascular disease, certain cancers and gestational hypertension are associated with high levels of Hcy in the blood [9–13]. Therefore, the detection of Hcy has received extensive attention in the fields of drug research, medical diagnosis and disease monitoring. Currently, there are numerous detection methods for detecting homocysteine, including enzyme-linked immunosorbent assay (ELISA), gas chromatography-mass spectrometry (GC-MS), high-performance liquid chromatography

(HPLC), capillary electrophoresis, and fluorescence polarization immunoanalysis [14–21]. Although these techniques can provide reliable Hcy detection results, they still present several limitations, such as complex pretreatment, high operational costs, and the requirement for specialized instruments and trained personnel. Therefore, it is highly necessary to develop a faster, more convenient, and lower-detection-limit Hcy determination technology. Due to their advantages such as low cost, reliability, excellent selectivity, high sensitivity, and portability, molecularly imprinted sensors have become a promising candidate for the development of novel Hcy detectors.

Molecular imprinting technology (MIT) is a well-established technique that involves copolymerization and cross-linking of functional monomers with template molecules, followed by template removal to create specific recognition sites [22–24]. Molecularly imprinted hydrogels (MIHs) are a novel functional material that combines MIT with hydrogel matrices [25]. By incorporating specific molecular recognition sites into the hydrogel network, MIHs not only retain the high water content, swelling capacity, and biocompatibility of conventional hydrogels but also exhibit highly selective and specific adsorption capabilities for target molecules [26–28]. Due to their intelligent molecular recognition and responsive properties, MIHs demonstrate broad application prospects in biomedical fields, food, and industrial separation [29–33]. However, during conventional MIH preparation, template molecules tend to become entrapped or embedded within the gel network, leading to difficult template removal and mass transfer limitations. These issues adversely affect the adsorption performance and specificity of MIHs, significantly hindering their practical applications.

Quantum dots (QDs) hold significant application value in sensor development due to their exceptional physical and optical properties, such as narrow emission spectra, high quantum yields, and size-tunable fluorescence characteristics [34–36]. The unique properties of QDs enable the development of highly sensitive sensing platforms. The novel intelligent sensing platform constructed by integrating QDs with molecularly imprinted hydrogels combines the superior signal transduction of QDs with the specific molecular recognition advantages of MIHs [37–39]. The molecularly imprinted hydrogel not only effectively protects quantum dots (QDs) from environmental quenching and enhances their stability, but its environmental responsiveness (such as pH and temperature) also enables intelligent regulation of detection conditions [40,41]. Furthermore, the molecularly imprinted cavities within the hydrogel can specifically capture target molecules, significantly improving detection selectivity.

In this study, quantum dots were integrated with molecularly imprinted hydrogels to fabricate a QD-based MIH fluorescence sensor for the detection of homocysteine, employing acrylamide and methacrylic acid as dual-functional monomers. The QD@MIPHs not only retain the conventional advantages of molecularly imprinted polymers, including excellent physical stability, high selectivity, low cost, and broad operating conditions, but also demonstrate additional merits such as a fast mass transfer rate, easy elution/adsorption, and a low detection limit. The developed sensor exhibits high sensitivity and accuracy in Hcy quantification, enabling reliable clinical assessment of cardiovascular disease risk and facilitating early intervention. Furthermore, the QD@MIH system demonstrates broad applicability in biomarker detection, environmental monitoring, and food safety analysis, offering enhanced sensitivity and specificity while paving the way for portable, real-time sensing devices.

2. Results and Discussion

2.1. Fabrication of Hcy Molecularly Imprinted Hydrogel

QD@MIHs were prepared through surface molecular imprinting technology by copolymerizing dual-functional monomers (AAM and MAA) on *L*-cysteine-modified Mn^{2+}-doped ZnS quantum dots to construct a molecularly imprinted hydrogel system. The specific preparation process is illustrated in Figure 1. First, water-soluble manganese-doped ZnS quantum dots (QDs) were employed as the signal transduction unit and substrate nanomaterial. ZnS QDs exhibit narrow emission bands, and doping with Mn^{2+} can further enhance their fluorescence quantum yield and photochemical stability. Meanwhile, the ZnS QDs were surface-modified with L-cysteine to improve their biocompatibility while enhancing their optical stability and aqueous dispersibility. Second, AAm and MAA were selected as dual-functional monomers to construct a molecularly imprinted hydrogel layer for Hcy on L-cysteine-modified ZnS quantum dots via surface imprinting technology. MAA provided pH sensitivity to the imprinted gel while AAm regulated the gel network elasticity and swelling rate by harnessing their synergistic effects. Finally, after eluting the Hcy molecules, complementary binding sites matching Hcy in terms of structure, size, shape, and functional groups were formed in the molecularly imprinted hydrogel on the prepared QD@MIHs. The constructed molecularly imprinted hydrogel coating on the QDs surface not only provided selectivity for Hcy but also prevented other interfering substances from binding to the QD@MIHs surface. Furthermore, the constructed QD@MIH exhibited pH-responsive characteristics, enabling rapid binding of Hcy molecules in samples through pH adjustment. In this study, QD@MIHs exhibited characteristic orange-red fluorescence emission at 594 nm in the absence of homocysteine (Hcy). Upon Hcy addition, the molecularly imprinted hydrogel layer on the QD@MIHs surfaces selectively captured Hcy molecules through specific binding interactions, leading to significant fluorescence quenching. Stern-Volmer analysis confirmed that the quenching efficiency showed a positive linear correlation with Hcy concentration. The fluorescence quenching mechanism involves photoinduced electron transfer from the excited state of quantum dots to Hcy molecules, introducing a new nonradioactive decay pathway for the excited-state energy [42]. This dynamic quenching process ultimately converts the molecular recognition event into analyzable optical signals, enabling rapid detection of the target molecule in the samples.

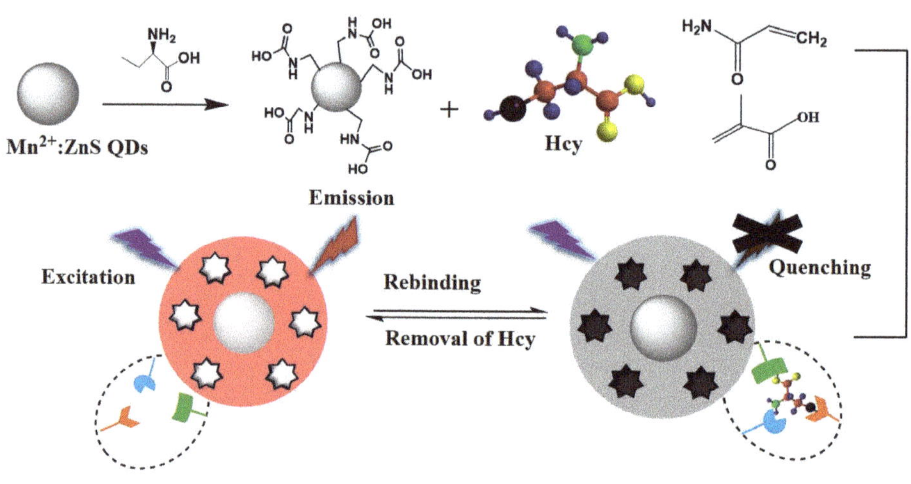

Figure 1. Schematic of the QD@MIHs preparation process.

2.2. Characterization

High-resolution transmission electron microscope (TEM) characterization was performed on both L-cysteine-functionalized ZnS quantum dots (QDs) and the QD@MIHs (Figure 2). The prepared nanoparticle diameters were measured from the TEM images using NanoMeasurer 1.2.5, with subsequent statistical analysis performed in OriginPro 2021 (v9.8.0.20) including Gaussian fitting of size distributions. The TEM images (Figure 2a) reveal well-defined lattice structures of the ZnS QDs with uniform particle size distribution, and the average diameter of the QDs is 3.12 ± 0.18 nm. The QD@MIH nanoparticles (Figure 2b) exhibit good dispersity with a moderately increased average diameter of 3.75 ± 0.31 nm. This size expansion results from the successful surface imprinting process, where the molecularly imprinted hydrogel coating endows molecular-recognition functionality to the QDs. The tailored imprinting cavities enable both high-affinity binding and efficient adsorption of homocysteine molecules.

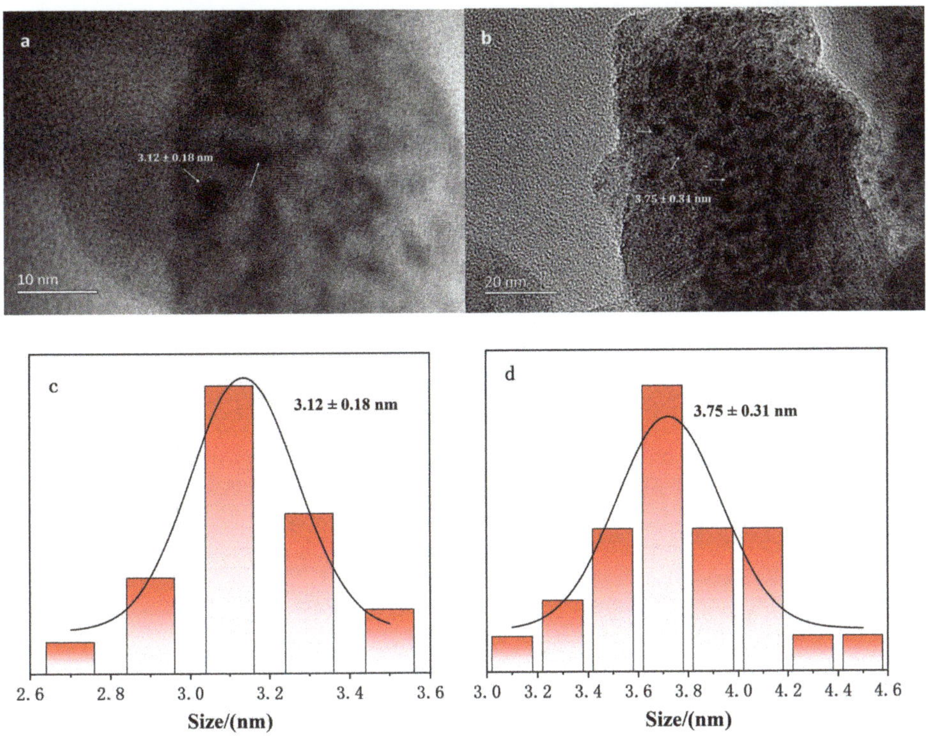

Figure 2. TEM images of (**a**) L-cysteine-modified QDsand (**b**) QD@MIHs, with corresponding size distribution of (**c**) L-cysteine-modified QDs and (**d**) QD@MIHs.

2.3. pH-Dependent Effects on QD@MIHs

Figure 3 demonstrates the changes in fluorescence intensity and quenching degree of QD@MIHs before and after Hcy adsorption under different pH conditions. As illustrated in Figure 3, the as-prepared QD@MIHs exhibit obvious pH-dependent fluorescence behavior in the absence of Hcy. Under acidic conditions (pH 3.5–5.0), the fluorescence intensity is relatively low. The emission intensity gradually increases with rising pH values, reaching its maximum at pH 7.0. However, further increasing the pH to alkaline conditions (7.0–9.0) leads to a slight decrease in fluorescence intensity. This phenomenon can be explained by (1) acidic hydrolysis of QD@MIHs generating H_2S_2, which quenches fluorescence [43], and (2) alkaline-induced aggregation or precipitation of quantum dots that which affects both material stability and fluorescence efficiency. In contrast, after the addition of Hcy, QD@MIHs exhibited significant fluorescence quenching with increasing pH (3.5–7.0). The maximum fluorescence quenching is achieved at pH 7.0, coinciding with the peak quenching efficiency ($F_0/F - 1$). This phenomenon can be attributed to the pH-responsive properties imparted by the AAm-MAA copolymerized hydrogel layer on the QD surfaces during QD@MIHs fabrication. At pH 7.0, the hydrogel layer swells, facilitating Hcy's entry into the binding cavities. This enhanced accessibility enables more effective Hcy capture by QD@MIHs, followed by electron transfer between QDs and Hcy that induces pronounced fluorescence quenching. These experimental results demonstrate that pH 7.0 provides maximum quenching efficiency ($F_0/F - 1$) for Hcy detection by QD@MIHs. Therefore, pH 7.0 was selected as the optimal condition for Hcy detection in subsequent experiments.

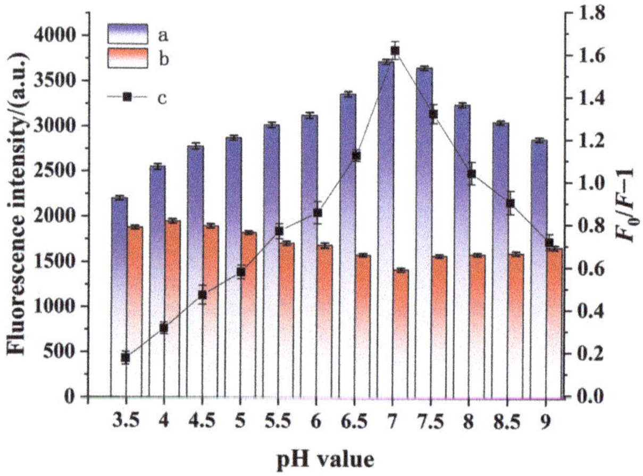

Figure 3. Fluorescence response of QD@MIHs at different pH values (a) without Hcy and (b) with Hcy, (c) Changes in fluorescence quenching efficiency. Experimental conditions: acetic acid–sodium acetate buffer at pH 3.5–5.5; sodium phosphate buffer at pH 6.0–8.0; boric ac-id-borax buffer at pH 8.0–9.0, room temperature.

2.4. Rebinding Experiments

2.4.1. Binding Kinetics

The adsorption kinetics of the prepared QD@MIHs and QD@NIHs were investigated by incubating them in homocysteine solutions and recording the time-dependent fluorescence intensity variations. As shown in Figure 4, when Hcy was present in the sample, the fluorescence intensity of QD@MIHs decreased rapidly within the first 3 min and then gradually stabilized over the remaining 7 min, ultimately achieving adsorption equilibrium within 5 min. To further investigate the effect of nonspecific adsorption on the prepared materials, the adsorption kinetics of QD@NIHs were measured under same conditions. It can be clearly observed that the fluorescence intensity of QD@NIHs decreased during the initial 2 min, with a slight change occurring in the subsequent 8 min. This phenomenon occurs because of QD@NIHs lacks specific Hcy recognition sites, and the QD@NIHs bind Hcy through nonspecific physical adsorption, resulting in fluorescence quenching. However, due to its limited binding capacity, the system quickly reaches equilibrium, after which the fluorescence intensity of QD@NIHs remains essentially unchanged. In contrast, QD@MIHs feature a molecularly imprinted hydrogel coating that creates tailored recognition cavities during imprinting. These cavities exhibit complementarity to Hcy in term of molecular size, functional group orientation, and three-dimensional structure. Hcy molecules are selectively captured and bound to the QDs surfaces, resulting in pronounced fluorescence quenching and a longer equilibration time. These experimental results demonstrate that the Hcy adsorption equilibrium time of QD@MIHs is 5 min.

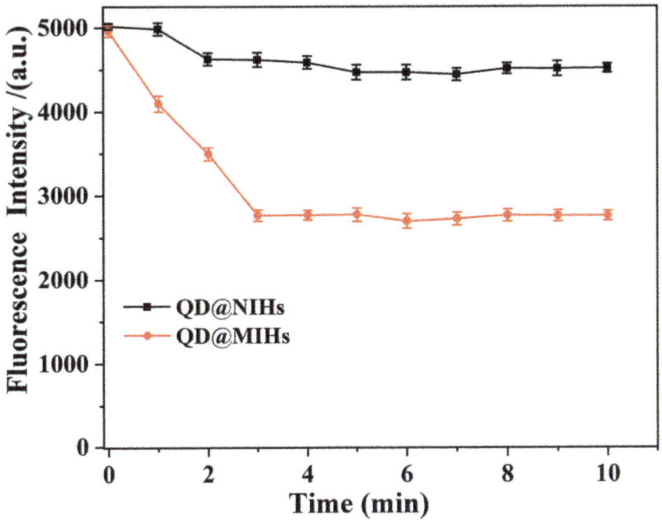

Figure 4. Binding kinetics of QD@MIHs and QD@NIHs in Hcy sample solution.

2.4.2. Adsorption Isotherm Experiments

The adsorption behavior of the prepared quantum dot-based molecularly imprinted hydrogels toward homocysteine was systematically investigated through rebinding experiments. As shown in Figure 5, the Hcy adsorption isotherms of QD@MIHs and QD@NIHs for Hcy were determined. The results demonstrate that the Hcy adsorption capacity of QD@MIHs increased rapidly with increasing Hcy concentrations. Notably, QD@MIHs exhibited significantly enhanced adsorption capacity compared to their non-imprinted counterparts (QD@NIHs). This remarkable performance can be attributed to the precisely constructed three-dimensional imprinted cavities within the molecularly imprinted hydrogel matrix coating the quantum dots, which provide numerous specific binding sites for effective Hcy recognition and capture. The molecular imprinting technology endowed the QD@MIHs with superior molecular recognition capability, thereby achieving substantially improved adsorption capacity for the target molecule (Hcy). The experimental adsorption isotherm was fitted using both Scatchard and Langmuir models. The Scatchard analysis displayed two distinct linear regressions with different slopes. The corresponding fitting equations were $Q_e/C_e = 0.00105\ Q_e - 0.01175$ ($R^2 = 0.9786$) and $Q_e/C_e = 0.03140\ Q_e - 0.9212$ ($R^2 = 0.9850$), respectively. The experimental adsorption isotherm was fitted using the Langmuir equilibrium model, and the fitting results are presented in Figure 5. The Langmuir Hcy adsorption isotherm equation of QD@MIHs was $C_e/Q = 0.02083\ C_e + 0.02966$ ($R^2 = 0.9958$). The fitting results demonstrate that the adsorption behavior of the molecularly imprinted material conforms well to the Langmuir model ($R^2 = 0.9958$), indicating a monolayer adsorption process on homogeneous surfaces. This suggests that the adsorption sites are uniformly distributed on the molecularly imprinted hydrogel surface, and the three-dimensional imprinted cavities exhibit excellent spatial complementarity with Hcy molecules.

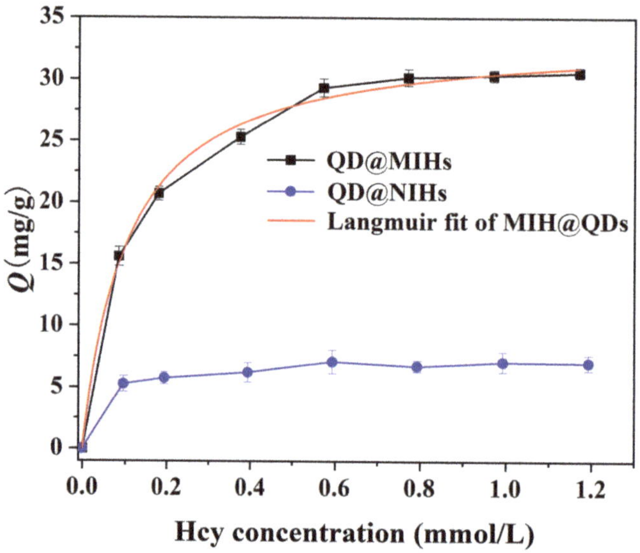

Figure 5. The adsorption isotherm of QD@MIHs and QD@NIHs and Langmuir fit of QD@MIHs.

2.5. Fluorescence Sensing of Hcy Using QD@MIHs

Figure 6 shows the changes in the fluorescence emission spectra of QD@MIHs at different Hcy concentrations in the samples. The synthesized QD@MIHs exhibit narrow and symmetric fluorescence emission with a large full width at half maximum (FWHM) and strong fluorescence intensity. After binding with Hcy molecules, the prepared QD@MIHs display significant fluorescence quenching, primarily attributed to the electron transfer process between the quantum dots and the template molecules. As shown in Figure 6, the fluorescence intensity of both QD@MIHs and QD@NIHs gradually decreased as the concentration of Hcy increased. Compared to QD@NIHs, QD@MIHs exhibited significant fluorescence quenching, demonstrating a much higher fluorescence quenching efficiency ($F_0/F - 1$) than QD@NIHs (Figure 6b). This pronounced fluorescence quenching of QD@MIHs can be attributed to the molecular imprinting process employed in QD@MIH synthesis. During imprinting process, non-covalent interactions including hydrogen bonding and van der Waals forces between functional monomers and Hcy molecules generated complementary binding cavities in the molecularly imprinted hydrogel following template removal. These imprinted cavities matched Hcy in term of spatial structure, size, shape, and functional groups, and facilitated more selective binding of Hcy molecules to the molecularly imprinted hydrogel layer on QD@MIHs. Subsequently, the electron transfer between the quantum dots and bound Hcy molecules resulted in the observed fluorescence quenching phenomenon. As a control, the adsorption of Hcy molecules by QD@NIHs mainly occured through nonspecific interactions, resulting in limited Hcy adsorption capacity and a lower degree of fluorescence quenching compared to QD@MIHs. Figure 6a demonstrates that as the Hcy concentration increases in the samples, the fluorescence intensity of QD@MIHs decreases proportionally, indicating that calculating the Hcy concentration in the solution based on fluorescence quenching is feasible and effective. Under optimal conditions, when the Hcy concentration ranges from 0.1 to 10.0 μM, the degree of fluorescence quenching ($F_0/F - 1$) of the QD@MIHs exhibits a good linear relationship with Hcy concentration, with a correlation coefficient of 0.9972. The corresponding method detection limit is 0.027 μM ($3\,\delta/S$). The detection method developed in this study demonstrates convenient operation, rapid detection, cost-effectiveness, and high selectivity.

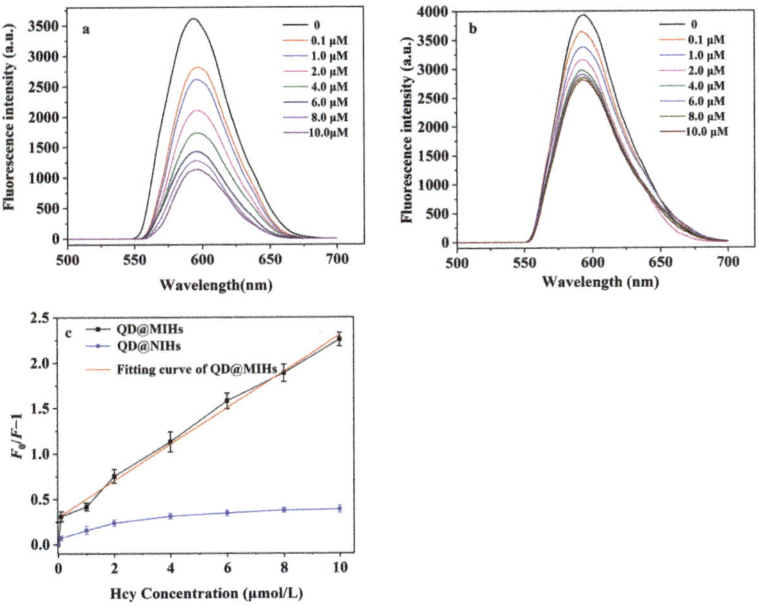

Figure 6. (**a**) Fluorescence quenching spectra of QD@MIHs and (**b**) QD@NIHs at different Hcy concentrations; (**c**) Fitting curve of QD@MIHs fluorescence quenching degree versus Hcy concentration.

2.6. Selective Experiments

To evaluate the specific Hcy recognition capability of QD@MIHs for Hcy, bovine serum albumin (BSA), lysozyme (Lyz), hemoglobin (Hb) and glutathione (GSH) were selected as reference molecules for comparative analysis. As shown in Figure 7, within the concentration range of 0.1–10.0 μM, Hcy exhibited significantly higher fluorescence quenching constants (*Ksv*) for QD@MIHs compared to other interfering molecule (BSA, Lyz, Hb and GSH). This phenomenon can be attributed to the numerous Hcy imprinting sites created on the molecularly imprinted hydrogels during the imprinting process. These binding sites demonstrated complementary interactions with Hcy molecules in terms of spatial configuration, size matching, functional groups and surface charge distribution, thereby enabling enhanced Hcy binding and more pronounced fluorescence quenching of QD@MIHs. On the other hand, the bovine serum albumin, lysozyme, Hb and GSH molecules did not match the imprinted sites on the QD@MIHs surface. Their adsorption primarily relied on non-specific interactions such as physical adsorption, resulting in low adsorption capacity for the target molecules and thus a weaker degree of fluorescence quenching. Furthermore, the quenching effect of the Hcy molecules and reference molecules on the QD@NIHs showed no significant difference, and their quenching constants were quite similar. This is mainly because the QD@NIHs were prepared without corresponding template molecules, resulting in the absence of imprinted sites for the target analyte. The binding between the analyte molecules and QD@NIHs was primarily non-specific, leading to weak adsorption and thus an insignificant quenching effect. Experimental results demonstrated that the imprinting factor for Hcy was 6.08, significantly higher than those of the reference molecules (BSA: 1.39; Lyz: 1.18; Hb: 1.26; GSH: 1.59), indicating that the prepared QD@MIHs had high selectivity for Hcy molecules. The QD@MIHs prepared in this study were compared with other reported Hcy detection techniques, as shown in Table 1. Compared to other Hcy detection methods (such as HPLC, fluorescent probes, and Au NPs), QD@MIHs exhibited a good linear range, a lower detection limit, and faster response times for Hcy detection. The developed method is simple to operate, has low instrumental requirements, and does not require complex sample processing, while also demonstrating good selectivity.

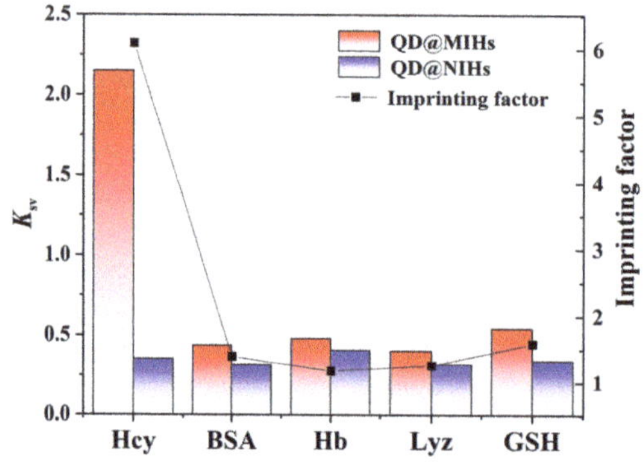

Figure 7. The imprinting factor (IF) and fluorescence quenching constant (K_{sv}) of QD@MIHs and QD@NIHs at different sample solution concentrations.

Table 1. Comparison of the performance of the QD@MIHs with previously reported methods for the determination of Hcy.

Analysis Technique	Linearity (μM)	LOD	Detection Time (min)	References
HPLC	0.15–22.2	0.037	30.0	[16]
Terahertz spectroscopy	10.0–150.0	10.0	7.0	[44]
Electrochemical biosensor	5.0–150	1.2	10.0	[45]
Two-photon fluorescent probe	0–10	0.018	60.0	[46]
Aptasensor based on aptamer/Au NPs	1–100	1.0	30.0	[47]
Magnetic imprinted polymer	1.0–2.0	0.03	90.0	[48]
QD@MIHs	0.1–10	0.027	5.0	This work

2.7. Applications

This experiment adopted the standard addition recovery method to validate the accuracy and reliability of the prepared molecularly imprinted hydrogel for detecting Hcy in urine samples. Since all samples were collected from healthy volunteers with no detectable endogenous Hcy in their urine, Hcy standards at varying concentrations were spiked into the urine samples to validate the accuracy of QD@MIHs detection. The recovery rates are presented in Table 2. As shown in Table 2, the recovery rates of Hcy ranged from 94.34% to 104.1%, with relative standard deviations (RSD, $n = 3$) between 3.56% and 7.17%, demonstrating satisfactory performance. The results indicate that the fabricated quantum dot-based molecularly imprinted hydrogel can effectively detect Hcy in real samples. The method is accurate, reliable, highly sensitive, and suitable for the rapid analysis of Hcy in practical applications.

2.8. Reusability and Stability of QD@MIHs

This experiment evaluated the reusability of the prepared QD@MIHs. the changes in fluorescence intensity after five consecutive elution-adsorption cyclesare shown in Figure 8. As depicted in Figure 8, the fluorescence intensity of QD@MIHs showed no significant variation during the first three cycles. After the fourth cycle, the fluorescence intensity decreased by 10.5%. Repeated QD@MIH regeneration cycles lead to gradual ligand loss from the QDs surface and structural damage to the molecularly imprinted hydrogel coating, ultimately resulting in performance decline. These results indicate that the prepared

QD@MIHs maintain good reusability within three operational cycles. Additionally, after 30 days of storage at 4 °C in the dark, the QD@MIHs had excellent fluorescence performance with no significant change in their intensity (Figure 9), demonstrating their high fluorescence stability.

Table 2. The results of the experiments on the Hcy recovery rate in real samples.

Sample	Detected (μM)	Added (μM)	Measured (μM)	Recovery Rates (%)	RSD (n = 3, %)
urine sample 1	Nd [1]	0.1	0.0952	95.2	4.25
		0.5	0.5128	102.6	5.67
		1.0	0.9838	98.4	3.56
urine sample 2	nd	0.1	0.0974	97.4	5.72
		0.5	0.5204	104.1	6.19
		1.0	1.015	101.5	4.23
urine sample 3	nd	0.1	0.0943	94.34	7.17
		0.5	0.5178	103.6	5.21
		1.0	1.012	101.2	5.25

[1] no Hcy detected.

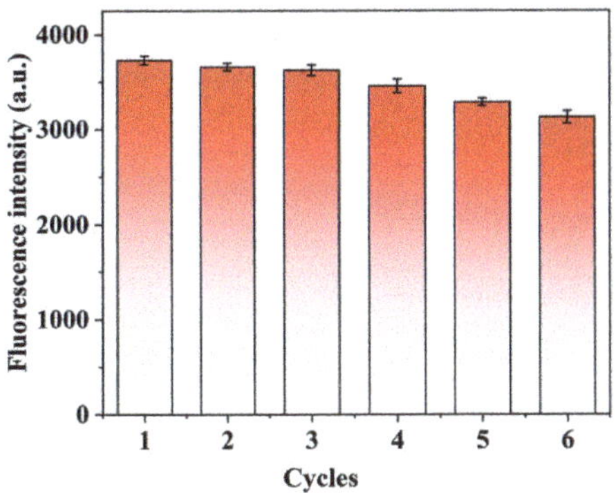

Figure 8. The reusability of QD@MIHs.

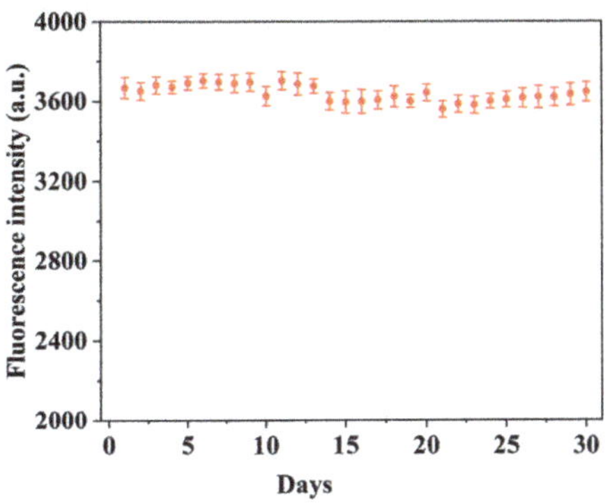

Figure 9. The fluorescence stability of QD@MIHs.

3. Conclusions

This study successfully developed a water-soluble quantum dot-based molecularly imprinted hydrogel sensor (QD@MIHs) for highly efficient detection of Hcy molecules. As advanced fluorescent biosensors, QD@MIHs integrate the optical properties of quantum dots with the high selectivity of molecularly imprinted hydrogels, significantly enhancing the selectivity and accuracy of Hcy detection in complex samples. The QD@MIHs demonstrates user-friendly operation, a rapid response, and greatly improved detection efficiency. The Experimental results demonstrate that QD@MIHs can effectively identify and detect Hcy in samples with a rapid response time and excellent selectivity. Furthermore, the QD@MIHs exhibit reliable accuracy in real sample analysis, along with good stability and reusability. As fluorescent biosensor, QD@MIHs enable real-time monitoring of Hcy concentrations, showing significant potential for early disease screening and point-of-care diagnostics, with broad applications in preventive medicine and biomedical research.

4. Materials and Methods

4.1. Instruments and Reagents

Zinc sulfate ($ZnSO_4{\cdot}7H_2O$), manganese chloride ($MnCl_2{\cdot}4H_2O$), sodium sulfide ($Na_2S{\cdot}9H_2O$), ammonium persulfate, L-homocysteine (Hcy), tris (2-carboxyethyl)phosphine hydrochloride (TCEP), L-cysteine, bovine serum albumin (BSA), lysozyme (Lyz), hemoglobin (Hb) and glutathione (GSH) were purchased from Maclin Biochemical Technology Co., Ltd. (Shanghai, China). Acrylamide (AAm), methacrylic acid (MAA), *N,N′*-methylene diacrylamide (MBAAm), tetramethylenediamine (TEMED), and potassium persulfate (KPS) were obtained from Aladdin Biochemical Technology Co., Ltd. (Shanghai, China). Acetic acid and anhydrous ethanol were purchased from Sinopharm Group Chemical Reagent Co., Ltd. (Shanghai, China). All of the reagents were of analytical grade, and the water used in experimental water was ultra-pure water.

The fluorescence spectra were measured by an FL-970 spectrofluorometer (Techcomp, Shanghai, China). The composition of the nanomaterials was analyzed using a JEM F200 field emission transmission electron microscope (JEOL, Tokyo, Japan). The UV/vis adsorption spectra were determined with a Specord 210 plus spectrophotometer (Analytik, Jena, Germany).

4.2. Synthesis of L-Cysteine-Modified Quantum Dots

The synthesis of L-cysteine-modified quantum dots was performed via a sequential aqueous-phase reaction [49]. Firstly, zinc sulfate heptahydrate (12.5 mmol) and manganese chloride tetrahydrate (1.0 mmol) were co-dissolved in 90 mL of deionized water. The precursor solution was stirred for 3 h at 25 °C under nitrogen protection. Secondly, a freshly prepared sodium sulfide solution (15.0 mmol in 10 mL H_2O) was added dropwise (0.5 mL/min) to the reaction mixture, which was maintained at 60 °C for 10 h. Thirdly, L-cysteine (0.5 mmol in 5 mL H_2O) was introduced to functionalize the nanoparticle surfaces during a 12 h dark-phase reaction. Finally, the resulting colloidal products were purified through three cycles of centrifugation (8000 rpm) and redispersion in deionized water to remove the residual reactants. The purified precipitate was collected and vacuum-dried for subsequent experiments.

4.3. Fabrication of Molecularly-Imprinted-Hydrogel-Capped QDs

Surface imprinting technology was employed to coat the homocysteine molecule-imprinted hydrogel onto the L-cysteine-modified QDs, constructing a QD@MIHs fluorescence sensor as illustrated in Figure 1. First, 3.6 mmol AAm, 1.2 mmol MAA, and 1.0 mmol Hcy were sequentially added to 50 mL of pure water and ultrasonically dispersed for 20 min. Next, 200 mg of L-cysteine-modified QDs were added, followed by 5 min of ultrasonic dispersion and the addition of0.18 mmol MBAAm were added. After stirring for 30 min, 15 mg KPS and 8 μL TEMED were added to initiate polymerization. The mixed solution was reacted at room temperature under nitrogen protection for 20 h. As a control, non-imprinted hydrogels (QD@NIHs) were prepared using the same protocol without Hcy molecules. The products were washed with water and ethanol to remove residual reactants. The QD@MIHs were then eluted with an SDS/acetic acid solution (1%: 10%, *w*/*v*) until their fluorescence intensity was the same as that of the QD@NIHs. Finally, the product was vacuum-dried and stored in darkness at 4 °C. The QD yields of the Mn: ZnSQDs, QDs@MIHs, and QDs@NIHs in ethanol which were 38.3%, 22.5%, and 23.7%, respectively.

4.4. Effect of pH on the QD@MIHs

In a 10 mL calibrated test tube, 1 mL of 0.1 g/L QD@MIHs and QD@NIHs dispersions were prepared in 9 mL buffer solutions across varying pH ranges (acetic acid–sodium acetate buffer at pH 3.5–5.5; sodium phosphate buffer at pH 6.0–8.0; boric acid–borax buffer at pH 8.0–9.0) and sonicated for 5 min. After 5 min of incubation at 25 °C, the change in fluorescence intensity of QD@MIHs in the presence and absence of Hcy in different buffer solutions was measured using an FL-970 spectrofluorometer.

4.5. Adsorption Experiments

4.5.1. Adsorption Kinetics

The adsorption kinetics of the QD@MIHs in Hcy solution were first investigated. A standard Hcy solution was prepared by dissolving 0.135 g of Hcy in 100 mL of phosphate buffer (pH 7.0), with 1.2 mmol TCEP added to prevent oxidative degradation. For the adsorption experiments, QD@MIHs or QD@NIHs were ultrasonically dispersed in 10 µmol/L Hcy solution. The mixtures were incubated at 25 °C with orbital shaking (150 rpm) for varying durations, and the time-dependent fluorescence intensity changes in both the QD@MIHs and QD@NIHs were recorded.

4.5.2. Binding Isotherm Experiments

In the rebinding experiments, QD@MIHs or QD@NIHs were dispersed in 10 mL of phosphate buffer (pH 7.0) containing varying concentrations of Hcy (0–1.2 mmol/L) at 25 °C. Binding isotherm studies were conducted by determining the adsorption capacities of QD@MIHs and QD@NIHs across an Hcy concentration range of 0.1–1.2 mmol/L. The adsorbed protein quantity (Q, mg/g) was calculated using the equation

$$Q = (C_0 - C_e)V/W \tag{1}$$

where C_0 and C_e represent the initial and equilibrium concentrations of Hcy, respectively; V is the solution volume; and W denotes the mass of QD@MIHs or QD@NIHs.

4.6. Determination of Homocysteine Using QD@MIHs

At room temperature (25 °C), homocysteine (Hcy) solutions were prepared by dissolving Hcy in phosphate buffer (pH 7.0). TCEP was then added as a reducing agent, followed by nitrogen (N_2) purging for 15 min to prevent oxidative degradation. A series of Hcy standard solutions with concentrations ranging from 0 to 10.0 µmol/L were prepared. QD@MIHs were sequentially added to these solutions, achieving a final concentration of 10 mg/L in all reaction systems. After thorough mixing, the solutions were incubated on a shaker at room temperature for 5 min. the fluorescence emission spectra of the QD@MIHs were recorded at an excitation wavelength of 310 nm, with QD@NIHs as the control. All experiments were performed in triplicate. The fluorescence quenching of the QD@MIHs followed the Stern–Volmer equation, as expressed below:

$$F_0/F = 1 + K_{SV}[Q] \tag{2}$$

Here, F_0 represents the initial fluorescence intensity, where F denotes the fluorescence intensity with the quencher (Hcy); K_{sv} is the Stern–Volmer constant; and $[Q]$ is the concentration of the quencher (Hcy).

4.7. Selective Experiments Methods

In this experiment, we selected BSA, Lyz, Hb, and GSH as competing substances for Hcy to evaluate the selective recognition capability of the prepared QD@MIHs. The choice of competing analytes was based on the following biological rationale: (i) glutathione (GSH) was included as a potential metabolic interferent due to its similar sulfhydryl structure to homocysteine (Hcy); (ii) bovine serum albumin (BSA), the most abundant protein in plasma, was used to simulate the matrix environment; (iii) hemoglobin (Hb) was in-cluded because it is a key interferent released during red blood cell lysis; and (iv) lysozyme (Lyz) was included as it is commonly present in secretions at inflammatory sites. A series of sample solutions with varying concentrations (0–10.0 μmol/L) of Hcy, BSA, lysozyme, Hb, and GSH were prepared. The prepared QD@MIHs and QD@NIHs were then added to these sample solutions to achieve a final QD@MIH concentration of 10 mg/L in all samples. After incubation at room temperature for 5 min, the changes in fluorescence intensity of QD@MIHs and QD@NIHs were measured and recorded. The imprinting factor (IF) was used to evaluate the selectivity of QD@MIHs and QD@NIHs toward each substance, and the calculation formula is as follows:

$$\mathrm{IF} = K_{\mathrm{SV,MIP}} / K_{\mathrm{SV,NIP}} \tag{3}$$

where $K_{\mathrm{sv,MIP}}$ and $K_{\mathrm{sv,NIP}}$ are the quenching constants for QD@MIHs and QD@NIHs for different sample solutions, respectively.

4.8. Application in Real Samples

To validate the practical application of the fabricated QD@MIHs sensor, urine samples were employed as real samples to evaluate the practical Hcy detection performance of the prepared QD@MIHs. Because urine contains negligible protein-bound Hcy, the developed QD@MIHs-based sensor primarily aims to detect free-form homocysteine. Urine samples collected from healthy volunteers were filtered through 0.4 μm membranes and stored at 4 °C in the dark. For analytical measurements, 100 μL of the prepared QD@MIHs (1.0 g/L) was dispersed into 9 mL of pretreated urine sample (filtered and reduced with 1 mM TCEP). The mixture was adjusted to pH 7.0 using phosphate buffer (NaH_2PO_4/Na_2HPO_4), and the final volume was increased to 10 mL with ultrapure water. After mixing, the solution was incubated at 25 °C for 5 min under dark conditions. The changes in fluorescence intensity of QD@MIHs were measured using a spectrofluorometer. To further verify the accuracy of the developed method, a standard addition approach was employed by spiking different levels of homocysteine (0.1, 0.5, 1.0 μmol/L) into the samples for recovery rate determination.

4.9. Stability and Reusability

The fluorescence stability of the prepared QD@MIHs was evaluated under dark storage conditions. The QD@MIHs were stored at 4 °C, and their fluorescence intensity was measured continuously for 30 days. Additionally, the reusability of QD@MIHs was systematically investigated. The prepared QD@MIHs underwent consecutive adsorption–de-sorption–adsorption cycles, with fluorescence intensity recorded after each cycle to evaluate their reusability. The specific cycling procedure was as follows: The QD@MIHs were incubated in Hcy samples for 5 min followed by fluorescence measurement. Then, bound homocysteine molecules were removed using SDS/acetic acid solution (1: 10,

m/v), and the QD@MIHs were washed with buffer until a neutral pH was achieved for subsequent reuse.

Author Contributions: Conceptualization, X.Z.; methodology, X.Z. and J.L.; software, X.Z.; validation, B.Z., P.J. and Q.X.; investigation, X.Z., J.L. and B.Z.; data curation, X.Z. and J.L.; writing—original draft preparation, X.Z.; writing—review and editing, J.L. and X.Z.; funding acquisition, X.Z. and Q.X. All authors have read and agreed to the published version of the manuscript.

Funding: This research was funded by the Key Scientific and Technological Projects in Henan Province (No. 242102310366); the Key Scientific and Technological Projects of Henan Province (No. 232102310198). Key Scientific Research Projects of Higher Education Institutions in Henan Province of China (No. 24A150028) and the Special Project for Key R & D and Promotion of Science and Technology of the Department of Henan Province (No. #231111310900).

Institutional Review Board Statement: Not applicable.

Informed Consent Statement: Not applicable.

Data Availability Statement: All the data generated by this research is included in the article.

Conflicts of Interest: The authors declare no conflicts of interest.

Abbreviations

The following abbreviations are used in this manuscript:

QDs	Quantum dot
Hcy	Homocysteine
MIHs	Molecularly imprinted hydrogel
MIT	Molecular imprinting technology
GC	Gas chromatography
HPLC	High-performance liquid chromatography
IF	Imprinting factor
NIHs	Non-imprinted hydrogels
QD@MIHs	Quantum dot (QD)-based molecularly imprinted hydrogels

References

1. Wu, D.F.; Yin, R.X.; Deng, J.L. Homocysteine, hyperhomocysteinemia, and H-type hypertension. *Eur. J. Prev. Cardiol.* **2024**, *31*, 1092–1103. [CrossRef]
2. Hu, D.F.; Yu, Y.; Wang, G.Y.; Wang, P.F.; Pu, J. Aberrant Human Epididymal Protein 4 in Heart Failure Patients' Serum and its Association with C-Reactive Protein, Uric Acid and Homocysteine. *Clin. Lab.* **2024**, *70*, 740. [CrossRef]
3. McCully, K.S. Homocysteine, vitamins, and vascular disease prevention. *Am. J. Clin. Nutr.* **2007**, *86*, 1563S–1568S. [CrossRef]
4. Smith, A.D.; Refsum, H. Homocysteine–from disease biomarker to disease prevention. *J. Intern. Med.* **2021**, *290*, 826–854. [CrossRef]
5. Clarke, R.; Halsey, J.; Bennett, D.; Lewington, S. Homocysteine and vascular disease: Review of published results of the homocysteine-lowering trials. *J. Inherit. Metab. Dis.* **2021**, *34*, 83–91. [CrossRef]
6. Hermann, A.; Sitdikova, G. Homocysteine: Biochemistry, molecular biology and role in disease. *Biomolecules* **2021**, *11*, 737. [CrossRef]
7. Koklesova, L.; Mazurakova, A.; Samec, M.; Biringer, K.; Samuel, S.M.; Büsselberg, D.; Kubatka, P.; Golubnitschaja, O. Homocysteine metabolism as the target for predictive medical approach, disease prevention, prognosis, and treatments tailored to the person. *EPMA J.* **2021**, *12*, 477–505. [CrossRef] [PubMed]
8. Pervez, W.; Yin, C.; Huo, F. Homocysteine fluorescent probes: Sensing mechanisms and biological applications. *Coord. Chem. Rev.* **2025**, *522*, 216202. [CrossRef]
9. Zhou, L. Homocysteine and Parkinson's disease. *CNS Neurosci. Ther.* **2024**, *30*, e14420. [CrossRef] [PubMed]
10. Zuliani, G.; Brombo, G.; Polastri, M.; Romagnoli, T.; Mola, G.; Riccetti, R.; Seripa, G.; Trentini, A.; Cervellati, C. High plasma homocysteine levels predict the progression from mild cognitive impairment to dementia. *Neurochem. Int.* **2024**, *177*, 105763. [CrossRef]

11. Zheng, H.; Chen, H.; Cai, Y.; Shen, M.; Li, X.; Han, Y.; Zong, L.; Zhang, Y. Hydrogen sulfide-mediated persulfidation regulates homocysteine metabolism and enhances ferroptosis in non-small cell lung cancer. *Mol. Cell.* **2024**, *84*, 4016–4030. [CrossRef]
12. Ding, C.; Li, J.; Wei, Y.; Fan, W.; Cao, T.; Chen, Z.; Shi, Y.; Yu, C.; Yuan, T.; Zhao, P.; et al. Associations of total homocysteine and kidney function with all-cause and cause-specific mortality in hypertensive patients: A mediation and joint analysis. *Hypertens. Res.* **2024**, *47*, 1500–1511. [CrossRef]
13. Tawfik, A.; Mohamed, R.; Elsherbiny, N.M.; DeAngelis, M.M.; Bartoli, M.; Al-Shabrawey, M. Homocysteine: A potential biomarker for diabetic retinopathy. *J. Clin. Med.* **2019**, *8*, 121. [CrossRef]
14. Wang, W.; Rusin, O.; Xu, X.; Kim, K.K.; Escobedo, J.O.; Fakayode, S.O.; Fletcher, K.A.; Lowry, M.; Schowalter, C.M.; Lawrence, C.M.; et al. Detection of homocysteine and cysteine. *J. Am. Chem. Soc.* **2005**, *127*, 15949–15958. [CrossRef]
15. Piechocka, J.; Wieczorek, M.; Głowacki, R. Gas chromatography–mass spectrometry based approach for the determination of methionine-related sulfur-containing compounds in human saliva. *Int. J. Mol. Sci.* **2020**, *21*, 9252. [CrossRef]
16. Li, J.S.; Huang, D.; Qiu, H.M.; Jiang, Q.S.; Liu, Y.H.; Du, T.T.; Jiang, X.H. A study on the determination of two related aminothiols in the brain of diabetes rats by HPLC-ECD. *J. Liq. Chromatogr. Relat. Technol.* **2020**, *43*, 725–732. [CrossRef]
17. Mikaliunaite, L.; Green, D.B. Using a 3-hydroxyflavone derivative as a fluorescent probe for the indirect determination of aminothiols separated by ion-pair HPLC. *Anal. Methods* **2021**, *13*, 2915–2925. [CrossRef] [PubMed]
18. Greño, M.; Salgado, A.; Castro-Puyana, M.; Marina, M.L. Nuclear magnetic resonance to study the interactions acting in the enantiomeric separation of homocysteine by capillary electrophoresis with a dual system of γ-cyclodextrin and the chiral ionic liquid EtCholNTf2. *Electrophoresis* **2019**, *40*, 1913–1920. [CrossRef] [PubMed]
19. Muzaffar, R.; Khan, M.A.; Mushtaq, M.H.; Nasir, M.; Khan, A.; Haq, I.U.; Muhammad, J. Hyperhomocysteinemia as an independent risk factor for coronary heart disease. Comparison with conventional risk factors. *Braz. J. Biol.* **2021**, *83*, e249104. [CrossRef] [PubMed]
20. Gaweł, M.; Głowacki, R.; Piechocka, J. First HPLC-UV method for the determination of homocysteine thiolactone in human urine after derivatization with 1-benzyl-2-chloropyridinium bromide. *Sci. Rep.* **2025**, *15*, 7310. [CrossRef]
21. Piechocka, J.; Głowacki, R. Comprehensive studies on the development of HPLC-MS/MS and HPLC-FL based methods for routine determination of homocysteine thiolactone in human urine. *Talanta* **2024**, *272*, 125791. [CrossRef] [PubMed]
22. Haupt, K.; Linares, A.V.; Bompart, M.; Bui, B.T.S. Molecularly imprinted polymers. *Mol. Imprint.* **2011**, *325*, 1–28.
23. Liu, Y.; Wang, L.; Li, H.; Zhao, L.; Ma, Y.; Zhang, Y.; Liu, J.; Wei, Y. Rigorous recognition mode analysis of molecularly imprinted polymers—Rational design, challenges, and opportunities. *Prog. Polym. Sci.* **2024**, *150*, 101790. [CrossRef]
24. Li, Y.; Luo, L.; Kong, Y.; Li, Y.; Wang, Q.; Wang, M.; Li, Y.; Davenport, A.; Li, B. Recent advances in molecularly imprinted polymer-based electrochemical sensors. *Biosens. Bioelectron.* **2024**, *249*, 116018. [CrossRef]
25. Byrne, M.E.; Park, K.; Peppas, N.A. Molecular imprinting within hydrogels. *Adv. Drug Deliv. Rev.* **2002**, *54*, 149–161. [CrossRef]
26. Fan, J.P.; Lai, J.H.; Huang, C.B.; Lai, Z.T.; Xie, C.F.; Chen, H.P.; Liu, Y.D. Synthesis of a gelatin based molecularly imprinted hydrogel with high selectivity on adsorbing bovine serum albumin. *Sep. Purif. Technol.* **2024**, *328*, 124999. [CrossRef]
27. Ivaskiene, T.; Kaspute, G.; Ramanavicius, A.; Prentice, U. Molecularly imprinted polymer advanced hydrogels as tools for gastrointestinal diagnostics. *Gels* **2025**, *11*, 269. [CrossRef] [PubMed]
28. Liu, C.; Kubo, T.; Otsuka, K. Specific recognition of a target protein, cytochrome *c*, using molecularly imprinted hydrogels. *J. Mater. Chem. B* **2022**, *10*, 6800–6807. [CrossRef]
29. Pan, M.; Gao, M.; Cui, J.; Gao, R.; Li, H.; Sun, J.; Chen, W.; Wang, S. Fluorescent molecularly imprinted hydrogel sensing strip based on nitrogen-doped carbon dots and inverse opal photonic crystals applying for effective detection for imidacloprid in fruits and vegetables. *Food Chem.* **2025**, *477*, 143497. [CrossRef] [PubMed]
30. Benito-Pena, E.; Gonzalez-Vallejo, V.; Rico-Yuste, A.; Barbosa-Pereira, L.; Cruz, J.M.; Bilbao, A.; Alvarez-Lorenzo, C.; Moreno-Bondi, M.C. Molecularly imprinted hydrogels as functional active packaging materials. *Food Chem.* **2016**, *190*, 487–494. [CrossRef]
31. Kakkar, V.; Narula, P. Role of molecularly imprinted hydrogels in drug delivery—A current perspective. *Int. J. Pharm.* **2022**, *625*, 121883. [CrossRef] [PubMed]
32. Völlmecke, K.; Afroz, R.; Bierbach, S.; Brenker, L.J.; Frücht, S.; Glass, A.; Giebelhaus, R.; Hoppe, A.; Kanememaru, K.; Lazarek, M.; et al. Hydrogel-based biosensors. *Gels* **2022**, *8*, 768. [CrossRef]
33. Cheng, L.; Guo, Z.; Lin, Y.; Wei, X.; Zhao, K.; Yang, Z. Bovine serum albumin molecularly imprinted electrochemical sensors modified by carboxylated multi-walled carbon nanotubes/CaAlg hydrogels. *Gels* **2023**, *9*, 673. [CrossRef] [PubMed]
34. Jing, L.; Kershaw, S.V.; Li, Y.; Huang, X.; Li, Y.; Rogach, A.L.; Gao, M. Aqueous based semiconductor nanocrystals. *Chem. Rev.* **2016**, *116*, 10623–10730. [CrossRef]
35. García de Arquer, F.P.; Talapin, D.V.; Klimov, V.I.; Arakawa, Y.; Bayer, M.; Sargent, E.H. Semiconductor quantum dots: Technological progress and future challenges. *Science* **2021**, *373*, eaaz8541. [CrossRef]
36. Sun, P.; Xing, Z.; Li, Z.; Zhou, W. Recent advances in quantum dots photocatalysts. *Chem. Eng. J.* **2023**, *458*, 141399. [CrossRef]

37. Azeez, K.F.; Salimi, A.; Hallaj, R. MOF and CdTe quantum dots entrapped hydrogel film as dual-signal ratiometric fluorometric-colorimetric sensing platform for erythromycin detection: Portable smartphone-assisted visual sensing in milk and water samples. *Food Chem.* **2025**, *482*, 143972. [CrossRef]
38. Yang, S.; Sarkar, S.; Xie, X.; Li, D.; Chen, J. Application of Optical Hydrogels in Environmental Sensing. *Energy Environ. Mater.* **2024**, *7*, e12646. [CrossRef]
39. Piloto, A.M.L.; Ribeiro, D.S.; Santos, J.L.; Sales, G. Development of a sensitive ratiometric imprinted hydrogel for the detection of matrix metalloproteinase 7 (MMP7) biomarker. *ACS Appl. Opt. Mater.* **2023**, *2*, 57–67. [CrossRef]
40. Culver, H.R.; Clegg, J.R.; Peppas, N.A. Analyte-responsive hydrogels: Intelligent materials for biosensing and drug delivery. *Acc. Chem. Res.* **2017**, *50*, 170–178. [CrossRef] [PubMed]
41. Toyoshima, Y.; Kawamura, A.; Takashima, Y.; Miyata, T. Design of molecularly imprinted hydrogels with thermoresponsive drug binding sites. *J. Mater. Chem. B* **2022**, *10*, 6644–6654. [CrossRef]
42. Tan, L.; Kang, C.; Xu, S.; Tang, Y. Selective room temperature phosphorescencesensing of target protein using Mn-doped ZnS QDs-embedded molecularlyimprinted polymer. *Biosens. Bioelectron.* **2013**, *48*, 216–223. [CrossRef]
43. Zhao, Y.; Ma, Y.; Li, H.; Wang, L. Composite QDs@MIP nanospheres for specific recognition and direct fluorescent quantification of pesticides in aqueous media. *Anal. Chem.* **2012**, *84*, 386–395. [CrossRef]
44. Wang, L.; Wu, X.; Peng, Y.; Yang, Q.; Chen, X.; Wu, W.; Zhu, Y.; Zhuang, S. Quantitative analysis of homocysteine in liquid by terahertz spectroscopy. *Biomed. Opt. Express* **2020**, *11*, 2570–2577. [CrossRef]
45. Wen, X.H.; Zhao, X.F.; Peng, B.F.; Yuan, K.P.; Li, X.X.; Zhu, L.Y.; Lu, H.L. Facile preparation of an electrochemical aptasensor based on Au NPs/graphene sponge for detection of homocysteine. *Appl. Surf. Sci.* **2021**, *556*, 149735. [CrossRef]
46. Wei, F.; Ding, Y.; Ou, J.; Chen, X.; Li, L.; Zhou, Q.; Chen, Q.; Wang, Q.; Feng, Y.; Meng, X. Accurate detection of hcy in human serum and two-photon visualization of atherosclerosis using a highly specific fluorescent probe. *Anal. Chem.* **2023**, *95*, 9173–9181. [CrossRef] [PubMed]
47. Kongintr, U.; Lertanantawong, B.; Promptmas, C. A label-free electrochemical biosensor for homocysteine detection using molecularly imprinted polymer and nanocomposite-modified electrodes. *Polymers* **2023**, *15*, 2241. [CrossRef] [PubMed]
48. da Conceição, P.; dos Santos Neto, A.G.; Khan, S.; Tanaka, A.A.; Santana, A.E.G.; del Pilar Taboada-Sotomayor, M.; Goulart, M.O.F.; Santos, A.C.F. Extraction-assisted voltammetric determination of homocysteine using magnetic nanoparticles modified with molecularly imprinted polymer. *Microchim. Acta* **2023**, *190*, 159. [CrossRef] [PubMed]
49. Zhang, X.; Wang, M.; Zhang, Y.; Zhao, P.; Cai, J.; Yao, Y.; Liang, J. Preparation of Molecularly Imprinted Cysteine Modified Zinc Sulfide Quantum Dots Based Sensor for Rapid Detection of Dopamine Hydrochloride. *Molecules* **2023**, *28*, 3646. [CrossRef]

gels

MDPI

Article

Polymer–Silicate Composite Gel Systems for Enhanced Chloride Resistance of Cement-Based Materials

Tianhang Zhang [1,*], Yonggui Dai [1], Shuai Ren [1], Zhengqiang Huang [2,3], Chong Han [1] and Wencheng Ding [1]

[1] School of Water Conservancy and Transportation, Zhengzhou University, Zhengzhou 450001, China; daiyg@gs.zzu.edu.cn (Y.D.); rs301077@163.com (S.R.); hanchong@gs.zzu.edu.cn (C.H.); dwc4113@gs.zzu.edu.cn (W.D.)

[2] Zhongyuan Research Institute, Zhejiang University, Zhengzhou 450000, China; hzq124@gmail.com

[3] Henan Province Engineering Technology Research Center of Infrastructure Disease Monitoring and Treatment, Zhengzhou 450000, China

* Correspondence: zzzth@zzu.edu.cn; Tel.: +86-136-1382-3029

Abstract: To address the issues of insufficient protection and poor durability in concrete during service, this study developed a novel polymer–silicate composite gel system by combining silane with fluorocarbon resin emulsion and applied it to mortar specimens. The chloride ion resistance enhancement of mortar provided by the novel gel system was evaluated using the RCM method and natural chloride ion penetration tests, with SEM images employed to analyze its anti-permeation mechanism. Results indicate that the chloride ion migration coefficient of the novel composite gel system is 4.91×10^{-12} m^2/s, representing a 63.97% reduction compared to the single fluorocarbon gel system. Within the 0–5 mm depth range, free chloride ion contents at 14, 28, and 56 days decreased by 55.35%, 50.10%, and 43.64%, respectively, demonstrating excellent resistance to chloride penetration. Acid and alkali resistance tests demonstrated that the system retained the inherent corrosion resistance of the fluorocarbon component. Carbonation tests demonstrated that the system exhibited a slight decrease in carbonation resistance compared with the pure fluorocarbon gel system, while still maintaining a satisfactory performance level. Overall, the polymer-silicate composite gel system significantly enhanced the mortar's resistance to chloride ion penetration.

Keywords: polymer–silicate composite gel system; silane; fluorocarbon; chloride ion resistance

1. Introduction

Concrete, a typical cement-based gel material, is highly susceptible to attack by harmful ions due to surface pores and cracks, particularly in marine, chemical, and saline-alkali environments, where acid and alkali ions can severely impact its structure [1–3]. Excessive concentrations of Cl^-, SO_4^{2-}, and OH^- compromise the calcium silicate hydrate (C-S-H) gel, resulting in severe structural damage. Moreover, anions can infiltrate the interior via diffusion, permeation, and capillary absorption, ultimately inducing steel corrosion [4–7]. A practical and effective way to enhance the durability of concrete is the application of surface protective materials [8]. Currently, surface protection for concrete mainly relies on polymer emulsions and silane-based coupling agents [9,10]. Polymer emulsions include epoxy, acrylic, polyurethane, fluorocarbon, and other types. These protective materials form a polymer-silicate gel system with concrete, creating a dense protective layer on the surface that effectively hinders water molecules and harmful ions introduced by water from penetrating the matrix [11–13]. Silane coupling agents mainly consist of silanes and siloxanes. These materials can penetrate into the concrete structure and react with C-S-H gel in the concrete to form a hydrophobic layer, preventing the penetration of water molecules and various harmful ions [14,15]. Numerous studies have confirmed that both types of protective materials can effectively improve the durability of concrete.

Almusallam et al. [16] compared five types of polymer emulsions—polyurethane, epoxy resin, chlorinated rubber, acrylic, and polyethylene—on improving the durability of concrete. The results indicated that all these polymers significantly reduced the penetration of water and chloride ions, with epoxy and polyurethane being most effective in enhancing substrate hydrophobicity. Vipulanandan et al. [17] evaluated the performance of two polyurethanes in a sulfuric acid environment and found that both effectively prolonged the service life of concrete. Merah et al. [18] compared acrylic and epoxy for carbonation resistance, revealing that epoxy more effectively decreased the carbonation depth of the matrix. Zheng et al. [19] evaluated the effects of waterborne fluorocarbon resin and silicone-acrylic emulsions on the water absorption and chloride ion resistance of concrete. The findings demonstrated a marked enhancement in chloride ion resistance and a significant decrease in water absorption. However, epoxy resins have poor toughness and are susceptible to aging [20]. Polyurethane exhibits excellent corrosion resistance, but its application demands high technical standards and it has relatively poor thermal stability [21]. Acrylics possess good weather and UV resistance but show poor water and chemical corrosion resistance, making them unsuitable for marine environments [15]. Fluorocarbons offer excellent weather and corrosion resistance, but their high rigidity makes them prone to cracking and peeling [22,23]. Although polymer-silicate gel systems can effectively enhance the matrix's durability, they have inherent drawbacks that hinder long-term structural protection.

Silane coupling agents have received wide attention due to their film-forming penetration properties, and their applications in concrete mainly focus on silanes and their derivatives [24,25]. Studies have shown that silanes can penetrate the micro-pores of concrete and, through de-alcoholization reactions with water as well as chemical reactions with hydroxyl groups in the concrete, form a three-dimensional cross-linked network of organosiloxane resin. This network achieves tight bonding with the C-S-H gel in the structure, preventing the ingress of water and various harmful ions [26–28]. Zhu et al. [29] systematically investigated the anti-corrosion performance of silanes in offshore concrete structures. Their results indicated that silanes could penetrate 2–3 mm into the surface layer of the structure, and silane-impregnated concrete exhibited significantly reduced water absorption and chloride ion uptake. Li et al. [30] incorporated different amounts of silanes into cement-based materials. Experiments demonstrated that silanes enhance crack resistance, increase contact angle, and improve impermeability, while reducing capillary water absorption, thereby generally strengthening water resistance. SEM and nitrogen adsorption tests revealed that the silane–silicate gel system exhibited higher maximum adsorption capacity and total pore volume compared to the control group, indicating that the silane component generated hydrophobic silicone resin within the pore network of the C–S–H gel in the matrix, converting a large number of internal pore surfaces into hydrophobic interfaces. However, after penetrating into the interior of the concrete, the hydrophobic layer formed by silanes only coats the surfaces of the internal pores without sealing them and cannot establish a dense protective layer on the concrete surface. Such materials are limited in enhancing carbonation resistance and weather durability [31].

The limitations of polymer–silicate gel systems are closely associated with the intrinsic structure of the cementitious substrate. The protective layer formed by the polymer emulsion effectively mitigates the detrimental effects of ultraviolet radiation, rainfall, and other environmental exposures on the substrate. However, concrete, as a highly porous material, contains water molecules and various mobile ions within its pore network, which can adversely influence the structure and durability of the film-forming coating. Fluctuations in ambient temperature and humidity cause volumetric expansion of internal moisture and gases, generating pressure on the protective film and eventually leading to reduced adhesion or even cracking. In addition, aggressive ions—particularly chlorides—react with other species during migration to form crystalline products, inducing volumetric expansion and microcracking that accelerate surface degradation and compromise the long-term durability of the coating. To overcome the inherent limitation of polymer–silicate gel systems in addressing the internal pore structure of concrete, numerous studies have been conducted. For instance, the incorporation of fluoroalkyl chains ($–(CH_2)_nCF_3$ or $–(CF_2)_n–$) into silane molecules has been shown to markedly reduce surface energy and enhance the overall weatherability of the system [32–34]. Silane-functionalized nano-silica effectively enhances coating hydrophobicity and weather resistance, thereby reducing chloride ion ingress [35,36]. However, although such modified silane systems can improve the internal pores of concrete and reduce the impact of water, oil, or ultraviolet radiation on the surface of the structure, they do not enhance carbonation resistance, and therefore the service life of the protective system remains limited. Some researchers have attempted to incorporate silane into polymer–silicate gel systems. Huang et al. [37] reported that silane-modified acrylic resin coatings improved interfacial bonding, hydrophobicity, and UV aging resistance, while Pramualkijja et al. [38] demonstrated that siloxane-modified polyacrylate coatings exhibited superior hydrophobicity, self-cleaning properties, and interfacial adhesion. Although these modifications enhance interfacial adhesion, they involve complex and costly procedures and fail to adequately address the potential deterioration induced by ion migration within the concrete or the synergistic corrosion mechanisms arising from both internal and external environments.

In this study, a novel polymer–silicate composite gel system was developed to protect concrete by integrating silane and fluorocarbon components. Compared with the previously mentioned modified silane coatings, this system preserves the excellent weathering and corrosion resistance of fluorocarbon coatings while overcoming the durability limitations of purely penetrating coatings. Compared with chemically silane-modified polymer coatings, the silane component in this system can penetrate the internal pores of the concrete and coat their surfaces, effectively preventing potential damage to the surface layer caused by the migration of harmful ions within the concrete, and it can be easily prepared through simple mechanical mixing. This study systematically evaluated the chloride ion protection performance of a silane-modified fluorocarbon–silicate composite gel system and analyzed the substrate's microstructure at the microscopic level using scanning electron microscopy. The vulnerability of single-film coatings to internal and external harmful ions was examined, and the synergistic protective mechanisms of the composite system were investigated. Furthermore, the effects of strong acidic and alkaline environments on the substrate were assessed to determine its corrosion resistance under harsh conditions, and carbonation tests were conducted to compare the carbonation resistance of different systems. This work provides important theoretical insights into the degradation mechanisms of concrete coatings and offers a solid foundation for the practical application of this novel protective system in concrete structures.

2. Results and Discussion

2.1. Chloride Ion Migration Coefficient

Figure 1 presents the measured chloride ion penetration depths from the RCM test, where the silvery-white regions indicate the extent of chloride penetration. Specifically, Figure 1a shows the blank control group, Figure 1b represents the silane/fluorocarbon-silicate composite gel system (hereafter SF/Si), and Figure 1c depicts the fluorocarbon-silicate gel system (hereafter F/Si). It is evident that both systems exhibit markedly lower chloride ion penetration depths than the blank control group. The penetration depth of SF/Si is reduced by 57% relative to F/Si, demonstrating that silane modification substantially improves the coating's impermeability. Furthermore, hydrophobic layer traces formed by silane infiltration are visible on both the side and top surfaces of SF/Si, offering stronger protective performance than F/Si.

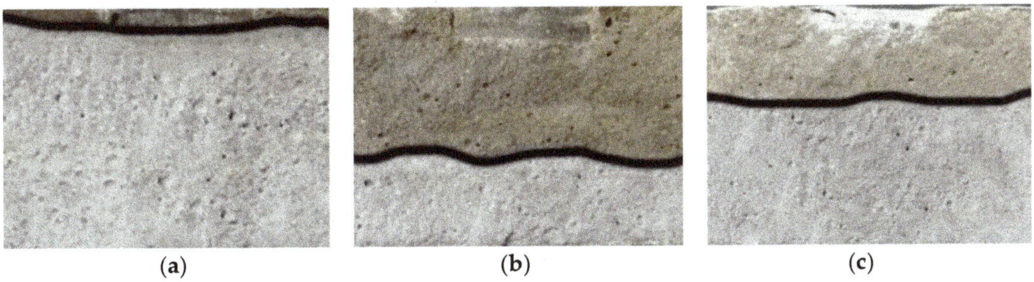

Figure 1. Measured depth of chloride penetration of mortar specimens: (**a**) Blank; (**b**) SF/Si; (**c**) F/Si.

Table 1 presents the chloride ion migration coefficients of the two gel systems. Statistical analyses were first performed using Levene's test to verify homogeneity of variance ($p > 0.05$). One-way ANOVA was then applied to assess the effect of different systems on chloride penetration depth and DRCM values, revealing statistically significant differences ($p < 0.05$). To further identify which groups differed, Tukey HSD post-hoc tests were conducted. The results confirmed that the silane-modified fluorocarbon–silicate gel system exhibited a significantly lower chloride penetration coefficient compared with the pure fluorocarbon system ($p < 0.05$). These analyses demonstrate that variations in system composition are the primary factor responsible for the observed differences in chloride resistance. Compared with the blank control, the chloride ion migration coefficients of SF/Si and F/Si were significantly reduced, with DRCM values decreasing by 88.1% and 67.1%, respectively. The D_{RCM} value of SF/Si was 63.97% lower than that of F/Si, indicating that silane significantly enhances the fluorocarbon's barrier effect against chloride ions, exerting a stronger restriction on their migration. The D_{RCM} value of SF/Si was 63.97% lower than that of F/Si, indicating that silane modification greatly enhanced the fluorocarbon's chloride ion barrier properties, effectively restricting chloride ion migration. As a surface film-forming coating, fluorocarbon blocks the pores of the mortar surface, isolating it from external chloride ions and forming an effective chloride ion barrier. However, its protection is limited to the surface; once the barrier is penetrated, chloride ion infiltration into the mortar follows a similar pattern to that in the untreated control, thereby restricting its long-term protective capacity. Chloride ion penetration is usually accompanied by water molecule movement. Silane molecules penetrate the specimen, where they hydrolyze to form silanol, which subsequently reacts with hydroxyl groups in silicates to generate siloxane chains. These siloxane structures condense and deposit onto the mortar pore surfaces, forming a hydrophobic silicone resin layer that effectively impedes chloride ion migration [39,40]. Therefore, adding a small amount of silane emulsion enhances the hydrophobicity of the fluorocarbon component, thereby improving the system's resistance to chloride ion penetration. The silane/fluorocarbon-silicate composite gel system demonstrates both the sealing effect of the fluorocarbon and the hydrophobic effect of the silane. The synergistic interaction between silane and fluorocarbon not only decreases the chloride ion migration coefficient but also enhances the durability of the mortar.

Table 1. Comparison of chloride migration coefficients of different materials.

Systems Type	Depth of Penetration (mm)	D_{RCM} (10^{-12} m^2/s)	D_{RCM} Decline Rate (%)
blank	44.2 ± 1.1	41.1 ± 1.8	--
SF/Si	14.8 ± 0.8	4.9 ± 0.2	88.1
F/Si	35.0 ± 1.5	13.6 ± 0.4	67.1

Notes: Data are presented as mean ± standard deviation (SD), n = 3.

Figure 2 shows the SEM images of SF/Si and F/Si after the RCM test. The images show that NaCl crystals are present in the membrane structures of both SF/Si and F/Si. This phenomenon indicates that during chloride ion penetration, both membrane structures have developed varying degrees of penetration pathways. The amount of NaCl crystals in the structure reflects the extent of membrane penetration. It can be observed that the number of NaCl crystals in Figure 2b is significantly greater than in Figure 2a. This indicates that SF/Si exhibits higher impermeability compared to F/Si, making it more difficult for chloride ions to penetrate. This observation is consistent with the RCM test results.

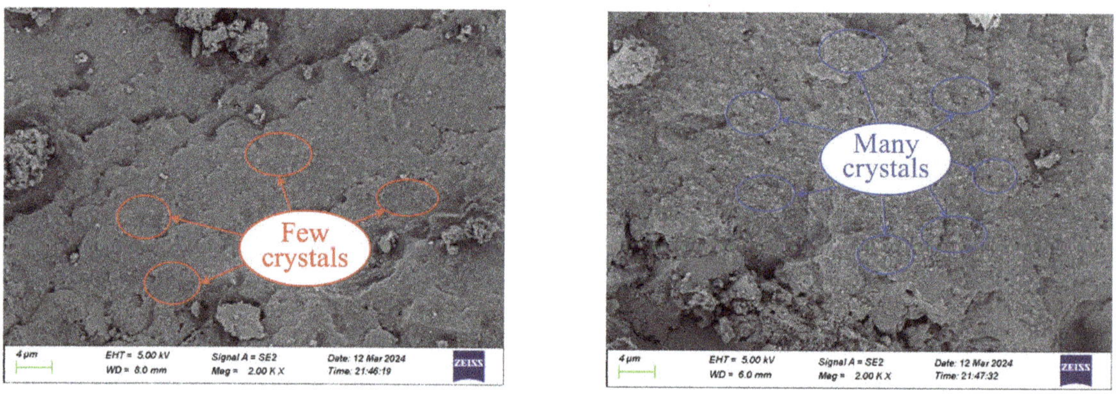

(**a**) (**b**)

Figure 2. SEM images of the two gel systems after undergoing the RCM test: (**a**) SF/Si; (**b**) F/Si.

2.2. Chloride Ion Content Distribution

The distribution pattern of chloride ion content in mortar under the same immersion time is shown in Figure 3. The chloride ion content is highest within the depth range of 0–5 mm, as the surface layer of the mortar is relatively looser than the interior. This results in lower penetration resistance for chloride ions, causing them to accumulate in the superficial layer and form a high-concentration region. Levene's test was performed to verify the homogeneity of variance ($p > 0.05$). A two-way ANOVA was conducted to assess the effects of coating system type and immersion time on free chloride ion content. The ANOVA results indicated a significant main effect of coating system type ($p < 0.05$). Subsequently, a simple effects analysis (Tukey HSD) was performed to compare the specific differences among coating systems at each immersion time. The results confirmed that the silane-modified fluorocarbon coating significantly reduced free chloride ion content compared with other systems ($p < 0.05$), supporting the enhanced chloride resistance of the proposed coating. Compared with the blank control group, the free chloride ion content in SF/Si decreased by 84.22%, 78.28%, and 68.23% after 14, 28, and 56 days of immersion, respectively, while that in F/Si decreased by 64.67%, 51.64%, and 43.64%, respectively. Compared with F/Si, the free chloride ion content in SF/Si decreased by 55.35%, 50.10%, and 43.64%, respectively. F/Si forms a dense protective layer between the chloride salt environment and the test block. However, due to its poor hydrophobicity, a small number of chloride ion penetration pathways may form within the protective layer. SF/Si integrates the impermeability of silane and the density of fluorocarbon to form a comprehensive protective system. The silane dispersed within the coating layer reduces the formation of penetration pathways through its intrinsic hydrophobicity, limiting both the inward penetration and lateral migration of chloride ions that have reached the surface layer. Consequently, its resistance to chloride ion penetration is superior to that of F/Si.

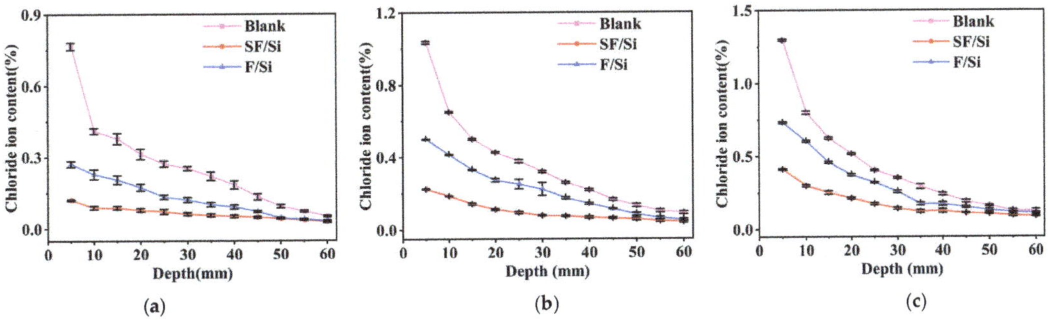

Figure 3. Distribution pattern of internal chloride ion content of mortar under the same soaking time: (**a**) 14d; (**b**) 28d; (**c**) 56d.

Figure 4 shows the variation of free chloride ion content in mortar for each coating system under different immersion times. Two-way ANOVA results indicated a significant interaction between coating system and immersion time ($p < 0.05$), demonstrating that the temporal variation of chloride ion content differed significantly among the coating systems. To further investigate specific differences, simple effects analyses (Tukey HSD) were conducted at each immersion time to compare coating systems. The results indicated that, overall, the SF/Si coating consistently exhibited significantly lower chloride ion content than the F/Si coating and the uncoated control at all time points ($p < 0.05$). Overall, the chloride ion concentration in the F/Si system fluctuated more noticeably over time compared to SF/Si. Meanwhile, by comparing the chloride ion content at a depth of 5–15 mm in Figure 4a,b, it can be observed that at a depth of 5–10 mm, the chloride ion concentration in both materials decreases significantly. However, at a depth of 10–15 mm, the rate of decline in chloride ion concentration for SF/Si slows down, especially at 14 days, where there is almost no reduction in chloride ion concentration within this depth range. In contrast, the decline in chloride ion concentration for F/Si at 10–15 mm remains nearly the same as at 5–10 mm, indicating that the reduction in chloride ion concentration in SF/Si slows earlier than in F/Si. This distribution pattern indicates that most chloride ions penetrating into the test block in SF/Si are confined to its surface layer, while F/Si, lacking an internal barrier, allows a greater accumulation of chloride ions in the deeper layers of the test block. This further demonstrates the barrier effect of silane against chloride ions.

The chloride ion penetration resistance mechanism of the two gel systems is shown in Figure 5. Since the protective effect of F/Si is mainly concentrated on the mortar surface, it cannot effectively restrict the inward diffusion of chloride ions passing through the membrane structure. The silane components in SF/Si can penetrate into the test block, forming a barrier zone, which slows the intrusion of water molecules and chloride ions, resulting in a high chloride ion concentration on the test block surface, while the internal chloride ion concentration is significantly reduced [39].

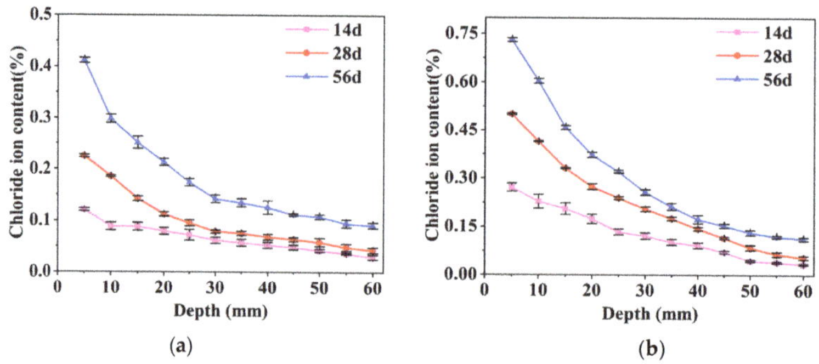

Figure 4. Change rule of internal chloride ion content of mortar under different soaking times: (**a**) SF/Si; (**b**) F/Si.

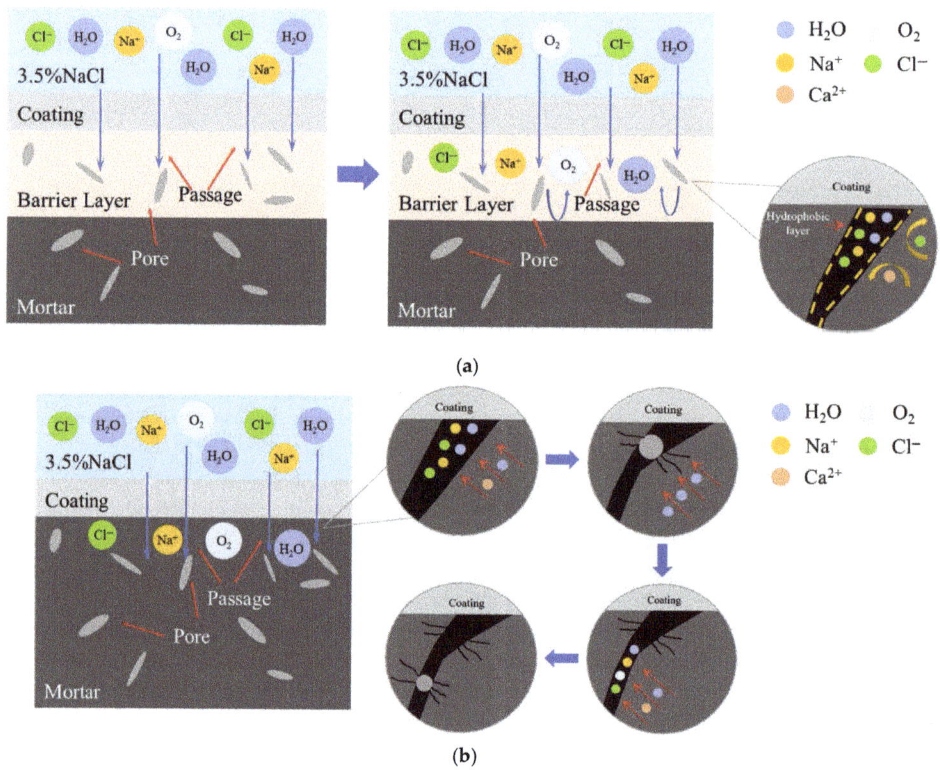

Figure 5. Schematic diagram of the mechanism of chloride ion impermeability of the two systems: (**a**) Mechanism of silane barrier to chloride ions; (**b**) Pore crystallization damage process of F/Si.

The barrier zone created by silane not only mitigates the penetration of external water molecules and chloride ions but also acts as an internal seal, preventing the migration of chloride ions and water molecules within the mortar, thereby offering internal protection. As mortar inherently contains some moisture, chloride ions migrate freely through its pores, using water as a carrier. During migration, these ions interact with internal Ca^{2+} and Na^{+} ions, precipitating as crystals. Table 2 presents the size data of typical ions and crystals in cement-based materials. The unit cell, as the basic geometric unit of the crystal structure, has a parameter *a* representing one edge length, which can be used to reflect the specific size of the unit cell. According to the data in the table, the unit cell parameter *a* of calcium carbonate is 5 times the radius of the calcium ion and 2.8 times the radius of the carbonate ion. For sodium chloride, the unit cell parameter *a* is 3.11 times the radius of the chloride ion and 5.5 times the radius of the sodium ion. The ionic radius is much smaller than the unit cell parameter of the corresponding crystal, indicating that significant volume expansion occurs during the process of ions combining to form crystals. The mortar is damaged due to the volume expansion caused by the transformation of ions into crystals within its pores. Meanwhile, ions continue to migrate via water molecules into other pores, crystallizing and inducing further damage, as shown in Figure 5b. This crystallization-induced deterioration, similar to freeze-thaw cycles, compromises the integrity of the concrete. If crystallization occurs within the pores near the pores at the material–matrix interface, it weakens adhesion and undermines the durability of the coating [41]. In Figure 5a, the barrier zone formed by silane can block internal ions near the mortar surface, preventing freeze-thaw cycle-like crystallization damage inside the mortar. While enhancing the mortar's resistance to chloride ions, it also improves its durability.

Table 2. Ionic radius and crystalline cell parameter data (pm).

Chloride Ion Radius	Calcium Ion Radius	Sodium Ion Radius	Carbonate Ion Radius	$CaCO_3$ Unit Cell Parameters a	NaCl Unit Cell Parameters a
181	100	102	178	499	564

The SEM images of chloride ion natural erosion after 56 days for the blank control group, SF/Si, and F/Si are shown in Figure 6. As shown in Figure 6a, the internal structure of the blank mortar is relatively dense, mainly due to the formation of abundant hydration products during the soaking process, which reduces the surface porosity of the mortar. This trend is consistent with the observation that the increase in chloride ion content slows down as soaking time increases [41]. As shown in Figure 6b,c, the surface of F/Si is smoother than that of SF/Si, due to the hydrophobicity provided by the silane molecules, which slowed down the hydration reaction at the silane-impregnated layer of the specimen. This resulted in SF/Si having a lower density compared to F/Si. The effect of SF/Si on the chloride ion resistance of the mortar can be attributed to its permeability resistance. Compared to F/Si, SF/Si has a more significant waterproof effect and can effectively prevent chloride ion penetration, indicating better chloride ion resistance.

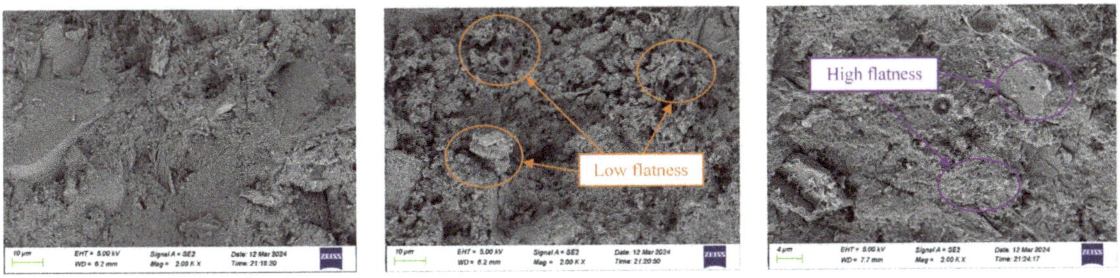

(a) (b) (c)

Figure 6. SEM images after 56 d of natural erosion by chloride ions: (**a**) Blank; (**b**) SF/Si; (**c**) F/Si.

2.3. Mass Loss Under Acid and Alkali Corrosion

The mass loss rate of mortar after acid and alkali exposure indicates its resistance to corrosion. Figure 7 shows the mass loss rates of mortars under different gel systems [42,43].

To evaluate the protective performance of different coating systems, Levene's test and two-way ANOVA were conducted on the mass loss rate. The results of Levene's test indicated that the data satisfied the assumption of homogeneity of variance ($p > 0.05$). The two-way ANOVA revealed that the coating system had a significant main effect on the mass loss rate under acidic and alkaline corrosion conditions ($p < 0.05$). The Tukey HSD post hoc test further showed that the differences between the coated groups and the blank control group were statistically significant ($p < 0.05$).

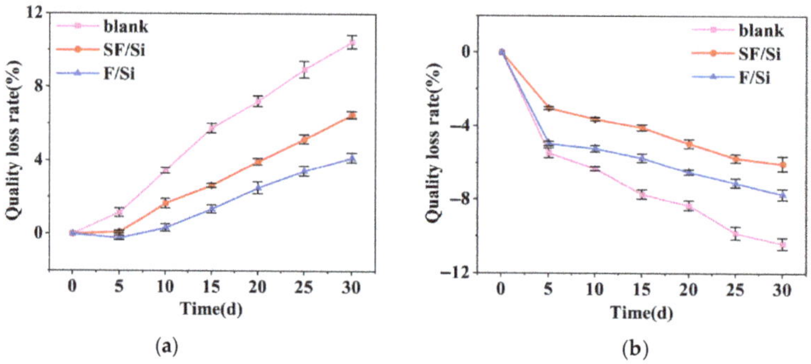

Figure 7. Mass loss rate curves of mortar under acid and alkali exposure: (**a**) Acid exposure, (**b**) Alkali exposure.

As shown in Figure 7a, SF/Si and F/Si exhibit significantly lower mass loss rates under acid erosion compared to the untreated control. Due to direct exposure to the acidic environment, the untreated control shows a linear increase in mass loss, exceeding 10% after 30 days of acid attack. The high content of F–C bonds in SF/Si and F/Si enables them to largely retain their protective properties in acidic environments, with mass loss rates of approximately 6% and 4%, respectively, after 30 days of acid exposure. The addition of silane emulsion reduces the original compactness of the fluorocarbon film in SF/Si, resulting in a mass loss rate approximately 2% higher than that of F/Si.

As shown in Figure 7b, all mortar samples exhibit negative mass loss rates, with the untreated control showing a substantially higher mass gain than the two mortars. At this stage, the change in mortar mass mainly depends on water absorption and the formation of internal gel products. Due to the absence of a protective coating, the untreated control exhibits higher internal moisture content and more abundant gel formation. In addition, the lower water absorption of SF/Si results in reduced internal moisture and less gel formation compared to F/Si. Consequently, under alkaline attack, SF/Si shows a slightly lower mass change rate than F/Si.

2.4. Compressive Strength Loss Under Acid and Alkali Corrosion

Figure 8 illustrates the relationship between the compressive strength loss rate of mortars and corrosion time for the two gel systems. Differences among coating systems were evaluated using Levene's test and two-way ANOVA. Levene's test confirmed that the compressive strength loss data under both acidic and alkaline conditions satisfied the assumption of homogeneity of variance ($p > 0.05$). The two-way ANOVA indicated that both the coating system type and corrosion time had significant main effects on the compressive strength loss rate ($p < 0.05$). Tukey HSD post hoc tests further revealed that the compressive strength loss in both coating groups was significantly lower than that of the blank control group at all tested time points ($p < 0.05$).

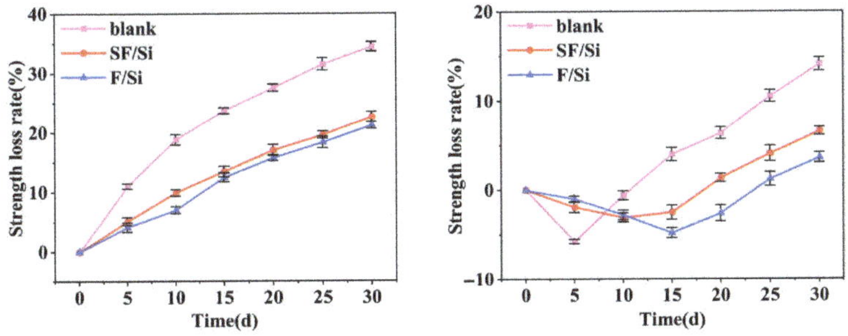

Figure 8. Variation curves of compressive strength loss rate of mortar: (**a**) Acid exposure; (**b**) Alkali exposure.

As shown in Figure 8a, under acid attack, the compressive strength loss of all mortars increased progressively over time. At the same exposure duration, the loss rates of SF/Si and F/Si were considerably lower than those of the blank group. Throughout the acid erosion process, the compressive strength loss rates of SF/Si and F/Si were nearly identical, differing by only 1–2%. Both gel systems markedly slowed the early-stage strength loss during acid erosion. The blank group exceeded a 20% loss after 15 days, whereas SF/Si and F/Si reached the same level only after 30 days. This demonstrates their superior acid resistance, with only minor differences between the two.

As shown in Figure 8b, the compressive strength of all mortars subjected to alkaline corrosion initially increased and then decreased. The time at which peak strength was reached differed among the coating systems, further confirming a significant time-dependent effect of coating type (two-way ANOVA, $p < 0.05$). Post-hoc Tukey HSD tests indicated that the compressive strength loss rate of the coated groups was significantly lower than that of the control group ($p < 0.05$), demonstrating that the coating systems effectively enhanced the compressive performance of mortar under alkaline corrosion. At 5 days of alkali exposure, the blank group exhibited a higher strength increase than SF/Si and F/Si. This was due to the higher OH^- concentration in the blank mortar, which generated more gel products and enhanced its compactness [44,45]. This observation already reflected the superior alkali resistance of the coated mortars. The strength peaks of SF/Si and F/Si were delayed to around 15 days, further indicating that OH^- intrusion into the mortar was effectively mitigated. Beyond 5 days of alkali exposure, the excessive formation of gel products disrupted the internal structure of the mortars. The strength loss rate of the blank mortar increased continuously, far surpassing that of SF/Si and F/Si, while the latter two still exhibited rising strength, further confirming their superior alkali resistance. At 30 days of alkali exposure, the strength loss rate of the blank mortar approached 15%. The compressive strength loss rate of SF/Si remained around 5%, differing from F/Si by only about 2%. This indicates that the incorporation of silane had little influence on the alkali resistance of the fluorocarbon–silicate gel system. In summary, under both acidic and alkaline environments, SF/Si exhibited comparable protective performance to F/Si, suggesting that silane had minimal influence on the acid and alkali resistance of the fluorocarbon–silicate gel system.

In summary, under both acidic and alkaline environments, SF/Si exhibited comparable protective performance to F/Si, suggesting that silane had minimal influence on the acid and alkali resistance of the fluorocarbon–silicate gel system.

2.5. Carbonation Depth

As indicated by the preceding results, the SF/Si coating exhibited outstanding resistance to chloride ion ingress. Likewise, carbonation resistance represents another critical parameter governing the durability of concrete structures [46]. To further assess the barrier efficiency of the coating against CO_2 ingress, an accelerated carbonation test was performed. The carbonation depths of the mortars at various curing ages are presented in Figure 9.

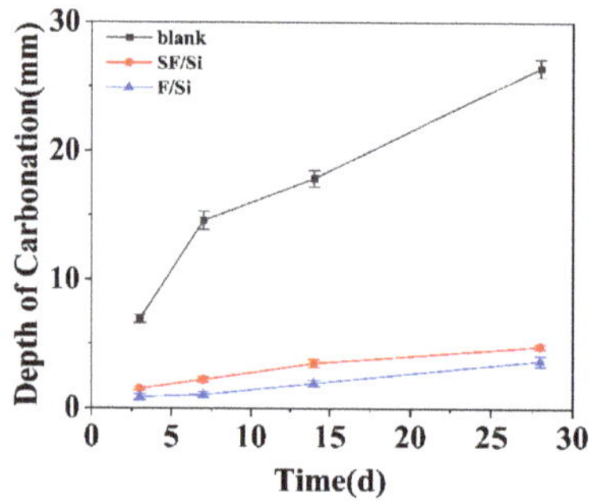

Figure 9. Carbonation depth of mortar at different curing ages.

Essentially, carbonation involves the diffusion of CO_2 gas through the coating into the concrete substrate, where chemical reactions occur; the resulting carbonation depth effectively reflects the coating's protective capability against CO_2 ingress [47,48]. To examine the statistical significance of inter-system differences, the carbonation depth data were analyzed using Levene's test for homogeneity of variance, one-way ANOVA, and the Tukey HSD post-hoc comparison. The Levene test confirmed that the data satisfied the assumption of homogeneity of variance ($p > 0.05$). The one-way ANOVA revealed a statistically significant influence of protective system type on the carbonation depth ($p < 0.05$). Subsequent Tukey HSD post-hoc analysis demonstrated that the SF/Si and F/Si coating systems exhibited significantly different carbonation performance compared with the uncoated control ($p < 0.05$).

As illustrated in Figure 9, both protective systems markedly reduced the carbonation depth of the mortars at identical carbonation ages compared with the uncoated control, indicating a pronounced enhancement in carbonation resistance. After 28 days of carbonation exposure, the carbonation depth reached 26.44 mm for the uncoated control, whereas the SF/Si and F/Si systems exhibited depths of 4.82 mm and 3.71 mm, representing reductions of approximately 82% and 86%, respectively, relative to the control. In terms of carbonation depth, the order followed F/Si < SF/Si << uncoated control. According to the Standard for Inspection and Evaluation of Concrete Durability (JGJ/T193-2009) [49], the SF/Si coating exhibited a carbonation depth of 4.82 mm after 28 days of accelerated carbonation testing, corresponding to a carbonation resistance rating of Grade T-IV, which denotes a good performance level, as shown in Table 3. Although the carbonation protection of SF/Si was slightly inferior to that of F/Si, it still satisfied the standard requirements.

Table 3. Classification of concrete carbonation resistance levels.

Grade	T-I	T-II	T-III	T-IV	T-V
Carbonation Depth d (mm)	$d \geq 30$	$20 \leq d < 30$	$10 \leq d < 20$	$0.1 \leq d < 10$	$d < 0.1$

Compared with the F/Si system, the SF/Si coating exhibited a marginal reduction in carbonation resistance. This difference is presumed to originate primarily from the limited compatibility between the silane component and the fluorocarbon resin. During the film-formation process, interfacial discontinuities or microdefects may have developed between the two phases, providing additional pathways for CO_2 diffusion and consequently diminishing the overall gas-barrier efficiency of the coating.

As illustrated in Figure 10, a distribution model of silane within the modified protective system was proposed to elucidate its influence on the coating densification and carbonation resistance. Silane species distributed on the coating surface tend to disrupt the continuity of the fluorocarbon film, which primarily accounts for the slight reduction in coating densification and carbonation resistance. In contrast, silane molecules embedded within the coating matrix and deposited near the substrate interface can react with the cementitious phase to form a siloxane network, thereby establishing the dual protective structure proposed in this study, which serves as an essential mechanism underlying the superior chloride-ion impermeability of the composite coating.

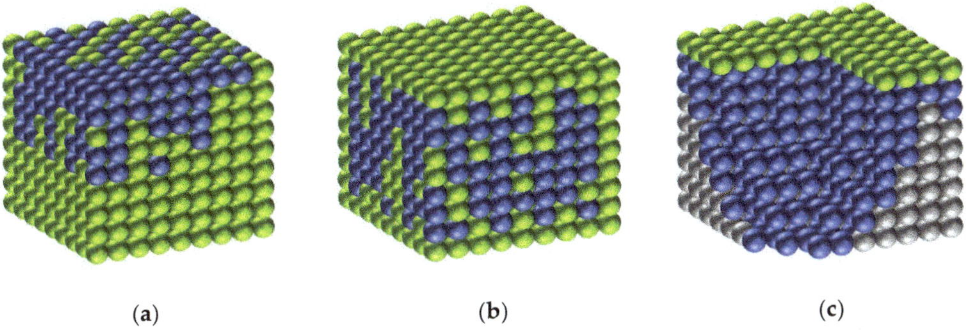

Figure 10. Form of silane emulsion in the SF/Si system: (**a**) Silane components floated on the fluorocarbon surface; (**b**) Silane components embedded within the fluorocarbon matrix; (**c**) Silane components deposited beneath the fluorocarbon coating. Blue spheres represent the fluorocarbon component, green spheres represent the silane component, and gray spheres correspond to the mortar specimens.

Subsequent SEM observations further validated the proposed model. Figure 11 displays the surface morphologies of the two protective systems. As shown, the F/Si coating developed a continuous and uniform dense film. The region highlighted in Figure 11a corresponds to the phase associated with the silane component. In the SF/Si coating, the incorporation of silane induced localized microphase separation, leading to interfacial defects within the otherwise homogeneous fluorocarbon matrix and thereby reducing the overall compactness of the coating. This microstructural feature provides direct experimental evidence for the slight reduction in gas-barrier efficiency of the composite coating and accounts for its intermediate carbonation resistance between the pure fluorocarbon coating and the uncoated control.

In summary, the incorporation of silane alters the compactness of the fluorocarbon film, thereby affecting the carbonation resistance of the overall protective system. Nevertheless, the hybrid structure formed by silane and fluorocarbon maintains the superior weathering resistance and chemical stability of the outer fluorocarbon film while markedly enhancing the system's ability to resist chloride-ion ingress from both directions. Although the presence of silane slightly reduces the compactness of the outer fluorocarbon layer and consequently its carbonation resistance, the coating still satisfies the engineering specifications and exhibits outstanding comprehensive protective performance.

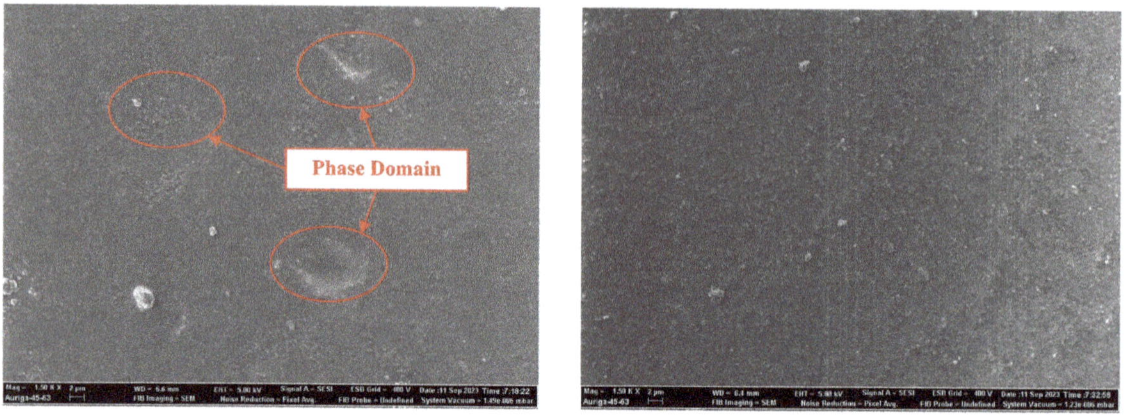

(a) (b)

Figure 11. Surface micro-morphology of the two protective systems: (**a**) SF/Si; (**b**) F/Si.

2.6. Comprehensive Performance Comparison and Analysis

The aforementioned findings indicate that the combination of silane and fluorocarbon resin forms a comprehensive protective system with complementary characteristics and synergistic effects, rather than a simple superposition of individual properties. This section aims to compare the performance of the composite coating system proposed in this study with representative existing protective systems by focusing on key indicators such as chloride ion penetration resistance and carbonation resistance, thereby further validating its protective advantages and application potential. The corresponding results are presented in Tables 4 and 5.

Table 4 presents a comparison of the chloride migration coefficients of the protective systems developed in this study and those of commonly reported coating systems in the literature. SF/Si exhibits a reduction in chloride migration of 88.1% relative to the blank control, markedly surpassing conventional fluorocarbon (67.1%), polyurethane (47.8%), and acrylic resin (54.7%) coatings [50,51]. The corresponding chloride migration coefficient (4.9×10^{-12} m^2/s) demonstrates excellent chloride resistance. Although SF/Si shows slightly lower chloride-ion protection than some silane systems, the enhancement in substrate protection achieved by SF/Si (88.1%) is comparable to that of the silane systems (84.3%) [52].

Table 4. Comparison of chloride ion resistance between the coatings studied and existing coatings.

Ref.	Coating Type	Test Method	Control/Coating (10^{-12} m^2/s)	Reduction Rate (%)	Protective System Type
(SF/Si)	Fluorocarbon/Silane	RCM	41.1/4.9	88.1	inorganic-modified organic composite system
(F/Si)	Fluorocarbon	RCM	41.1/13.6	67.1	Organic system
[50]	Polyurethane	FT	9.0/4.7	47.8	Organic system
[51]	Acrylic	RCMT	14.4/6.53	54.7	Organic system
[52]	Nano-SiO_2 modified silane	RCPT	20.93/3.29	84.3	Inorganic-modified system

Table 5 compares the carbonation depths of SF/Si, F/Si, and several representative protective systems after 28 days of accelerated carbonation. The results indicate that the combination of silane and fluorocarbon does not substantially diminish the improvement in carbonation resistance provided by fluorocarbon coatings, with reduction rates of 81.8% and 86.0% for SF/Si and F/Si, respectively. SF/Si therefore retains a relatively good carbonation resistance. When compared with certain polymer-based protective systems, such as acrylic emulsion coatings (carbonation depth: 2.98 mm; reduction: 70.8%) and nano-SiO_2-modified polyurethane coatings (carbonation depth: 2.0 mm; reduction: 65.5%), SF/Si exhibits slightly weaker carbonation protection but still falls within the same protection grade, while offering a more pronounced overall improvement in performance [49,53,54]. In comparison, single silane coatings provide only limited enhancement in carbonation resistance, reflected by a reduction rate of approximately 13.6% [55].

Table 5. Comparison of carbonation resistance between the coatings studied and existing coatings.

Ref.	Coating Type	28d Carbonation Depth (mm)	Reduction Rate (%)	Protective System Type
(SF/Si)	Fluorocarbon/Silane	26.44/4.82	81.8	inorganic-modified organic composite system
(F/Si)	Fluorocarbon	26.44/3.71	86.0	Organic system
[53]	Acrylic	10.2/2.98	70.8	Organic system
[55]	Pure silane	23.6/20.4	13.6	Inorganic system
[54]	Nano-SiO_2 modified Polyurethane	5.8/2.0	65.5	Organic-modified system

In summary, SF/Si, a novel polymer–silicate composite gel system, demonstrates excellent performance in two critical durability metrics: resistance to chloride ion penetration and carbonation. Compared with silane-based systems, SF/Si maintains comparable chloride-ion resistance while exhibiting a significantly enhanced carbonation resistance. When compared with polymer-based protective systems, SF/Si shows slightly lower carbonation resistance but still meets equivalent protection-grade standards, while its chloride-ion resistance is notably superior. These differences reflect the fundamental distinctions in protective mechanisms between different coating systems. Although silane-based systems can penetrate the substrate, they lack the intrinsic density and durability characteristic of polymer-based systems. Single polymer films, as discussed in Section 2.2, are unable to effectively prevent the back-diffusion of harmful ions from the concrete pores, thereby limiting long-term protective performance. SF/Si integrates the inherent density of the polymer film with the protective layer formed through silane penetration, creating a dual-layer synergistic system. This structure provides a balanced enhancement of durability and demonstrates improved overall protective performance.

3. Conclusions

This study developed a novel polymer–silicate composite gel system based on silane and fluorocarbon resin. Through the synergistic effect of dual-layer protection, the system significantly enhances mortar resistance to chloride penetration while maintaining inherent chemical durability. The main conclusions are summarized as follows:

1. The RCM test indicated that the SF/Si composite gel system had a chloride penetration depth of only 14.9 mm, representing a 57% reduction compared to the F/Si gel system. Its DRCM value was 4.91×10^{-12} m^2/s, 63.97% lower than F/Si, demonstrating a more effective limitation of chloride ion migration.
2. Chloride natural diffusion tests demonstrated that after 14, 28, and 56 days of immersion, SF/Si contained less free chloride across the full depth compared to F/Si. Within the 0–5 mm range, SF/Si's free chloride content was 0.121%, 0.225%, and

0.412%, corresponding to reductions of 55.35%, 50.10%, and 43.64% relative to F/Si. This indicates that the novel polymer–silicate composite gel system exhibits superior resistance to chloride penetration compared to the fluorocarbon–silicate gel system.

3. SEM images revealed that SF/Si exhibited fewer surface NaCl crystal precipitations and a slower hydration reaction, suggesting enhanced hydrophobicity. This effectively restricted chloride transport, allowing SF/Si to resist chloride penetration more efficiently than F/Si.
4. The incorporation of silane had minimal impact on the inherent acid and alkali resistance of the F/Si gel system, with SF/Si maintaining comparable performance to F/Si under acidic and alkaline conditions.
5. The incorporation of silane components decreased the compactness of the coating, resulting in a carbonation resistance slightly lower than that of the pure fluorocarbon coating. Nevertheless, according to the JGJ/T193-2009 standard, the 28-day carbonation depth of SF/Si (4.82 mm) still corresponds to Class T-IV, indicating a satisfactory engineering performance.

This study verified the effectiveness of the silane–fluorocarbon composite system in improving the chloride ion resistance of concrete, providing a feasible technical approach for enhancing the durability of concrete structures under harsh environments. From a lifecycle perspective, the fluorocarbon component, due to its excellent chemical stability and dense film-forming characteristics, can significantly extend the service life of structures and reduce maintenance frequency, which has positive significance for engineering sustainability. However, as a recalcitrant material, fluoropolymers still face certain controversies regarding their environmental sustainability. Therefore, under the premise of maintaining protective performance, further research on reducing the fluorocarbon content or using alternative green resins (such as waterborne acrylic and waterborne epoxy resins) is necessary for the effective application of the protective system in this study. At the same time, a comprehensive assessment of the lifecycle performance of the coating system, including durability, sustainability, and environmental impact, should be conducted to provide theoretical support for the development of future green concrete protective materials from the perspectives of service performance and ecological benefits.

4. Materials and Methods

4.1. Experimental Materials

The cement used in this study was ordinary Portland cement (P·O 42.5) produced by China Resources Cement Co., Ltd., China. River sand with a fineness modulus of 2.8, sourced from Xinyang, Henan, China, was used as the fine aggregate. A silane emulsion was supplied by Henan Juyan Co., Ltd., China. The fluorocarbon emulsion was prepared following the formulation provided by Henan Juyan Co., Ltd., with the main raw material composition summarized in Table 6. All water used in the experiments was obtained from the laboratory.

Table 6. Fluorocarbon component main raw material ratio.

Name	Dosage (g)	Mass Fraction (%)
Deionized water	90	30
Hydroxyethyl cellulose	0.75	0.25
Dispersant	1.8	0.6
pH adjuster	0.45	0.15
Wetting agent	0.4	0.13
Antifreeze agent	3	1
Titanium dioxide R-699	60	20
Film-forming additive	11	3.67
Liquid Fluorocarbon	135	45

4.2. Preparation of Mortar Specimens

Following the guidelines outlined in the "Standard Test Method for Strength of Cement Mortar" (GB/T17971-2021) [56], two types of mortar specimens, Φ100 mm × 100 mm, 100 mm × 100 mm × 100 mm and 40 mm × 40 mm × 160 mm, were prepared and placed in a constant-temperature curing chamber for curing.

4.3. Preparation of Test Materials

The preparation process of the silane/fluorocarbon–silicate (SF/Si) gel system is illustrated in Figure 12: Deionized water was poured into a container, and a mixer was started. HEC was slowly added while stirring for 10 min to ensure full mixing with water. pH adjuster, dispersing agent, wetting agent, antifreezing agent, and titanium dioxide were sequentially added and stirred continuously for 40 min. Then, the film-forming aid and liquid fluoropolymer were added and stirred for another 10 min. Finally, a thickener, biocide, 0.3% carbon black pigment, and defoamer were added and stirred for 10 min to form a fluorocarbon emulsion. Silane emulsion and fluorocarbon emulsion were weighed at a mass ratio of 1:3 and thoroughly stirred for 3 min to obtain the silane-modified fluorocarbon coating. The resulting coating was evenly applied to the surface of cement mortar specimens to form the SF/Si gel system. For comparison, a fluorocarbon emulsion was applied to the specimens to prepare the fluorocarbon–silicate (F/Si) gel system.

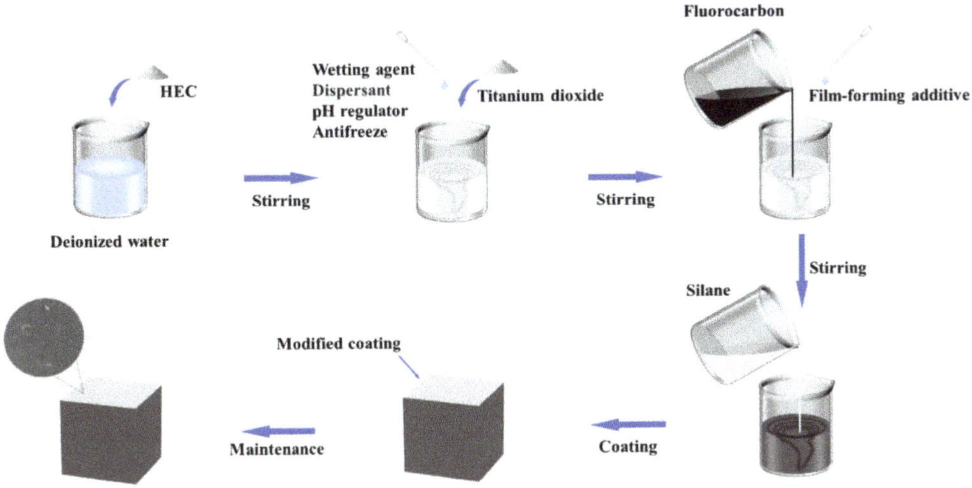

Figure 12. Preparation process of silane/fluorocarbon–silicate gel system.

4.4. Test Method

4.4.1. RCM Test

Following the guidelines specified in the "Standard Test Method for Long-Term Performance and Durability of Ordinary Concrete" (GB/T50082-2009) [57], the rapid chloride migration (RCM) method was employed to determine the chloride penetration depth and migration coefficient in mortar. The specimens were placed in a vacuum saturation apparatus (VJH, Beijing Kangluda Experimental Instrument Co., Ltd., Beijing, China). Vacuum saturation was conducted at 0.013 MPa for 3 h, followed by a pressure saturation for 1 h and subsequent immersion for 18 h, resulting in a total saturation duration of 22 h. After saturation, the specimens were removed, surface moisture was wiped off, and the specimens were mounted on a rapid chloride migration (RCM) apparatus (RCM-6, Beijing Kangluda Experimental Instrument Co., Ltd., Beijing, China). The anode compartment was filled with 0.3 mol/L NaOH solution, while the cathode contained 10 wt% NaCl solution. An initial current was measured at 30 V to determine the appropriate voltage for the subsequent test. The applied voltage was then adjusted based on the measured initial current, and the test duration was determined accordingly.

4.4.2. Chloride Ion Natural Erosion Test

The specimens with dimensions of 100 mm × 100 mm × 100 mm were immersed in a 3.5% NaCl solution for 14, 28, and 56 days, with the solution replaced every 7 days. After the designated immersion period, the specimens were removed, and surface residual moisture was wiped off. Powder samples were collected by drilling at the test surface, with sampling conducted every 5 mm up to a depth of 60 mm. After drying, the powder samples were analyzed using a rapid chloride ion content tester (CLU-H, Beijing Kangluda Experimental Instrument Co., Ltd., Beijing, China) to determine the free chloride ion content (mass fraction of chloride ions relative to the specimen powder).

4.4.3. Acid and Alkali Corrosion Test

The 5% H_2SO_4 and 5% NaOH solutions were prepared, and mortar specimens with dimensions of 40 mm × 40 mm × 160 mm were immersed in the corresponding solutions. At 5, 10, 15, 20, 25, and 30 days of immersion, the specimens were removed, surface residues were cleaned, and the specimens were wiped dry. The visual condition and damage of each specimen were inspected, and the specimen mass was measured. Subsequently, the flexural strength was tested using a universal testing machine (DYE-600S-20, Wuxi Construction Testing Instrument Manufacturing Co., Ltd., Wuxi, China), and the two halves resulting from the flexural test were further used for compressive strength testing. A constant loading rate of 1500 N/s was applied until failure. The ultimate load at failure (N_u) was recorded, and the compressive strength was calculated using the conversion factor $K = 1.35$, thereby converting the strength of non-standard specimens to the equivalent standard cubic compressive strength [58].

4.4.4. Carbonation Test

The carbonation test was conducted according to the "Standard for Test Methods of Long-term Performance and Durability of Ordinary Concrete" GB/T 50082-2009 [57]. The test specimens included SF/Si, F/Si, and a blank control group, each in the form of 100 mm × 100 mm × 100 mm mortar cubes. All specimens were placed in a carbonation chamber (CCB-70, Beijing Kangluda Experimental Instrument Co., Ltd., Beijing, China) and subjected to accelerated carbonation under conditions of CO_2 concentration of (20 ± 3)%, relative humidity of (70 ± 5)%, and temperature of (20 ± 2) °C.

4.5. Statistical Analysis

All quantitative experimental data were subjected to statistical analysis, following the procedures below:

(1) Data presentation

All data are presented as mean ± standard deviation, with the number of replicates for each experimental group $n = 3$.

(2) Homogeneity of variance test

Prior to performing analysis of variance, Levene's test was used to verify the homogeneity of variances. All datasets satisfied the homogeneity assumption ($p > 0.05$).

(3) Significance tests

One-way analysis of variance (one-way ANOVA) was used to compare the differences in chloride migration coefficients among the control group, the fluorocarbon-coated group, and the silane-fluorocarbon composite-coated group.

Two-way analysis of variance (two-way ANOVA) was employed to compare differences in free chloride content, mass loss, and compressive strength loss under acid-base exposure among the same three groups.

Post-hoc Tukey HSD tests were performed to compare the specific differences between the two coating systems and the control group under each experimental condition, evaluating the extent to which the coatings improved mortar performance.

All statistical analyses were performed using Excel 2021 (Microsoft Corp., Redmond, WA, USA), along with SPSS Statistics 26.0 (IBM Corp., Armonk, NY, USA) for the ANOVA and post-hoc tests.

(4) Significance level

The significance level was set at $\alpha = 0.05$, and $p < 0.05$. was considered statistically significant. The raw experimental data are provided in the Supplementary Materials.

Supplementary Materials: The following supporting information can be downloaded at: https://www.mdpi.com/article/10.3390/gels11120936/s1, Table S1: Levene's Test and ANOVA results. Table S2: Post Hoc test.

Author Contributions: Conceptualization, T.Z. and Z.H.; Methodology, T.Z.; Validation, S.R., C.H. and W.D.; Formal analysis, Y.D. and C.H.; Investigation, Y.D., S.R., C.H. and W.D.; Resources, Z.H.; Writing—original draft, Y.D.; Writing—review & editing, T.Z. and Z.H.; Visualization, Y.D. and S.R.; Supervision, T.Z.; Project administration, S.R.; Funding acquisition, T.Z. and Z.H. All authors have read and agreed to the published version of the manuscript.

Funding: This research received no external funding.

Institutional Review Board Statement: Not applicable.

Informed Consent Statement: Not applicable.

Data Availability Statement: The original contributions presented in this study are included in the article. Further inquiries can be directed to the corresponding author.

Conflicts of Interest: The authors declare that they have no known competing financial interests or personal relationships that could have appeared to influence the work reported in this paper.

References

1. Fenaux, M.; Reyes, E.; Galvez, J.C.; Moragues, A. Modelling the transport of chloride and other ions in cement-based materials. *Cem. Concr. Compos.* **2019**, *97*, 33–42. [CrossRef]
2. Qu, F.; Li, W.; Dong, W.; Tam, V.W.Y.; Yu, T. Durability deterioration of concrete under marine environment from material to structure: A critical review. *J. Build. Eng.* **2021**, *35*, 102074. [CrossRef]
3. Liao, J.; Wang, Y.; Wang, Y.; Lai, X. Preparation and evaluation of TA/APTES-HDTMS hydrophobic nanocomposite coating for enhancing corrosion resistance of concrete. *Constr. Build. Mater.* **2023**, *408*, 133792. [CrossRef]
4. Glasser, F.P.; Marchand, J.; Samson, E. Durability of concrete—Degradation phenomena involving detrimental chemical reactions. *Cem. Concr. Res.* **2008**, *38*, 226–246. [CrossRef]
5. Michel, A.; Otieno, M.; Stang, H.; Geiker, M.R. Propagation of steel corrosion in concrete: Experimental and numerical investigations. *Cem. Concr. Compos.* **2016**, *70*, 171–182. [CrossRef]
6. Peng, J.; Hu, S.; Zhang, J.; Cai, C.S.; Li, L. Influence of cracks on chloride diffusivity in concrete: A five-phase mesoscale model approach. *Constr. Build. Mater.* **2019**, *197*, 587–596. [CrossRef]
7. Rodrigues, R.; Gaboreau, S.; Gance, J.; Ignatiadis, I.; Betelu, S. Reinforced concrete structures: A review of corrosion mechanisms and advances in electrical methods for corrosion monitoring. *Constr. Build. Mater.* **2021**, *269*, 121240. [CrossRef]
8. Zhang, A.; Wang, Y.; Wang, H. Preparation of inorganic-polymer nano-emulsion inhibitor for corrosion resistance of steel reinforcement for concrete. *Alex. Eng. J.* **2023**, *66*, 537–542. [CrossRef]

9. Guo, S.-Y.; Luo, H.-H.; Tan, Z.; Chen, J.-Z.; Zhang, L.; Ren, J. Impermeability and interfacial bonding strength of TiO_2-graphene modified epoxy resin coated OPC concrete. *Prog. Org. Coat.* **2021**, *151*, 106029. [CrossRef]
10. Dorado, F.; Toledo, L.; de la Osa, A.R.; Esteban-Arranz, A.; Sacristan, J.; Pellegrin, B.; Steck, J.; Sanchez-Silva, L. Adhesion enhancement and protection of concrete against aggressive environment using graphite-Fe_2O_3 modified epoxy coating. *Constr. Build. Mater.* **2023**, *379*, 131179. [CrossRef]
11. Duan, Y.; Zhao, Y.; Liu, J.; Chen, B.; Zhao, Q.; Li, J.; Sun, Y.; Ma, X. Preparation of Fluorine—Containing Acrylate Coatings and Its Application in Concrete Protection. *Paint Coat. Ind.* **2016**, *46*, 72–77.
12. Sassani, A.; Arabzadeh, A.; Ceylan, H.; Kim, S.; Gopalakrishnan, K.; Taylor, P.C.; Nahvi, A. Polyurethane-carbon microfiber composite coating for electrical heating of concrete pavement surfaces. *Heliyon* **2019**, *5*, e02359. [CrossRef] [PubMed]
13. Ajir, K.; Toufigh, V.; Ghaemian, M. Protecting ordinary cement concrete against acidic and alkaline attacks utilizing epoxy resin coating. *Constr. Build. Mater.* **2025**, *472*, 141003. [CrossRef]
14. Vipulanandan, C.; Parihar, A.; Issac, M. Testing and Modeling Composite Coatings with Silanes for Protecting Reinforced Concrete in Saltwater Environment. *J. Mater. Civ. Eng.* **2011**, *23*, 1602–1608. [CrossRef]
15. Pan, X.; Shi, Z.; Shi, C.; Ling, T.-C.; Li, N. A review on surface treatment for concrete—Part 2: Performance. *Constr. Build. Mater.* **2017**, *133*, 81–90. [CrossRef]
16. Almusallam, A.; Khan, F.; Dulaijan, S.; Al-Amoudi, O. Effectiveness of surface coatings in improving concrete durability. *Cem. Concr. Compos.* **2003**, *25*, 473–481. [CrossRef]
17. Vipulanandan, C.; Liu, J. Performance of polyurethane-coated concrete in sewer environment. *Cem. Concr. Res.* **2005**, *35*, 1754–1763. [CrossRef]
18. Merah, A.; Khenfer, M.M.; Korichi, Y. The effect of industrial coating type acrylic and epoxy resins on the durability of concrete subjected to accelerated carbonation. *J. Adhes. Sci. Technol.* **2015**, *29*, 2446–2460. [CrossRef]
19. Zheng, Y.; Mao, Q.J.; Wang, Y.L.; Wang, Z.M.; Cui, S.P. Study on the influence of painting processes on the protective property of concrete coating. In Proceedings of the 3rd Mainland, Taiwan and Hong Kong Conference on Green Building Materials, Wuhan, China, 25–27 November 2011; pp. 88–92.
20. Li, G.; Hu, W.; Cui, H.; Zhou, J. Long-term effectiveness of carbonation resistance of concrete treated with nano-SiO_2 modified polymer coatings. *Constr. Build. Mater.* **2019**, *201*, 623–630. [CrossRef]
21. Hong, Z.; Jiang, H.; Xue, M.; Ke, C.; Luo, Y.; Yin, Z.; Xie, C.; Zhang, F.; Xing, Y. SiC-enhanced polyurethane composite coatings with excellent anti-fouling, mechanical, thermal, chemical properties on various substrates. *Prog. Org. Coat.* **2022**, *168*, 106909. [CrossRef]
22. Li, W.; Liao, X.; Ji, T.; Wu, S. Effects of Fluorocarbon Coating on Resistance to Chloride Ion Penetration of Concrete in Marine Environment. *Surf. Technol.* **2017**, *46*, 43–47. [CrossRef]
23. Pan, Y.; Zhou, R.; Zhu, X.; Zhao, B.; Li, W. Development of Elastic Fluorocarbon Coatings for Concrete Structures in Marine Environment. *Paint Coat. Ind.* **2019**, *49*, 27–32. [CrossRef]
24. Cai, Y.; Hou, P.; Duan, C.; Zhang, R.; Zhou, Z.; Cheng, X.; Shah, S. The use of tetraethyl orthosilicate silane (TEOS) for surface-treatment of hardened cement-based materials: A comparison study with normal treatment agents. *Constr. Build. Mater.* **2016**, *117*, 144–151. [CrossRef]
25. Moradllo, M.K.; Sudbrink, B.; Ley, M.T. Determining the effective service life of silane treatments in concrete bridge decks. *Constr. Build. Mater.* **2016**, *116*, 121–127. [CrossRef]
26. Sudbrink, B.; Moradllo, M.K.; Hu, Q.; Ley, M.T.; Davis, J.M.; Materer, N.; Apblett, A. Imaging the presence of silane coatings in concrete with micro X-ray fluorescence. *Cem. Concr. Res.* **2017**, *92*, 121–127. [CrossRef]
27. Hou, D.; Wu, C.; Yin, B.; Hua, X.; Xu, H.; Wang, X.; Li, S.; Zhou, Y.; Jin, Z.; Xu, W.; et al. Investigation of composite silane emulsion modified by in-situ functionalized graphene oxide for cement-based materials. *Constr. Build. Mater.* **2021**, *304*, 124662. [CrossRef]
28. Jiang, J.; Li, S.; Shen, J.; Hu, J.; Geng, Y.; Hou, D.; Wang, M.; Yuan, M.; Shi, J. Microscopic mechanism of corrosion inhibition in cementitious materials by silane coatings in sulfuric acid: Experimental and theoretical insights. *Constr. Build. Mater.* **2025**, *471*, 140751. [CrossRef]
29. Zhu, Y.; Chen, Y.; Gan, W. Effects of organism silanes on anti-corrosion properties of high-performance marine concrete. *Concrete* **2007**, *30*, 77–80.
30. Li, S.; Zhang, W.; Liu, J.; Hou, D.; Geng, Y.; Chen, X.; Gao, Y.; Jin, Z.; Yin, B. Protective Mechanism of Silane on Concrete upon Marine Exposure. *Coatings* **2019**, *9*, 558. [CrossRef]
31. Aguiar, J.B.; Junior, C. Carbonation of surface protected concrete. *Constr. Build. Mater.* **2013**, *49*, 478–483. [CrossRef]
32. Szubert, K.; Wojciechowski, J.; Karasiewicz, J.; Maciejewski, H.; Lota, G. Corrosion-protective coatings based on fluorocarbosilane. *Prog. Org. Coat.* **2018**, *123*, 374–383. [CrossRef]
33. Gonzalez-Coneo, J.; Zarzuela, R.; Luna, M.; Mosquera, M. Water-soluble fluorosilane supplemented with fumed silica as admixture for producing hydrophobic concrete: Effects on cement hydration, mechanical properties and water protection properties. *Dev. Built Environ.* **2024**, *17*, 100317. [CrossRef]

34. Szubert, K.; Dutkiewicz, A.; Nowicki, M.; Maciejewski, H. Fluorocarbosilane-Based Protective Coatings for Concrete. *Materials* **2022**, *15*, 5994. [CrossRef] [PubMed]
35. Boutamart, M.; Rafqah, S.; Hadri, A.; Nouneh, K.; Zaidi, S.; Bichara, H.; Briche, S. Design of fluorine-free superhydrophobic coating for fibred architectonic concrete. *Constr. Build. Mater.* **2024**, *425*, 136086. [CrossRef]
36. Ibrahim, A.; Bassuoni, M.; Carroll, J.; Ghazy, A. Performance of concrete superficially treated with nano-modified coatings under sulfuric acid exposures. *J. Build. Eng.* **2024**, *86*, 108957. [CrossRef]
37. Huang, H.; Fang, S.; Luo, S.; Hu, J.; Yin, S.; Wei, J.; Yu, Q. Multiscale modification on acrylic resin coating for concrete with silicon/fluorine and graphene oxide (GO) nanosheets. *Constr. Build. Mater.* **2021**, *305*, 124297. [CrossRef]
38. Pramualkijja, W.; Jiratumnukul, N. The preparation of hydrophobic hybrid film coatings from siloxane-modified polyacrylate associated with nano-fumed silica and organo-modified clay. *J. Coat. Technol. Res.* **2022**, *19*, 1467–1492. [CrossRef]
39. Tian, J.; Li, Y.; Yang, G.; Su, M.; Yang, Z. Silane-nanoSiO_2 composite surface modification of steel fibres: A multiscale experimental study of fibre-UHPC interfaces. *Compos. Part B Eng.* **2026**, *308*, 112999. [CrossRef]
40. Liu, W.; Song, J.; Zhao, H.; Cui, Z.; Zhang, S.; Qiao, Y.; Cao, C.; Li, W. Mechanically stable and superhydrophobic nano-SiO_2@silane/silicate coating for enhanced impermeability of mortar. *Constr. Build. Mater.* **2025**, *470*, 140541. [CrossRef]
41. Ji, Y.; Wendt, K.; Pel, L.; Stephan, D. Insights into Cl-binding and phase evolution during the early hydration of cement pastes prepared with NaCl solutions: A study using high-field NMR and in situ XRD. *Cem. Concr. Compos.* **2025**, *164*, 106266. [CrossRef]
42. Pramanik, S.; Bhuiyan, M.; Robert, D.; Roychand, R.; Gao, L.; Cole, I.; Pramanik, B. Functional Polymer-Clay Composite Coating for Corrosion Protection in Concrete Sewer Structures. *ACS Appl. Eng. Mater.* **2025**, *3*, 2979–2994. [CrossRef]
43. Liu, J.; Wu, L.; Zhu, J.; Jia, H.; Liu, L.; Zhang, S.; Yang, C.; Chen, Z.; Shi, C. Effect of silica fume on corrosion resistance of cement-based materials under carbonic acid water environment. *Cem. Concr. Compos.* **2025**, *157*, 105949. [CrossRef]
44. Zheng, Y.; Zhong, H.; Sun, K.; Shen, B.; Cui, K.; Zhao, Y.; Xiong, G.; Qin, Q. Effect of composite activator on hydration kinetics and micromechanical properties of alkali-activated slag. *Cem. Concr. Compos.* **2025**, *160*, 106047. [CrossRef]
45. Leemann, A. Alkali-silica reaction—The mechanism leading to concrete deterioration. *Can. J. Civ. Eng.* **2025**, *52*, 1615–1629. [CrossRef]
46. Thissen, P.; Bogner, A.; Dehn, F. Surface treatments on concrete: An overview on organic, inorganic and nano-based coatings and an outlook about surface modification by rare-earth oxides. *RSC Sustain.* **2024**, *2*, 2092–2124. [CrossRef]
47. Nguyen, M.; Nakarai, K. An enhanced air permeability model based on stable moisture conditions for nondestructive durability assessment. *Mater. Struct.* **2025**, *58*, 164. [CrossRef]
48. Mottl, M.; Pazderka, J.; Reiterman, P. Crystalline Coating and Its Influence on Chloride Ion Diffusion Resistance of Carbonated Concrete. *Coatings* **2025**, *15*, 163. [CrossRef]
49. *JGJ/T193-2009*; Standard for Inspection and Assessment of Concrete Durability. Ministry of Housing and Urban-Rural Development of the People's Republic of China: Beijing, China, 2009.
50. Zhang, J.-Z.; Buenfeld, N. Chloride profiles in surface-treated mortar specimens. *Constr. Build. Mater.* **2000**, *14*, 359–364. [CrossRef]
51. Aguiar, J.; Camoes, A.; Moreira, P. Coatings for concrete protection against aggressive environments. *J. Adv. Concr. Technol.* **2008**, *6*, 243–250. [CrossRef]
52. Schueremans, L.; Van Gemert, D.; Giessler, S. Chloride penetration in RC-structures in marine environment—Long term assessment of a preventive hydrophobic treatment. *Constr. Build. Mater.* **2007**, *21*, 1238–1249. [CrossRef]
53. Lo, T.; Liao, W.; Wong, C.; Tang, W. Evaluation of carbonation resistance of paint coated concrete for buildings. *Constr. Build. Mater.* **2016**, *107*, 299–306. [CrossRef]
54. Qu, H.; Feng, M.; Li, M.; Tian, D.; Zhang, Y.; Chen, X.; Li, G. Enhancing the carbonation and chloride resistance of concrete by nano-modified eco-friendly water-based organic coatings. *Mater. Today Commun.* **2023**, *37*, 107284. [CrossRef]
55. Ibrahim, M.; Al-Gahtani, A.; Maslehuddin, M.; Dakhil, F. Use of surface treatment materials to improve concrete durability. *J. Mater. Civ. Eng.* **1999**, *11*, 36–40. [CrossRef]
56. *GB/T 17671-2021*; Test Method of Cement Mortar Strength (ISO Method). National Standardizationc Administration: Beijing, China, 2021.
57. *GB/T 50082-2009*; Standard for Test Methods of Long-Term Performance and Durability of Ordinary Concrete. Ministry of Housing and Urban-Rural Development of the People's Republic of China: Beijing, China, 2009.
58. *JGJT70-2009*; Standard for Test Method of Basic Properties of Construction Mortar. Ministry of Housing and Urban-Rural Development of the People's Republic of China: Beijing, China, 2009.

gels

MDPI

Article

Investigation of Toughening Mechanism of Virgin Asphalt by Blending with Waste Battery Powder

Chenze Fang [1,2,3,4,†], Xu Guo [1,†], Yuanzhao Chen [1,2,3,4,*], Hui Li [5,*], Naisheng Guo [6], Zhenxia Li [1,2,3,4], Zongyuan Wu [1], Jingyu Yang [1,2,3,4] and Tengteng Guo [1,2,3,4]

1 School of Civil Engineering and Transportation, North China University of Water Resources and Electric Power, Zhengzhou 450045, China; fangchenze@126.com (C.F.); gx20032025@126.com (X.G.); zhenxiali2009@ncwu.edu.cn (Z.L.); wuzongyuan@ncwu.edu.cn (Z.W.); yangjingyu@ncwu.edu.cn (J.Y.); guotth@ncwu.edu.cn (T.G.)

2 Electric Power-Henan Provincial Institute of Transportation Planning and Design Co., Ltd., Green, Low Carbon, and High Performance Road Materials Research and Development Center, North China University of Water Resources, Zhengzhou 450045, China

3 Technology Innovation Center of Henan Transport Industry of Utilization of Solid Waste Resources in Trafffc Engineering, North China University of Water Resources and Electric Power, Zhengzhou 450045, China

4 Henan Province Engineering Technology Research Center of Environment Friendly and High-Performance Pavement Materials, Zhengzhou 450045, China

5 Department of Transportation, Southeast University, Nanjing 210096, China

6 Department of Transportation Engineering, Dalian Maritime University, Dalian 116026, China; naishengguo@126.com

* Correspondence: cyz740513@ncwu.edu.cn (Y.C.); huili94@seu.edu.cn (H.L.)

† These authors contributed equally to this work.

Abstract

Waste battery powder (WBP) can effectively enhance the service performance of virgin asphalt with sol–gel structures; however, its toughening mechanism for sol–gel virgin asphalt still lacks rigorous mechanical characterization. Therefore, the objective of this study is to investigate the toughening of WBP-modified asphalt based on the mechanical parameter of cracking area. First, a 12% content of WBP was incorporated into the sol–gel 70# virgin asphalt to prepare WBP-modified asphalt and its fatigue performance was evaluated through linear amplitude, non-damage, and damage time sweep tests. Then, energy–mechanics balance equations were used to establish a cracking area model. Furthermore, the asphalt cracking area was employed to quantify its induced damage and determine the representative rate for the cracking damage process (k_{cd}). Finally, the activation energy for cracking damage (E_{acd}) was used to quantify the difficulty of the cracking damage process. The scanning electron microscope test was employed to examine the microstructure of WBP-modified asphalt and the E_{acd} and microscopic morphology of WBP-modified asphalt were analyzed to reveal the toughening effect of WBP on virgin asphalt. The results showed that WBP-modified asphalt exhibits three nonlinear cracking stages, with a lower cracking rate than virgin asphalt. Its cracking damage generally increases over time, and the damage evolution parameter β serves as k_{cd}. The micro-grooves and wrinkles of WBP improve bonding to asphalt, increasing the E_{acd} of sol–gel 70# virgin asphalt from 10.6 to 23.88 kJ·mol^{-1}, thus achieving toughening. In summary, the fatigue damage process of WBP-modified asphalt can be characterized by the kinetic parameters β and E_{acd}.

Keywords: road engineering; waste battery powder; asphalt toughening; cracking area; damage variables; activation energy

https://doi.org/10.3390/gels12020117

1. Introduction

The rapid development of new energy battery technology has significantly improved people's living standards. However, the issue of discarded batteries as household waste has increasingly troubled people's daily lives. According to incomplete statistics, over 95% of used batteries globally are treated as solid waste through incineration and landfill disposal, resulting in significant pollution to watershed soils, groundwater, and the ecological environment in 2024 [1–3]. Scientifically applying waste battery resources to transportation infrastructure construction can effectively promote the high-value utilization of waste battery resources and the development of low-carbon building material technologies.

According to classical colloid theory, conventional virgin asphalt without modified additives typically exhibits characteristic sol–gel structural features, which ensure its excellent high-temperature stability and low-temperature crack resistance. Its large-scale production and application in road engineering can reasonably be regarded as a key approach for the treatment and utilization of waste batteries [4–6]. The enhancement of asphalt material performance by the components of waste battery materials has been confirmed by many scholars. In general, the related asphalt modifiers can be categorized into two types. The corresponding first type of asphalt modifier is carbon materials [7–9]. Jiang et al. [10] described high-temperature pyrolysis and demonstrated that the high-temperature pyrolysis of waste tires can produce high-quality carbon black. Feng et al. [11] investigated the preparation process of the conductive asphalt mixture and proved that carbon fiber added to the mixture can reduce its deformation under loading. He et al. [12–14] evaluated the road performance of graphene-modified asphalt and the results showed that graphene can significantly improve the high-temperature stability of asphalt. However, as a modifier, graphene is prone to agglomeration and has a high manufacturing cost. The corresponding second type of asphalt modifier is metal oxide materials [15–17]. Zhu et al. [18] found that manganese dioxide improved the microwave heating performance more effectively than magnetite powder. Zhao et al. [19,20] developed a novel approach for value-added recycling of wood waste by constructing porous carbon structures (Pc-S) on aggregate surfaces. Compared to basalt materials, the carbon-modified granite produced via this method exhibits enhanced interfacial bonding properties, resulting in an over 78.9% improvement in resistance to water ingress. In summary, asphalt performance can be enhanced by the carbon materials and metal oxides in waste battery powder.

The above studies have extracted single-component materials from waste batteries with complex compositions for preparing modified asphalt, which is a complicated process [21–23] and obviously not easy to realize. Therefore, Fan [24] used the whole waste battery powder (WBP) as a modifier and verified the feasibility of preparing modified asphalt using whole waste battery powder. Based on rheological performance analysis, the optimal addition of the WBP was recommended to be 9%. Meng et al. [25,26] demonstrated that asphalt can exhibit a significant encapsulation effect on heavy metals in the WBP, effectively preventing pollution caused by the leaching of heavy metals. Meng et al. [27] employed microscopic techniques, including FTIR and SEM, and found that the carbon in WBP exhibited relatively high crystallinity and content. The incorporation of WBP enhanced the bond energy of the methylene groups, thereby strengthening the molecular interactions between the asphalt and WBP and consequently improving the pavement performance of the modified asphalt. In addition, the grooves and wrinkles observed on the microscopic surface of WBP were analyzed and confirmed to enhance the bonding strength between aggregates and asphalt effectively. In summary, WBP can be used as a safe and effective asphalt modifier.

Although the aforementioned studies have demonstrated that asphalt materials can serve as an effective carrier for recycling waste batteries, most of the related studies have

https://doi.org/10.3390/gels12020117

focused on the effect of waste battery powder materials on the asphalt's rheological behavior, particularly lacking systematic mechanical characterization of the cracking damage behavior of the asphalt modified by waste battery powder materials under cyclic loading. Furthermore, the damage variable definition methods based on traditional phenomenological indicators (such as modulus and strength attenuation) lack rigorous mechanical derivation [28], making it difficult to characterize the significant differences in mechanical response between damaged and undamaged asphalt, and challenging to accurately define the damage variables of waste battery material-modified asphalt. This results in a lack of scientifically rigorous mechanical explanations for the toughening mechanism of the WBP on virgin asphalt.

At the same time, the existing studies [29] indicate that the energy–mechanics method can accurately describe the damage behavior of asphalt in terms of its mechanical nature by establishing energy–mechanics equilibrium equations for damaged and undamaged asphalt. Given this, the objective of this study is to utilize the energy–mechanics method to derive a cracking area indicator with clear mechanical significance, and to investigate the toughening mechanism of the WBP on sol–gel virgin asphalt based on the cracking area. The significant contribution of this study lies in establishing a cracking-area-based damage model derived from energy–mechanical balance equations and further proposing a damage activation energy evaluation method based on kinetics theory, which provides a theoretical basis for extending the service life of asphalt pavements by utilizing waste battery resources. First, the energy–mechanics method was used to establish the cracking area model of WBP-modified asphalt for analyzing its cracking area response laws. Then, a damage model for the WBP-modified asphalt was developed to determine its representative rate for the cracking damage process (k_{cd}). Finally, the activation energy for cracking damage (E_{acd}) was used to quantify the difficulty of the cracking damage process, and the WBP's microscopic morphology and E_{acd} were utilized to analyze the toughening mechanism of WBP on sol–gel virgin asphalt.

2. Results and Discussion

2.1. Cracking Area Analysis of WBP-Modified Asphalt Based on Energy–Mechanics Method

2.1.1. Establishment of Asphalt Cracking Area Model Based on Energy–Mechanics Method

Figure 1 illustrates the asphalt specimen and its force distribution under cyclic shear loading. As shown in Figure 1a, the entire asphalt specimen (cylinder indicated by dashed lines) mainly consists of the crack-damaged asphalt section (annular region indicated by dashed and solid lines) and intact asphalt section (cylinder formed by solid lines) [30]. During loading, the crack-damaged asphalt propagates progressively from the outer periphery of the specimen toward its center.

The entire asphalt specimen and intact asphalt specimen are, respectively, referred to as the apparent asphalt and true asphalt and their mechanical responses are shown in Figure 1b. For the apparent asphalt during the cyclic shearing process, the stress and strain are shown in Equations (1) and (2).

$$\tau^A(t,r) = \tau_0^A(t_0,r)\sin(\omega t) \quad (1)$$

$$\gamma^A(t,r) = \gamma_0^A(t_0,r)\sin(\omega t - \delta) \quad (2)$$

where $\tau^A(t,r)$ and $\gamma^A(t,r)$ represent the stress and strain induced in the apparent asphalt, respectively; t denotes loading time; r denotes specimen radius length; t_0 denotes the initial time; $\tau_0^A(t_0,r)$ and $\gamma_0^A(t_0,r)$ denote shear stress amplitude and shear strain amplitude, respectively; ω denotes angular velocity; and δ denotes phase angle.

https://doi.org/10.3390/gels12020117

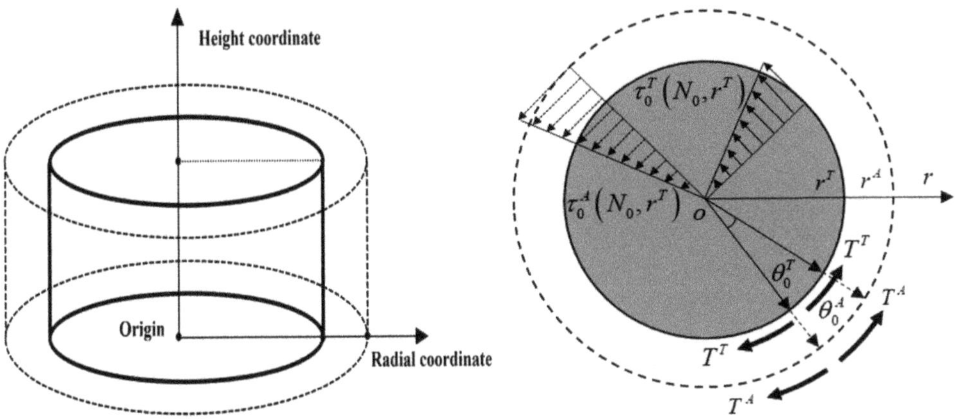

(**a**) Asphalt specimen (**b**) Mechanical response

Figure 1. Schematic diagrams of asphalt specimen and its mechanical response during cyclic loading process.

For the true asphalt during the cyclic shearing process, its stress and strain are expressed by Equations (3) and (4).

$$\tau^T(t,r) = \tau_0^T(t_0,r)\sin(\omega t) \tag{3}$$

$$\gamma^T(t,r) = \gamma_0^T(t_0,r)\sin(\omega t - \delta) \tag{4}$$

where $\tau^T(t,r)$ and $\tau_0^T(t_0,\mathbf{r})$ denote the shear stress and its amplitude in true asphalt, respectively; $\gamma^T(t,r)$ and $\gamma_0^T(t_0,r)$ denote the shear strain and its amplitude in true asphalt, respectively.

The energy–mechanics approach for establishing a cracking area model relies on two fundamental assumptions: First, the apparent asphalt consists of cracked asphalt and true asphalt. Second, an equilibrium exists between the true asphalt and apparent asphalt in terms of recoverable strain energy, dissipated strain energy, and torque. Although the crack-damaged asphalt can lead to significant differences in the mechanical response between true asphalt and apparent asphalt, relevant studies [26–28] indicate that the two exhibit energy–mechanical equilibrium equations in terms of recoverable strain energy, dissipated strain energy, and torque, as shown in Equations (5)–(7).

$$RSE^T = RSE^A \tag{5}$$

$$DSE^T = DSE^A \tag{6}$$

$$T^T = T^A \tag{7}$$

where RSE^T and RSE^A represent the recoverable strain energy of true asphalt and apparent asphalt, respectively; DSE^T and DSE^A represent the dissipated strain energy of true asphalt and apparent asphalt, respectively; T^T and T^A represent the torque of true asphalt and apparent asphalt, respectively.

By combining the three energy–mechanical equilibrium equations above, a cracking area model for asphalt can be derived, as shown in Equation (8). Equation (8) indicates that modulus decay can quantitatively reflect the cracking area of asphalt. Since the cracking

https://doi.org/10.3390/gels12020117

area provides an intuitive quantification of asphalt damage, this study will analyze the damage evolution of asphalt during repeated loading based on this cracking area model.

$$CA = \pi\left(r^A\right)^2\left\{1-\left[1-\left(1-G_r^{0.25}\right)^2\right]\right\} \tag{8}$$

where CA is the cracking area of the asphalt; r^A is the apparent asphalt radius, numerically equivalent to the radius of the entire asphalt specimen; G_r is the modulus ratio, numerically equal to the shear modulus corresponding to the apparent asphalt divided by that corresponding to the true asphalt.

According to the derived cracking area model shown in Equation (8), the cracking area results for WBP-modified and sol–gel 70# virgin asphalt are obtained, as depicted in Figure 2. It should be noted that the research subject, WBP-modified asphalt, in this paper refers to modified asphalt containing 12% waste battery powder, with its detailed preparation process described in Section 4.1.2. As observed in Figure 2, the cracking area curves of WBP-modified and sol–gel 70# virgin asphalt induced by cyclic loading exhibits the similar nonlinear cumulative trend under the intermediate temperatures of 15 °C, 20 °C, and 25 °C. A straightforward comparison between Figure 2a,b shows that, under identical temperature and stress conditions, WBP-modified asphalt exhibits a slower overall trend in crack area growth compared to virgin asphalt. This is particularly evident during the mid-to-late loading stages (corresponding to the second and third phases), where the crack area curve of the virgin asphalt remains below that of the virgin asphalt, indicating that the incorporation of waste battery powder can delay crack propagation.

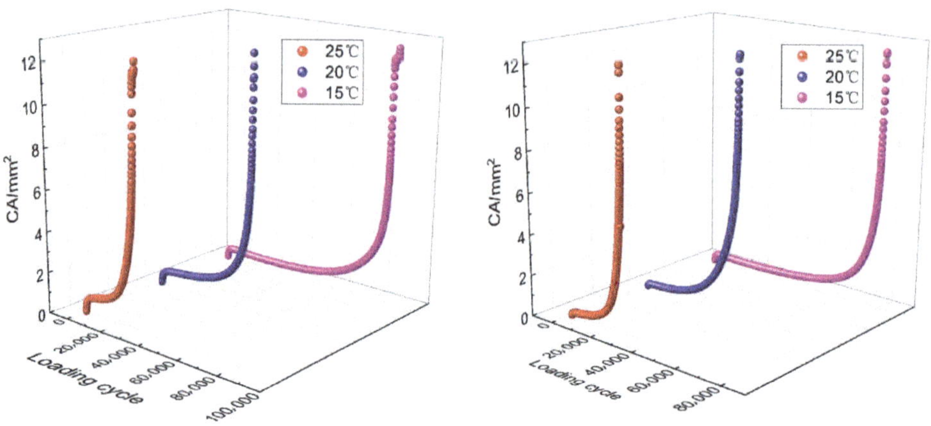

(**a**) WBP-modified asphalt (**b**) Sol–gel 70# virgin asphalt

Figure 2. Cracking area curves of tested asphalt.

2.1.2. Cracking Area Evolution Analysis of WBP-Modified Asphalt

To quantitatively analyze the evolution laws of cracking area in the WBP-modified asphalt, the rate of cracking area change ($RCAC$) is defined as shown in Equation (9). Based on Equations (8) and (9), the curve results of the cracking area and rate of cracking area change for WBP-modified and sol–gel 70# virgin asphalt are obtained, as shown in Figure 3.

$$RCAC = \frac{|CA_b - CA_a|}{CA_a(b-a)} \tag{9}$$

where $RCAC$ is rate of cracking area change; CA_a is cracking area of the asphalt in the a-th cycle; CA_b is the cracking area of the asphalt in the b-th cycle.

https://doi.org/10.3390/gels12020117

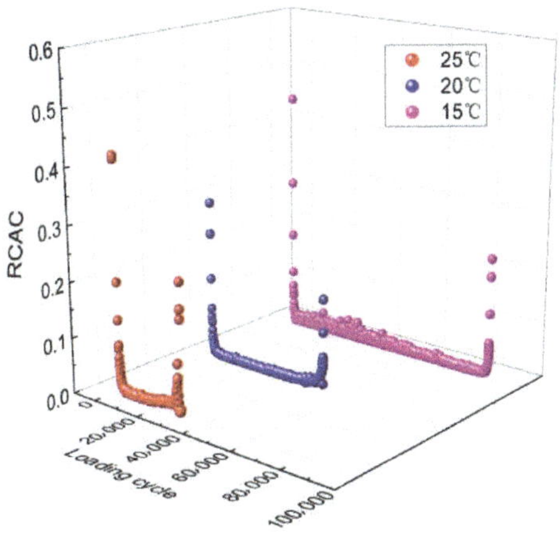

(a) WBP-modified asphalt

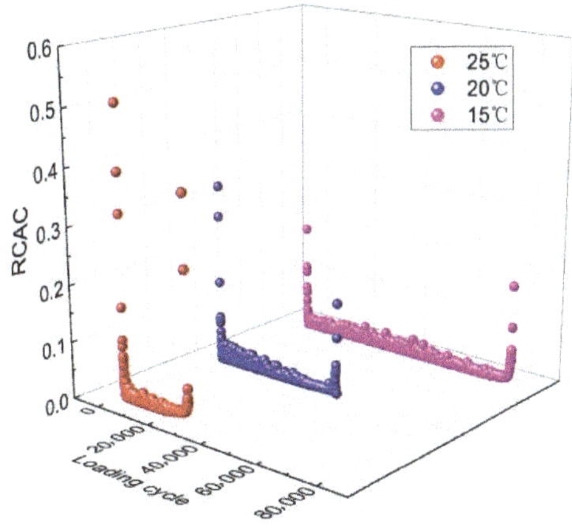

(b) Sol–gel 70# virgin asphalt

Figure 3. Curve results of cracking area and rate of cracking area change for WBP-modified asphalt.

As observed in Figure 3, the cracking area response of the WBP-modified and sol–gel 70# virgin asphalt can be divided into the first phase of sudden and rapid accumulation, the second phase of long-term constant speed fluctuation, and the third phase with a brief and rapid leap. During the first phase, the cracking area rapidly accumulates from 0 to a certain level of cracking area, but the rate of cracking area change gradually decreases. After the cracking area evolution enters the second phase, the cracking area continues to maintain a stable cumulative trend and the rate of cracking area change remains generally stable with slight fluctuations. At this phase, the WBP-modified and sol–gel 70# virgin asphalt exhibit stable crack resistance. During the final or third phase, the cracking area sharply accumulates and the rate of cracking area change rapidly increases. Finally, the WBP-modified and sol–gel 70# virgin asphalt nearly completely lose their cracking resistance and experience fatigue failure. The analysis above indicates that the rate of cracking area change can reflect the cracking resistance of the WBP-modified and sol–gel 70# virgin asphalt and that the two exhibit a negative correlation. Therefore, this study defines the loading cycle at the tangent intersection point corresponding to the second and third phases of the rate of cracking area change curves as the fatigue life. Compared to the WBP-modified asphalt, the RCAC curve of virgin asphalt enters the steeply rising third stage earlier. This phenomenon indicates that under identical cyclic loading, virgin asphalt loses its fatigue crack resistance more rapidly, thereby reaching fatigue failure sooner. In contrast, modified asphalt incorporating WBP delays the transition to the failure stage, exhibiting more enduring and stable crack resistance. This directly confirms that WBP incorporation effectively enhances the fatigue crack resistance of virgin asphalt.

The fatigue life results obtained through analysis of the rate of cracking area change are shown in Table 1. As indicated in Table 1, when the temperature–loading conditions are 15 °C–250 kPa, 20 °C–100 kPa, and 25 °C–80 kPa, the obtained fatigue life results corresponding to the sol–gel 70# virgin asphalt are 79,530, 45,140, and 25,890, respectively, which correspond to increased values for the WBP-modified asphalt of 87,880, 50,466, and 29,022, respectively. The average increase in asphalt fatigue life by waste battery powder is 11.5%, which indicates that waste battery powder added to sol–gel 70# virgin asphalt can delay the cracking process of asphalt and improve its service life. The above analysis indicates the waste battery powder exhibits a toughening effect on virgin asphalt, which is in good agreement with the results in references [24–27].

https://doi.org/10.3390/gels12020117

Table 1. Loading amplitudes and fatigue life of destructive time sweep test.

Asphalt Type	Temperature/°C	Loading Amplitude/kPa	Fatigue Life	Coefficients of Variation/%
Sol–gel 70# virgin asphalt	15	250	79,530	8.736
	20	100	45,140	8.698
	25	80	25,890	9.057
WBP-modified asphalt	15	250	87,880	11.468
	20	100	50,466	10.176
	25	80	29,022	10.797

2.2. Analysis of Representative Rate of Cracking Damage Process for WBP-Modified Asphalt

Compared to indirect indicators of asphalt damage, such as modulus decay and energy dissipation, the cracking area exhibits clear physical significance and quantifies the extent of asphalt damage. Therefore, this study defines the damage variable of WBP-modified and sol–gel 70# virgin asphalt as the ratio of the cracking area to the intact specimen area, as shown in Equation (10). It should be noted that damage variable definition methods based on traditional phenomenological indicators (such as modulus and strength attenuation) represent an indirect approach to quantifying damage, lacking rigorous mechanical derivation and a clear mechanical meaning. Damage definition methods based on crack area can directly quantify damage, thereby partially addressing these two shortcomings.

$$D = \frac{CA_N}{SA} \tag{10}$$

where D is the damage variable; CA_N is the specimen cracking area of the N-th cycle; SA is the intact area of the asphalt specimen, with a geometric size of r (radius) in this study, $SA = \pi(r^A)^2$.

The determined damage curve of WBP-modified and sol–gel 70# virgin asphalt using Equation (10) is shown in Figure 4. As observed in Figure 4, the damage of both WBP-modified and sol–gel 70# virgin asphalt produced by cyclic shear exhibits an overall evolution trend with increasing rate. The existing research indicates that dissipated energy evolution can be used to quantitatively describe asphalt damage evolution, as shown below:

$$\frac{dD}{dN} = \left(\frac{\partial W_N}{\partial N}\right)^{\beta} \tag{11}$$

where $\frac{dD}{dN}$ is the damage evolution; $\frac{\partial W_N}{\partial N}$ is the dissipated energy evolution; β is a material characteristic parameter that reflects the sensitivity of asphalt damage evolution to dissipated energy evolution. It should be noted that β quantifies the rate correlation between damage evolution and dissipated energy evolution: a larger β indicates that the asphalt damage process is more sensitive to the change of dissipated energy (i.e., a small change in dissipated energy will lead to a significant acceleration of damage); conversely, a smaller β means the damage evolution is less dependent on dissipated energy variation.

According to Equation (11), a damage model suitable for asphalt materials under cyclic loading can be derived, as shown in Equation (12) [31–34]. This damage model is used to match the damage curves of WBP-modified and sol–gel 70# virgin asphalt. The determined matching results are presented in Table 2 and Figure 4. As presented, the damage model expressed in Equation (12) can accurately capture the cracking damage process of WBP-modified and sol–gel 70# virgin asphalt under cyclic loading. Therefore, such a damage model will be used to quantitatively analyze the cracking damage process of WBP-modified and sol–gel 70# virgin asphalt.

https://doi.org/10.3390/gels12020117

$$D = 1 - \left(1 - \frac{N}{N_f}\right)^{\frac{1}{1+2\beta}} \tag{12}$$

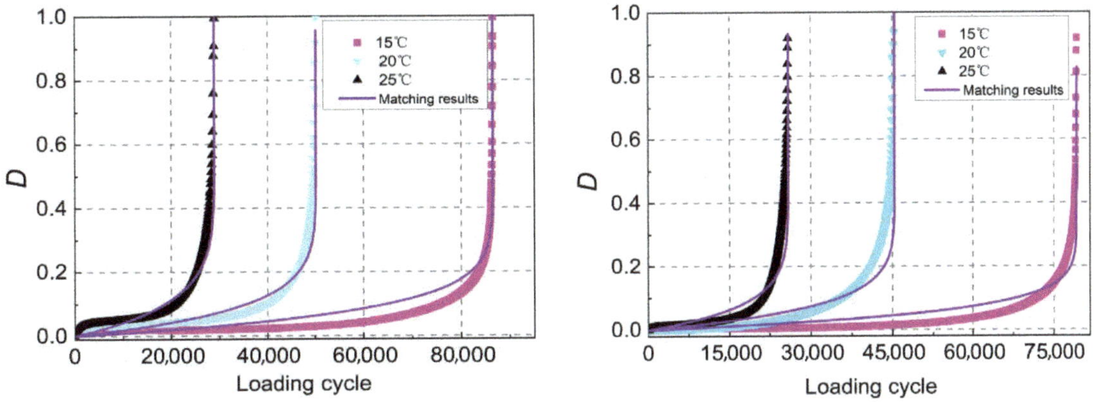

(**a**) WBP-modified asphalt (**b**) Sol–gel 70# virgin asphalt

Figure 4. Fatigue damage curves of WBP-modified and sol–gel 70# virgin asphalt.

Table 2. Matching results of damage model.

Asphalt	Temperature/°C	β	R^2
WBP-modified asphalt	15	6.14982	0.901
	20	5.38166	0.917
	25	4.40148	0.896
Sol–gel 70# virgin asphalt	15	7.11267	0.902
	20	6.55815	0.901
	25	6.13306	0.897

N_f refers to the total number of cyclic loading cycles when the asphalt specimen reaches the failure state.

The aforementioned cracking damage process is a complex rate-variable physical reaction. To quantify the corresponding reaction rate, taking the logarithm of Equation (13) yields the damage evolution equation in logarithmic coordinates, as shown below:

$$\ln\left(\frac{dD}{dN}\right) = \beta \ln\left(\frac{\partial W_N}{\partial N}\right) \tag{13}$$

Equation (13) reveals that $\ln\left(\frac{dD}{dN}\right)$ is linearly correlated with $\ln\left(\frac{\partial W_N}{\partial N}\right)$ and the corresponding slope is equal to β. This β can reflect the damage evolution rate of the material under specific operating conditions. As the fatigue life fraction increases from 0 to 1, damage gradually evolves toward the failure threshold. During this process, the damage results are output by $D = 1 - (1 - \frac{N}{N_f})^{\frac{1}{1+2\beta}}$ and are directly reflected by the β [30–32]. As illustrated in Tables 3 and 4, as the test temperature is sequentially decreased from 25 °C to 20 °C and then to 15 °C, both the β and N_f values for the WBP-modified and sol–gel 70# virgin asphalt exhibit an increasing trend. This indicates that lowering the temperature can delay the propagation rate of asphalt fatigue cracks and the overall rate for the cracking damage process of WBP-modified and sol–gel 70# virgin asphalt is positively correlated with β.

https://doi.org/10.3390/gels12020117

Table 3. Basic parameter indicators of sol–gel 70# virgin asphalt.

Indicators	Test Conditions	Results
Softening point/°C	135 °C	48
Viscosity/(m Pa·s)	-	27
Penetration/(0.1 mm)	25 °C	69

Table 4. Physical parameter indicators of WBP.

Technical Indices	Results
Specific surface area/($m^2 \cdot g^{-1}$)	0.045
Particle/mm	<0.075

2.3. Cracking Damage Activation Energy Analysis of WBP-Modified Asphalt

The representative rates for physical reaction processes at different temperatures can be accurately described by the *Arrhenius* kinetics equation, as shown in Equation (14) [35].

$$k = Ae^{\frac{-E_a}{RT}} \tag{14}$$

where k is the representative rate; E_a is the activation energy; A is a pre-exponential parameter factor; T is the absolute temperature; and R is a gas constant.

For the damage model shown in Equation (12), β can be utilized as the representative rate for asphalt cracking damage. By combining Equations (12) and (14), the kinetics model for asphalt cracking damage is obtained:

$$D = 1 - \left(1 - \frac{N}{N_f}\right)^{\frac{1}{1+2Ae^{\frac{-E_a}{RT}}}} \tag{15}$$

where E_a represents activation energy for cracking damage.

According to kinetics theory [35], the activation energy for cracking damage represents the minimum energy required for cracking damage to occur in asphalt. The higher its value, the higher the energy threshold for asphalt cracking damage, meaning the asphalt cracking process is less likely to occur. Therefore, the toughening effect of waste battery powder on sol–gel virgin asphalt can be characterized by comparing the activation energy differences between the WBP-modified and sol–gel 70# virgin asphalt during cracking damage.

To accurately obtain the activation energy for cracking damage in WBP-modified and sol–gel 70# virgin asphalt, the β at different temperatures were substituted into the *Arrhenius* kinetics equation in a double-logarithmic coordinate system as shown in Equation (16). The corresponding β were matched by Equation (16), as illustrated in Figure 5. It can be observed that the *Arrhenius* kinetics equation can accurately match the representative rates for the cracking damage of WBP-modified and sol–gel 70# virgin asphalt, further validating its effectiveness in quantifying the activation energy for cracking damage in WBP-modified and sol–gel 70# virgin asphalt. Taking the absolute value of the slope from the straight line in Figure 5 as the activation energy for cracking damage yields the results shown in Figure 5.

$$\ln\left(Ae^{\frac{-E_a}{RT}}\right) = \ln A - \frac{E_a}{RT} \tag{16}$$

As shown in Figure 6, the activation energy for cracking damage of sol–gel 70# virgin asphalt is 10.6 kJ·mol^{-1}, while that of the WBP-modified asphalt is 23.88 kJ·mol^{-1}. This indicates that the WBP-modified asphalt requires 13.28 kJ·mol^{-1} more energy than sol–gel 70# virgin asphalt to induce cracking damage. Thus, incorporating an appropriate amount of waste battery powder into sol–gel 70# virgin asphalt increases the difficulty of inducing

https://doi.org/10.3390/gels12020117

cracking damage and extends its service life. Analysis of the activation energy for cracking damage confirms that waste battery powder exhibits a toughening effect on virgin asphalt. Such results occur mainly because the microstructure of waste battery powder can increase the difficulty of asphalt cracking under cyclic loading by improving the bonding ability between the asphalt and waste battery powder.

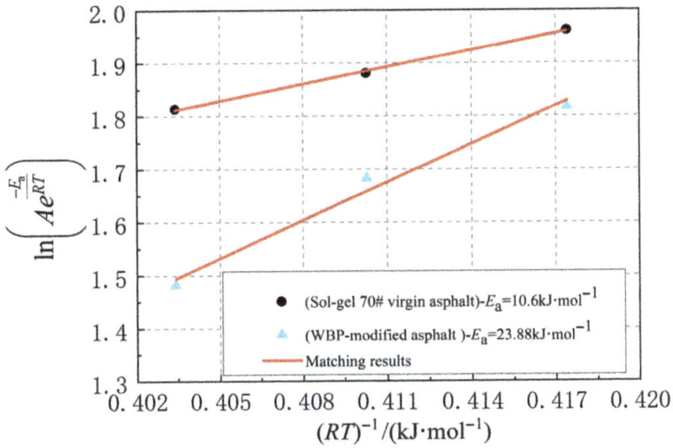

Figure 5. Representative rate for asphalt cracking damage.

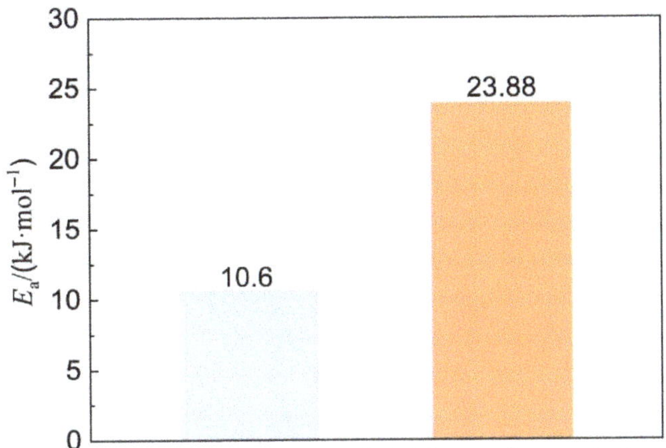

Figure 6. Activation energy for cracking damage.

2.4. Microscopic Morphology Analysis of Waste Battery Powder and WBP-Modified Asphalt

The microstructure of waste battery powder obtained from the SEM test is illustrated in Figure 7a–d. Figure 7a shows the relatively uniform spatial distribution and size level of waste battery powder particles, which can effectively ensure the uniform distribution of waste battery powder in asphalt. The varying degrees of wrinkles or grooves distributed across the waste battery powder surface are shown in Figure 7b–d. Such rough surfaces can significantly increase the specific surface area of the waste battery powder, indicating a large bonding area between the asphalt and waste battery powder.

https://doi.org/10.3390/gels12020117

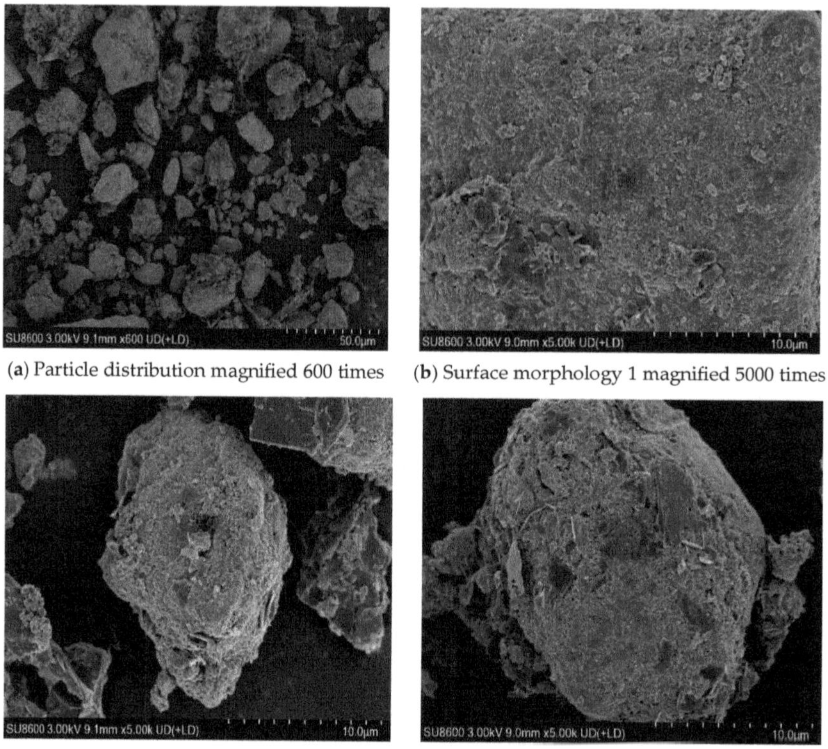

(**a**) Particle distribution magnified 600 times (**b**) Surface morphology 1 magnified 5000 times

(**c**) Surface morphology 2 magnified 5000 times (**d**) Overall surface morphology magnified 5000 times

Figure 7. Microscopic morphology of waste battery powder.

Figure 8 shows the microstructure of the tested WBP-modified and sol–gel 70# virgin asphalt. As presented in Figure 8, the added waste battery powder is distributed relatively evenly throughout the sol–gel 70# virgin asphalt, which can enhance the intermolecular forces between the waste battery powder and asphalt and improve the corresponding adhesion. When the waste battery powder is used to modify the sol–gel 70# asphalt at temperatures exceeding 100 °C, the asphalt adopts a sol–gel structure predominantly in the sol state. Its grooves and folds adsorb asphalt, while some asphalt flows into its pores. Subsequently, as the asphalt cools from high temperatures to 15 °C room temperature, the sol–gel structure undergoes a transformation, gradually shifting toward a predominantly gel-state sol–gel structure. This gel hardening produces an anchoring effect, thereby enhancing the asphalt's crack resistance under loading. In addition, existing research [27] indicates that the carbon in WBP exhibits relatively high crystallinity and content. The incorporation of WBP enhances the bond energy of methylene groups, thereby strengthening the molecular interactions between asphalt and WBP, and consequently improving the asphalt performance. The above microscopic analysis results are consistent with the analysis of activation energy for cracking damage, which validates the effectiveness of the analysis method proposed in this study for the toughening of waste battery powder on sol–gel 70# virgin asphalt.

https://doi.org/10.3390/gels12020117

(**a**) Surface morphology of sol–gel 70# virgin asphalt magnified 1000 times

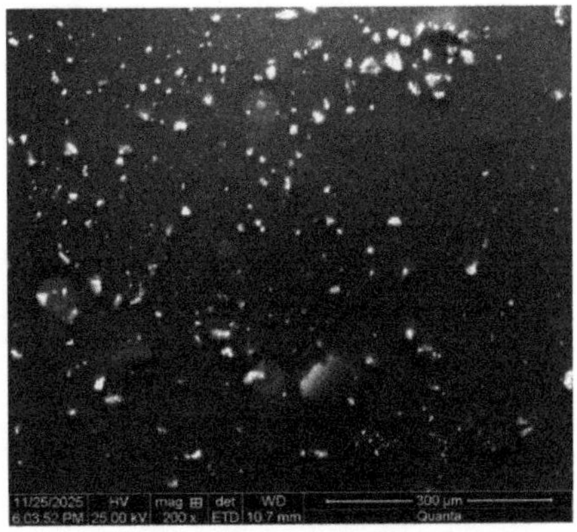

(**b**) Surface morphology of WBP-modified asphalt magnified 200 times

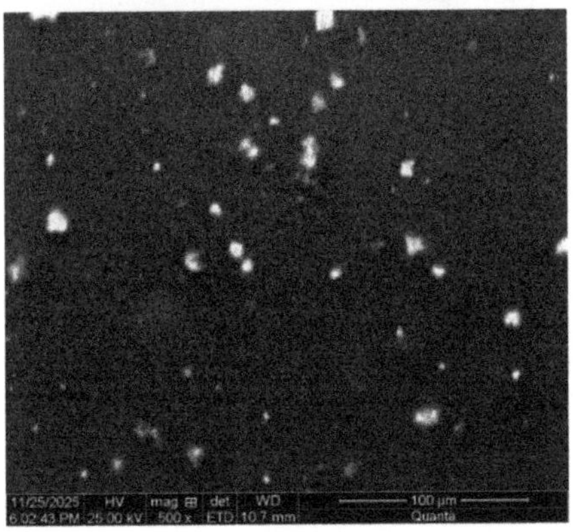

(**c**) Surface morphology of WBP-modified asphalt magnified 500 times

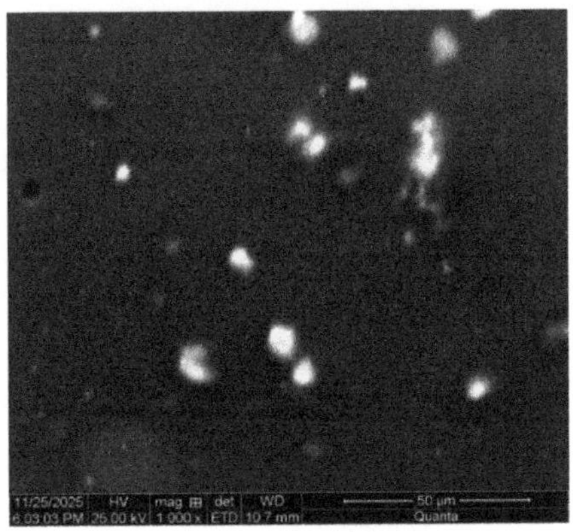

(**d**) Surface morphology of WBP-modified asphalt magnified 1000 times

Figure 8. Microscopic morphology of WBP-modified and sol–gel 70# virgin asphalt.

3. Conclusions

The significant contribution of this study lies in establishing a cracking area-based damage model derived from energy–mechanics balance equations, which enables accurate quantification and characterization of the fatigue damage behavior of the WBP-modified asphalt under cyclic loading. In addition, a damage activation energy evaluation method based on kinetics theory is proposed, which is expected to provide a new theoretical basis for the quantitative analysis of toughening mechanisms and performance optimization of the WBP-modified asphalt materials. The main conclusions are summarized as follows:

(1) The cracking area accurately characterizes the fatigue damage of the WBP-modified asphalt, which exhibits an overall trend of rate-increased evolution under stress-controlled conditions.

(2) The pronounced nonlinear characteristics of fatigue damage in the WBP-modified asphalt result in a variable-rate physical reaction process during asphalt fatigue damage. The parameter β in the damage evolution equation serves as a representative rate, quantifying the overall speed of the asphalt fatigue damage process.

(3) The kinetics equation can characterize the variable-rate fatigue damage process of the WBP-modified asphalt by correlating representative fatigue damage rates. The

https://doi.org/10.3390/gels12020117

Arrhenius kinetics equation becomes a linear equation in logarithmic coordinates, where the absolute value of the slope equals the activation energy for fatigue damage.

(4) The fatigue damage activation energy characterizes the minimum energy required for asphalt to sustain fatigue damage. A higher value indicates greater energy needed for fatigue damage to occur, signifying that the material is more resistant to fatigue damage. The micro-grooves and wrinkles on the surface of WBP modifiers increase the activation energy for fatigue damage, thereby improving the fatigue performance of the WBP-modified asphalt.

A method for analyzing the toughening effect of WBP on sol–gel virgin asphalt is proposed in this paper. The authors exclusively utilized 5# household mercury-free alkaline batteries and sol–gel 70# virgin asphalt as materials for preparing the WBP-modified asphalt. However, there are various types of waste batteries. Therefore, future research should validate the applicability of this method to other battery types. Subsequent studies will investigate the impact of different degrees of aging on the fatigue life of WBP-modified asphalt. Additionally, it is necessary to establish an intelligent decision-making system based on more extensive experimental data to determine the theory and technology for modified asphalt that takes into account factors such as environmental protection, performance, and economics.

4. Materials and Methods

4.1. Materials and Specimen Fabrication

4.1.1. Sol–Gel Virgin Asphalt

The 70# virgin asphalt, provided by Shandong High-speed Construction Materials Co., Ltd. (Jinan, Shandong Province, China). Based on classical colloid theory, the conventional 70# virgin asphalt typically demonstrates characteristic sol–gel structural features. At temperatures above 100 °C, it exhibits a sol–gel structure dominated by the sol state. As the temperature gradually decreases from 100 °C to 50 °C, the sol–gel structure undergoes a progressive transformation. When the temperature falls below 50 °C, the 70# virgin asphalt exhibits a sol–gel structure where the gel state becomes more pronounced than the sol state. Such sol–gel structural features can enable 70# virgin asphalt binders to maintain stable viscoelastic properties across a wide temperature range. Sol–gel 70# virgin asphalt has been widely applied in road engineering. Therefore, the sol–gel 70# virgin asphalt was used as the virgin asphalt for the preparation of the WBP-modified asphalt, and Table 3 presents its basic indicators.

4.1.2. Preparation Process of WBP-Modified Asphalt

According to the method in the literature of [15,24–27], the WBP was extracted from the recycled 5# household mercury-free alkaline batteries. First, the battery shell is removed, and the cathode material is ground into smaller particles using a grinder. Then, the battery particles are placed into the grinder for 20 min of grinding treatment, followed by screening with a 0.075 mm sieve to ensure a uniform particle size distribution of the waste battery powder. Finally, the screened WBP is placed into a 160 °C oven for 2 h to remove residual moisture and volatile impurities, ultimately yielding the final WBP. Table 4 shows the physical parameter indicators of the WBP.

According to the literature [24,27], the method of recycling waste batteries for preparing the WBP-modified asphalt can be described by Figure 9 and the optimal WBP content (by mass fraction) was found to be 12% through rheological performance testing. Therefore, in this study, the WBP content is set at 12% to prepare the WBP-modified asphalt according to the process. First, the 70 #VA is heated in an oven set to 165 °C until it reaches a molten state. Then, 12% by mass of WBP is added to the sol–gel 70# virgin asphalt and the mixture is sheared at 5000 r/min for 1 h at 155 °C. Next, the mixture is sheared at 1000 r/min for 10 min to remove any bubbles. Next, the asphalt is swollen

https://doi.org/10.3390/gels12020117

and developed in an oven at 160 °C for one hour, at which point it adopts a sol–gel structure predominantly in the sol state. Finally, the asphalt is cooled to approximately 15 °C to produce the WBP-modified asphalt. At this point, the asphalt exhibits a sol–gel structure where the gel state is more pronounced than the sol state.

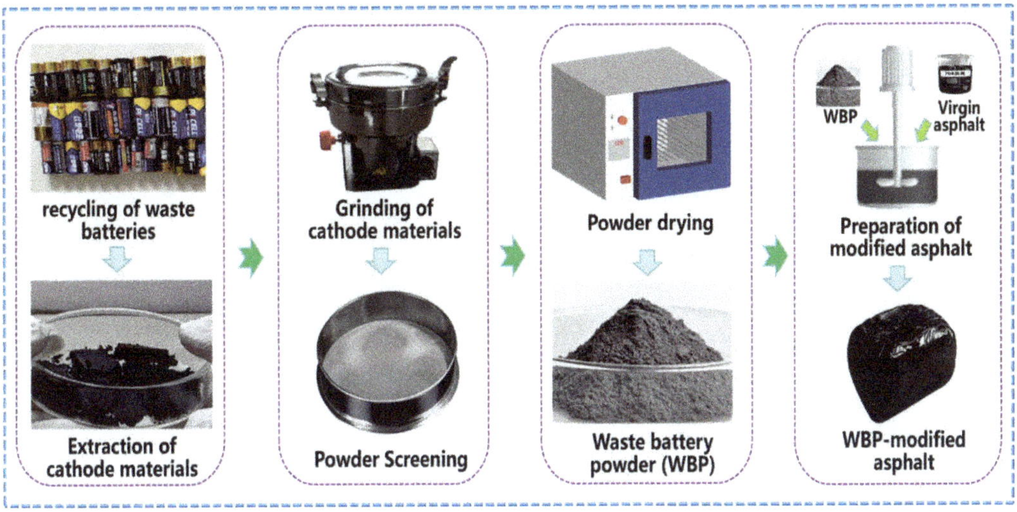
recycling of waste batteries
Extraction of cathode materials
Grinding of cathode materials
Powder Screening
Powder drying
Waste battery powder (WBP)
WBP
Virgin asphalt
Preparation of modified asphalt
WBP-modified asphalt

Figure 9. Recycling waste batteries for preparing WBP-modified asphalt.

4.1.3. Specimen Fabrication

A dynamic shear rheometer (DSR) was selected as the molding and loading equipment for the sol–gel 70# virgin asphalt and the WBP-modified asphalt.. The DSR selected in this paper was produced by Tianjin Gangyuan test instrument factory (Tianjin, China). First, the hot flowing asphalt is placed into a rubber mold for fabricating a cylindrical asphalt specimen. Then, the cylindrical specimen is placed into the DSR to form the final test specimens. The trimming gap and target gap of DSR are set as 2050 μm and 2000 μm, respectively. The molding diameter and height are set as 8 mm and 2 mm for fabricating the cylindrical specimens of the 70# virgin and the WBP-modified asphalt, as shown in Figure 10

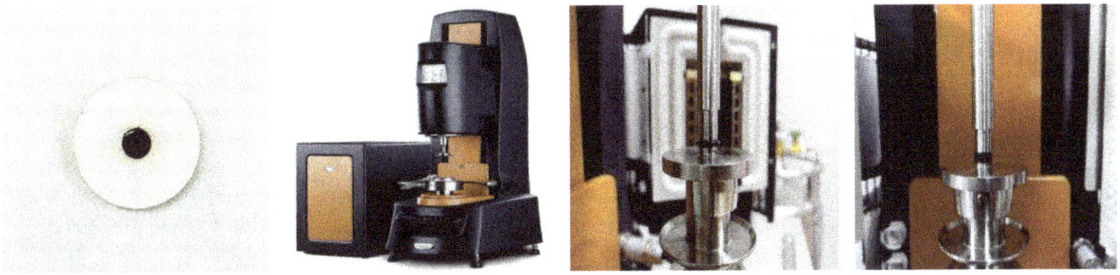

(a) Specimen in a rubber mold **(b)** DSR from Anton Paar **(c)** Trimming gap **(d)** Target gap

Figure 10. Preparation of 70# Virgin Asphalt and WBP Modified Asphalt Samples.

4.2. Test Methods

In this study, 10 Hz was selected as the loading frequency for the conducted tests of the WBP-modified and sol–gel 70# virgin asphalt, with five parallel tests set up. Existing

https://doi.org/10.3390/gels12020117

studies [36,37] have shown that asphalt fatigue cracking mainly occurs in the 15–25 °C intermediate temperature range, and related studies often conduct fatigue tests under intermediate temperature conditions. Therefore, the asphalt fatigue test temperatures selected for this study are 15 °C, 20 °C, and 25 °C. At these temperatures, the tested asphalt exhibits a sol–gel structure where the gel state is more pronounced than the sol state.

4.2.1. Linear Amplitude Time Sweep (LATS) Test

The LATS tests were performed for quantifying the nonlinear viscoelastic critical shear stress (τ_{cri}). The applied loading control mode is a strain-controlled standard sinusoidal loading and the shear strain level of the loading amplitude is linearly increased from 0.001 to 0.3. Taking the LATS test of the WBP-modified asphalt at 20 °C as an example, the method for determining the τ_{cri} is analyzed. The curves of phase angle (δ) and shear modulus (G^*) as functions of shear strain (γ) are shown in Figure 11.

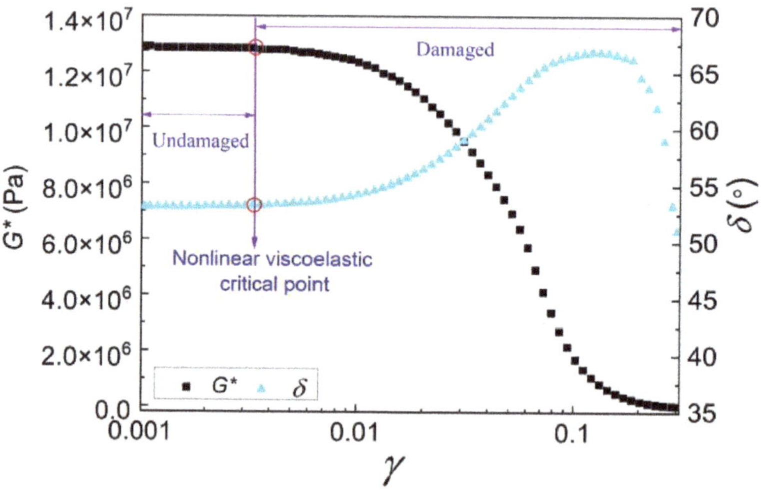

Figure 11. LATS test results of WBP-modified asphalt.

As presented, the loading amplitude is less than the nonlinear viscoelastic critical point corresponding to the nonlinear viscoelastic critical shear strain (γ_{cri}) and shear stress (τ_{cri}) with no damage accumulation, resulting in the δ and G^* remaining in an almost linear and steady state. As the loading level gradually increases, damage accumulates, causing the δ to first increase and then decrease, while the G^* decreases nonlinearly. The γ corresponding to the intersection point where the G^* rapidly decreases and the linear steady phase ends is taken as the γ_{cri}. The shear stress corresponding to the γ_{cri} is recorded as the τ_{cri}, and the obtained τ_{cri} of the WBP-modified asphalt at 20 °C is 95 kPa.

4.2.2. Non-Damage Time Sweep (NDTS) Test

The stress-controlled NDTS tests were utilized to analyze the non-damaging mechanical response of the tested asphalt. The loading waveform is set as a standard sinusoidal loading. The loading amplitude and loading time are τ_{cri} and 300 s, respectively. Figure 12 presents the results of δ and G^* for the WBP-modified asphalt at 20 °C. As observed, under cyclic loading with an amplitude of τ_{cri}, the WBP-modified asphalt exhibits δ and G^* values that do not produce significant changes, which is due to the fact that the WBP-modified asphalt tested by the τ_{cri} is in a non-destructive phase.

https://doi.org/10.3390/gels12020117

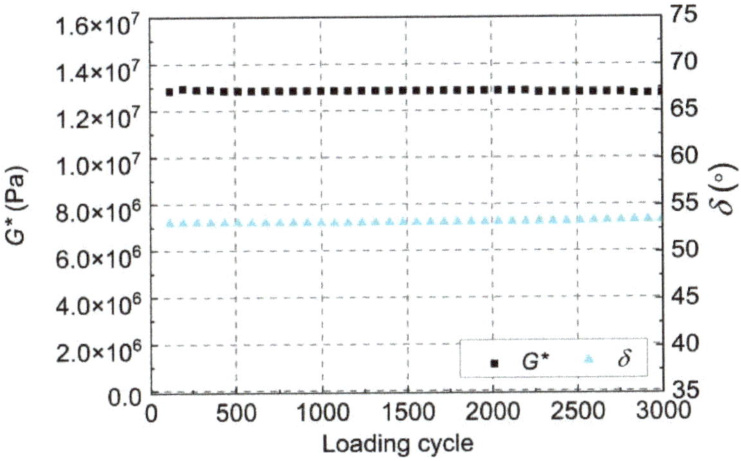

Figure 12. NDTS test results of WBP-modified asphalt.

4.2.3. Damage Time Sweep (DTS) Test

The damage mechanical response of the 70# virgin and the WBP-modified asphalt was analyzed by the DTS tests. First, the asphalt specimen tested by the NDTS test is allowed to recover for 300 s. Then, the stress-controlled standard sinusoidal loading with the amplitude shown in Table 5 is applied to the same asphalt specimen. Taking the tested WBP-modified and sol–gel 70# virgin asphalt under 20 °C and 100 kPa as an analysis example, their G^* decay trend is described. Figure 13 shows the corresponding G^* results. As can be seen, G^* gradually exhibits a nonlinear decay, which is due to the stress amplitude being greater than the τ_{cri}, resulting in the crack damage induced during cyclic loading. In addition, the G^* decay rate of the WBP-modified asphalt is less than that of the sol–gel 70# virgin asphalt, which indicates that the asphalt damage evolution rate can be delayed by the WBP.

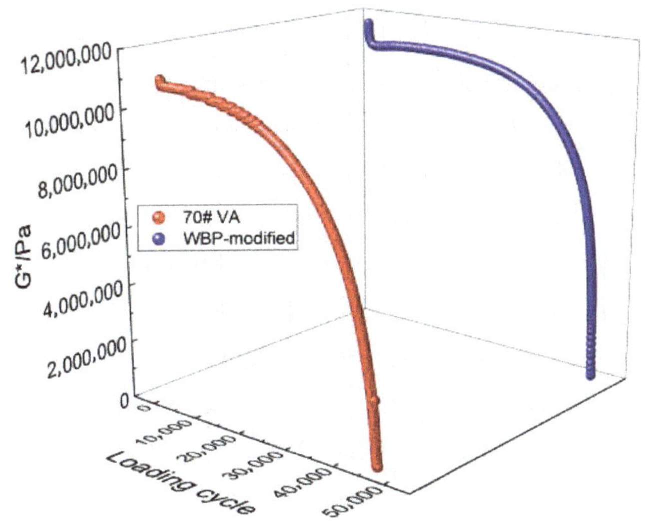

Figure 13. DTS test results of WBP-modified and sol–gel 70# virgin asphalt.

https://doi.org/10.3390/gels12020117

Table 5. Loading amplitudes of the DTS tests.

Asphalt Type	Temperature/°C	Loading Amplitude/kPa
sol–gel 70# virgin asphalt	15	250
	20	100
	25	80
WBP-modified asphalt	15	250
	20	100
	25	80

4.2.4. Scanning Electron Microscope (SEM) Test

The microstructures of WBP and the WBP-modified asphalt were measured using an IT300 SEM machine and Figure 14 illustrates the corresponding specimen preparation procedure. The SEM selected in this paper was produced by Chinainstru & Quantumtech (Hefei) Co., Ltd. (Hefei, Anhui Province, China). The WBP or asphalt was dried to remove moisture to obtain the test samples. Conductive adhesive was applied to the specimen stage. The WBP or asphalt specimen was placed onto the adhesive using a chemical spoon. The microstructures of WBP and the WBP-modified asphalt were then extracted and analyzed.

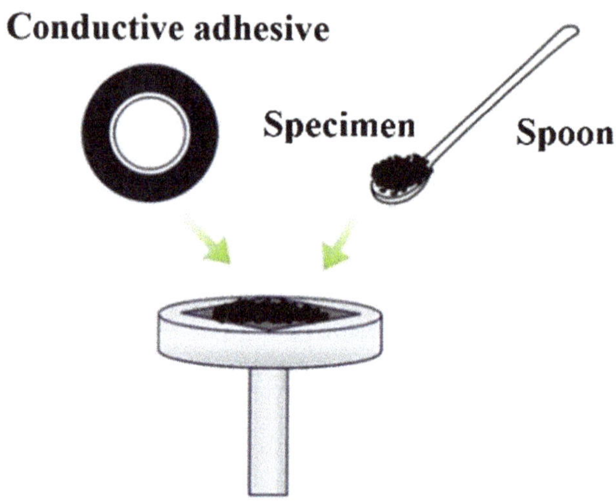

Figure 14. Specimen preparation procedure of the SEM test.

Author Contributions: Writing—original draft preparation, C.F., Y.C. and X.G.; writing—review and editing, N.G., H.L., Z.L., Y.C., C.F. and J.Y.; investigation, X.G., Z.W., T.G. and N.G.; data curation, C.F. and H.L. All authors have read and agreed to the published version of the manuscript.

Funding: This work was supported by the Planned project supported by the science and technology innovation teams of universities and colleges in the Henan province (24IRTSTHN011); the Central Plains Science and Technology Innovation Leader Project (244200510031); Key Scientific and Technological Projects in Henan Province (252102240031); Special Plan for Key Scientific Research Projects of Higher Education Institutions in Henan Province to Serve Industry Development (25CY022); Key Scientific Research Projects of Universities in Henan Province (26B580002; 26A580003); and the Henan Provincial Natural Science Foundation (252300423427).

Institutional Review Board Statement: Not applicable.

Informed Consent Statement: Not applicable.

https://doi.org/10.3390/gels12020117

Data Availability Statement: The data are contained within the article. Some or all of the data, models, or code that support the findings of this study are available from the corresponding author upon reasonable request.

Conflicts of Interest: Chenze Fang, Yuanzhao Chen, Zhenxia Li, Jingyu Yang, and Tengteng Guo were employed by the North China University of Water Resources and Electric Power-Henan Provincial Institute of Transportation Planning and Design Co., Ltd. Green, Low Carbon, and High Performance Road Materials Research and Development Center, Zhengzhou 450045, Henan, China. The remaining authors declare that the research was conducted in the absence of any commercial or financial relationships that could be construed as a potential conflict of interest.

References

1. Zhang, J.W.; Chen, M.Z.; Wu, S.P.; Chen, D.Y.; Zhao, Y.C.; Zhou, X.X. Characteristics of waste dry battery powder and its enhancement effect on the physicochemical properties of asphalt binder. *J. Clean. Prod.* **2023**, *426*, 139090. [CrossRef]
2. Sabbaghi, M.; Behdad, S. Estimating energy left in discarded alkaline batteries: Evaluating consumption and recovery opportunities. *Waste Manag.* **2024**, *189*, 58–67. [CrossRef]
3. Gao, W.F.; Wang, J.Q.; Wang, Z.Q.; Wang, Z.; Wang, Z.L.; Cui, H.; Zeng, X.J.; Wang, G.H.; Lv, L.Y.; Sun, Z. Analysis of the current status of national and local policies on the recycling of used power batteries in China. *Chem. Ind. Eng. Prog.* **2024**, *43*, 5820–5836. (In Chinese)
4. Ruan, D.S.; Wang, F.M.; Wu, L.; Du, K.; Zhang, Z.H.; Zou, K.; Wu, X.F.; Hu, G.R. A high-performance regenerated graphite extracted from discarded lithium-ion batteries. *New J. Chem.* **2020**, *45*, 1535–1540. [CrossRef]
5. Azam, M.G.; Kabir, M.H.; Shaikh, M.A.A.; Ahmed, S.; Mahmud, M.; Yasmin, S. A rapid and efficient adsorptive removal of lead from water using graphene oxide prepared from waste dry cell battery. *J. Water Process. Eng.* **2022**, *12*, 102597. [CrossRef]
6. Roy, D.; Neogi, S.; De, S. Adsorptive removal of heavy metals from battery industry effluent using MOF incorporated polymeric beads: A combined experimental and modeling approach. *J. Hazard. Mater.* **2021**, *403*, 123624. [CrossRef] [PubMed]
7. Roy, I.; Sarkar, G.; Mondal, S.; Rana, D.; Bhattacharyya, A.; Saha, N.R.; Adhikari, A.; Khastgir, D.; Chattopadhyay, S.; Chattopadhyay, D. Synthesis and characterization of graphene from waste dry cell battery for electronic applications. *RSC Adv.* **2016**, *6*, 10557–10564. [CrossRef]
8. Liu, G.N.; Yu, Y.J.; Hou, J.; Xue, W.; Liu, X.H.; Liu, Y.Z.; Wang, W.H.; Alsaedi, A.; Hayat, T.; Liu, Z.T. An ecological risk assessment of heavy metal pollution of the agricultural ecosystem near a lead-acid battery factory. *Ecol. Indic.* **2014**, *47*, 210–218. [CrossRef]
9. Liu, J.W.; Hao, P.W.; Dou, Z.S.; Wang, J.B.; Rheological, L.J.M. Healing and microstructural properties of unmodified and crumb rubber modified asphalt incorporated with graphene/carbon black composite. *Constr. Build. Mater.* **2021**, *305*, 124512. [CrossRef]
10. Jiang, H.; Shao, J.A.; Zhu, Y.J.; Yu, J.; Cheng, W.; Yang, H.P.; Zhang, X.; Chen, H.P. Production mechanism of high-quality carbon black from hightemperature pyrolysis of waste tire. *J. Hazard. Mater.* **2023**, *443*, 130350. [CrossRef]
11. Feng, X.J.; Zha, X.D.; Cheng, J. Preparation and properties of PAN-based carbon fiber conductive asphalt concrete. *China J. Highw. Transp.* **2012**, *25*, 27–32. (In Chinese)
12. He, J.; Hu, W.; Xiao, R.; Wang, Y.H.; Polaczyk, P.; Huang, B.S. A review on Graphene/GNPs/GO modified asphalt. *Constr. Build. Mater.* **2022**, *330*, 127222. [CrossRef]
13. Guo, F.; Li, X.Y.; Wang, Z.R.; Chen, Y.J.; Yue, J.C. Study on the Factors Affecting the Self-Healing Performance of Graphene-Modified Asphalt Based on Molecular Dynamics Simulation. *Polymers* **2024**, *16*, 2482. [CrossRef] [PubMed]
14. Liu, Z.Q.; Liang, K.; Cao, X.J.; Chen, J.C.; Ji, S.Z.; Shen, Q.R. Influence of graphene on the composite modified asphalt based on viscoelastic and elastic properties. *Constr. Build. Mater.* **2024**, *443*, 137671. [CrossRef]
15. Nie, F.H.; Chow, C.L.; Lau, D. Effect of functionalization and defects on thermal conductivity of graphene sheets modified asphalt nanocomposites. *Appl. Surf. Sci.* **2023**, *621*, 156804. [CrossRef]
16. Liu, S.T.; Cao, W.D.; Shang, S.J.; Qi, H.; Fang, J.G. Analysis and application of relationships between low-temperature rheological performance parameters of asphalt binders. *Constr. Build. Mater.* **2010**, *24*, 471–478. [CrossRef]
17. Hu, X.F.; Robles, A.; Vikstrom, T. A novel process on the recovery of zinc and manganese from spent alkaline and zinc-carbon batteries. *J. Hazard. Mater.* **2021**, *411*, 124928. [CrossRef]
18. Zhu, H.R.; Yu, M.M.; Zhang, Y.; Wang, W.F. Study on wave-absorbing and warming properties of asphalt mixtures doped with magnetite powder/manganese dioxide. *Highw. Eng.* **2022**, *47*, 160–165. (In Chinese)
19. Zhao, D.; Jiang, J.; Gu, X.; Liu, J.; Wang, J.; Yang, G. Value-added recycling of plant waste for modification of asphalt pavement used aggregates: Interface enhancement and carbon sequestration. *Chem. Eng. J.* **2025**, *505*, 159822. [CrossRef]
20. Liu, T.C.; Jiang, J.W.; Lu, G.Y.; Ding, J.T.; Ni, F.J. Adsorption-state test guided enhancement of asphalt emulsion–aggregate interface: From microscopic defects to macroscopic strengthening. *Constr. Build. Mater.* **2026**, *506*, 144909. [CrossRef]

https://doi.org/10.3390/gels12020117

21. Liu, K.F.; Zhang, K.; Shi, X.M. Performance evaluation and modification mechanism analysis of asphalt binders modified by graphene oxide. *Constr. Build. Mater.* **2018**, *163*, 880–889. [CrossRef]
22. Jahanbakhsh, H.; Karimi, M.M.; Jahangiri, B.F.; Moghadas, N. Induction heating and healing of carbon black modified asphalt concrete under microwave radiation. *Constr. Build. Mater.* **2018**, *174*, 656–666. [CrossRef]
23. Liu, Z.M.; Yang, X.; Wang, Y.D.; Luo, S. Engineering properties and microwave heating induced ice-melting performance of asphalt mixture with activated carbon powder filler. *Constr. Build. Mater.* **2019**, *197*, 50–62. [CrossRef]
24. Fan, L.P. *Evaluation of the Effect of Asphalt Modified by Waste Batteries, Micro-Mechanism and its Mixture Properties*; Guangxi University: Guangxi, China, 2023. (In Chinese)
25. Meng, Y.J.; Chen, P.Y.; Fan, L.P.; Rong, H.L.; Lai, J.; Zhang, C.Y.; Chen, J.P.; Li, Y.W. Investigation into the modification mechanism and performance assessment of waste battery powder modified bitumen. *Int. J. Pavement Eng.* **2024**, *25*, 2393310. [CrossRef]
26. Meng, Y.J.; Lai, J.; Fan, L.P.; Mo, S.Y.; Guo, C.L.; Zhang, C.Y. Recycling of the waste battery: Effect of waste battery on property of asphalt and environmental impact evaluation. *Sci. Total. Environ.* **2023**, *904*, 166983. [CrossRef] [PubMed]
27. Meng, Y.J.; Fan, L.P.; Chen, J.; Liao, Y.J.; Han, H.H. Microscopic characterization of waste battery powder modified bitumen and its performance. *China J. Highw. Transp.* **2021**, *34*, 34–44. (In Chinese)
28. Gan, X.L.; Chen, P.; Yu, B.; Zhang, W.G. Study on the performances of waste battery powder modified asphalt and asphalt mixture. *Polymers* **2023**, *14*, 5409. [CrossRef] [PubMed]
29. Fang, C.Z.; Guo, N.S.; Li, H.; Leng, Z.; Jiang, J.W. Investigating fatigue damage accumulation of asphalt binders considering amplitude sequence and loading interaction. *J. Mater. Civ. Eng.* **2024**, *36*, 04024142. [CrossRef]
30. Li, H.; Luo, X.; Yan, W.; Zhang, Y.Q. Pseudo energy-based kinetic characterization of fatigue in asphalt binders. *China J. Highw. Transp.* **2020**, *33*, 115.
31. Lv, S.T.; Liu, C.C.; Zheng, J.L.; You, Z.P.; You, L.Y. Viscoelastic Fatigue Damage Properties of Asphalt Mixture with Different Aging Degrees. *KSCE J. Civ. Eng.* **2018**, *22*, 2073–2081. (In Chinese) [CrossRef]
32. Zheng, J.L.; Lv, S.T.; Tian, X.G. Research on viscoelastic fatigue damage model of aging asphalt mixture. *Eng. Mech.* **2010**, *27*, 116–122. (In Chinese)
33. Lv, S.T.; Liu, C.C.; Lan, J.T.; Zhang, H.W.; Zheng, J.L.; You, Z.P. Fatigue equation of cement-treated aggregate base Materials under a true stress ratio. *Appl. Sci.* **2018**, *8*, 691. [CrossRef]
34. Lv, S.T.; Zhao, T.D.; Xia, C.D.; Zhao, S.G.; Liu, T.J.; Liu, Y.H.; Liu, B.; Cabrera, M.B. A new method for characterizing the fatigue performance of high-modulus asphalt mixtures. *J. Test. Eval.* **2022**, *50*, 1763–1776. [CrossRef]
35. Li, H.; Luo, X.; Zhang, Y.Q. A kinetics-based model of fatigue crack growth rate in bituminous material. *Int. J. Fatigue* **2021**, *148*, 106185. [CrossRef]
36. Fang, C.Z.; Tang, D.Q.; Li, Z.X.; Chen, Y.Z.; Guo, N.S.; Guo, T.T. A new fatigue equation for asphalt mixtures considering loading sequence effects. *Case Stud. Constr. Mater.* **2024**, *20*, e03286. [CrossRef]
37. Fang, C.Z.; Li, H.; Li, Z.X.; Chen, Y.Z.; Guo, T.T. Fatigue life prediction of asphalt binders under variable loading levels based on dissipated pseudo-strain energy. *Case Stud. Constr. Mater.* **2025**, *22*, e04321. [CrossRef]

https://doi.org/10.3390/gels12020117

gels

Review

A State-of-the-Art Review on the Freeze–Thaw Resistance of Sustainable Geopolymer Gel Composites: Mechanisms, Determinants, and Models

Peng Zhang [1,2], Baozhi Shi [1], Xiaobing Dai [1], Cancan Chen [1,*] and Canhua Lai [1]

[1] School of Water Conservancy and Transportation, Zhengzhou University, Zhengzhou 450001, China; zhangpeng@zzu.edu.cn (P.Z.); 15136736833@163.com (B.S.); daixb@zzu.edu.cn (X.D.); 13395998071@163.com (C.L.)
[2] State Key Laboratory of Tunnel Boring Machine and Intelligent Operation, Zhengzhou 450001, China
[*] Correspondence: ccchen1365@zzu.edu.cn

Abstract: Geopolymer, as a sustainable, low-carbon gel binder, is regarded as a potential alternative to cement. Freeze–thaw (F-T) resistance, which has a profound influence on the service life of structures, is a crucial indicator for assessing the durability of geopolymer composites (GCs). Consequently, comprehending the F-T resistance of GCs is of the utmost significance for their practical implementation. In this article, a comprehensive and in-depth review of the F-T resistance of GCs is conducted. This review systematically synthesizes several frequently employed theories regarding F-T damage, with the aim of elucidating the underlying mechanisms of F-T damage in geopolymers. The factors influencing the F-T resistance of GCs, including raw materials, curing conditions, and modified materials, are meticulously elaborated upon. The results indicate that the F-T resistance of GCs can be significantly enhanced through using high-calcium-content precursors, mixed alkali activators, and rubber aggregates. Moreover, appropriately increasing the curing temperature has been shown to improve the F-T resistance of GCs, especially for those fabricated with low-calcium-content precursors. Among modified materials, the addition of most fibers and nano-materials remarkably improves the F-T resistance of GCs. Conversely, the effect of air-entraining agents on the F-T resistance of GCs seems to be negligible. Furthermore, evaluation and prediction models for the F-T damage of GCs are summarized, including empirical models and machine learning models. In comparison with empirical models, the models established by machine learning algorithms exhibit higher predictive accuracy. This review promotes a more profound understanding of the factors affecting the F-T resistance of GCs and their mechanisms, providing a basis for engineering and academic research.

Keywords: geopolymer gel composites; freeze–thaw resistance; deterioration mechanisms; influence factors; prediction models

1. Introduction

Ordinary Portland cement (OPC) finds extensive applications in the realm of construction engineering. However, during the manufacturing process of OPC, excessive energy is consumed and the environment is damaged [1–3]. Since the production of OPC requires the calcination of limestone, approximately one ton of carbon dioxide is emitted for every ton of cement produced. The CO_2 emissions from OPC production account for about 8% of the total annual anthropogenic CO_2 emissions [4,5]. Therefore, it is urgent to develop new environmentally friendly binders to replace cement, which can alleviate serious issues such as environmental pollution [6,7]. Geopolymer, first proposed by Davidovits [8], is a novel aluminosilicate cementitious material that has attracted increasing attention in recent years. Geopolymer composites (GCs) are prepared from precursors such as fly ash (FA), ground granulated blast furnace slag (GGBFS), and metakaolin (MK), along with alkali activators [9]. By replacing cement with geopolymer, industrial by-products can be effectively recycled. Moreover, since calcination is not required in the production of GCs, CO_2 emissions can be significantly reduced. In addition, GCs possess excellent mechanical properties and chemical resistance. Thus, geopolymer has great potential as a substitute for traditional cementitious composites.

As a potential alternative to OPC, it is necessary to investigate the durability of GCs in complex environments, especially in high-latitude or cold regions, which is of great significance. The freeze–thaw (F-T) cycle gives rise to non-uniform cracks within the concrete matrix. These cracks have a significant detrimental impact on the safety and the service lifespan of concrete structures, potentially leading to structural integrity issues and premature deterioration [10,11]. Several studies have elucidated the F-T damage process of GCs. When subjected to F-T cycling, the free water in the pores of GCs generates repeated crystallization pressure [12] and water pressure [13]. Under the influence of crystallization pressure and water pressure, new microcracks form in the matrix. Such new microcracks allow more water to penetrate into the matrix, ultimately resulting in structural damage to, or even the destruction of, the GC [14,15]. The extent of F-T damage can be quantified using several indices. These include the relative dynamic modulus of elasticity (RDME), weight loss, compressive strength, and ultrasonic pulse velocity (UPV) [9,16–18].

The F-T resistance of GCs is significantly affected by a variety of raw materials, which play a crucial role in determining their performance under F-T conditions. Regarding raw materials, the calcium (Ca) content in the precursor is a crucial factor affecting the F-T resistance of GCs. More specifically, when the Ca content in the precursors of GCs is increased, their F-T resistance is significantly strengthened [19]. Additionally, the F-T durability of GCs shows a positive correlation with the increase in the Na/Al ratio, while it decreases as the Si/Al ratio increases. This indicates that a higher Na/Al ratio and a lower Si/Al ratio are beneficial for improving F-T resistance [20]. The properties of alkali activators, including their types, modulus, and dosage, also impact the F-T resistance of GCs [19,21–24]. For example, Sun et al. [25] found that the RDME loss of GCs activated solely by sodium hydroxide was 32% after 80 F-T cycles, while GCs prepared with a mixed solution of sodium hydroxide and sodium silicate exhibited a significantly lower RDME loss only of 1% after 80 F-T cycles. The properties of the aggregate also influence the F-T resistance of GCs [26–30]. The use of rubber particles (RPs) can significantly decrease the damage brought about by F-T cycles, primarily because of their excellent energy-dissipating ability [28]. Furthermore, the curing temperature is another critical factor affecting the F-T resistance of GCs. Studies have demonstrated that appropriately increasing the curing temperature improves the F-T resistance of these materials [31–33]. Research has shown that as the curing temperature increased from 23 °C to 50 °C, the compressive strength loss of a red mud, slurry class F, FA-based geopolymer decreased from 34.4% to 1.63% [31].

To improve the F-T resistance of GCs, many researchers incorporate modified materials such as fibers, nano-materials, and air-entraining agents (AEAs) into GCs [34–38]. Fibers improve the F-T resistance of GCs by restricting the propagation of cracks [39]. One study showed that when compared to a control group that did not contain any steel fibers (SF), GCs that incorporated 0.8% steel fibers (SFs) experienced a reduction in the loss of compressive strength. Specifically, after 200 F-T cycles, this reduction in the loss of compressive strength was roughly 50% [40]. The compressive strength loss in a GC with

0.1% polyethylene (PE) fibers was only 1.4% after 180 F-T cycles, while that of the control group without fibers reached 17.8% [41]. Nano-materials strengthen the F-T durability of GCs by filling matrix pores and facilitating the formation of hydration products [42,43]. For instance, when the graphene oxide (GO) content of a GC was 0.06%, its compressive strength loss was reduced by 41.1% compared to a sample without GO [44]. Ekinci et al. [18] reported that the incorporation of 1% nano-silica (NS) into a GC resulted in a 54% reduction in compressive strength loss after 300 F-T cycles compared to a control group.

Despite numerous reports on the F-T resistance of GCs, the related data is still rather scattered, and comprehensive reviews on this subject are scarce. Figure 1 represents a graphical map of the keywords that are relevant to existing reviews on GCs. The bubble sizes represent the frequency of keywords. From Figure 1, it can be seen that there are almost no existing reviews on the F-T resistance of GCs. Hence, the primary objective of this review is to summarize and conduct a comprehensive review of the relevant literature and data on the F-T resistance of GCs over the past decade. Figure 2 illustrates the process diagram for reviewing the F-T resistance of GCs. The F-T degradation process of GCs and common theories of F-T damage are presented by the review. The impacts of raw materials, curing conditions, and modified materials on the F-T durability of GCs are discussed. Moreover, this review summarizes the evaluation and prediction models for F-T damage of GCs, including empirical models and machine learning (ML) models. This review contributes to a more profound understanding of the factors influencing the F-T resistance of GCs and their underlying mechanisms, thereby providing a foundation for both engineering applications and academic research.

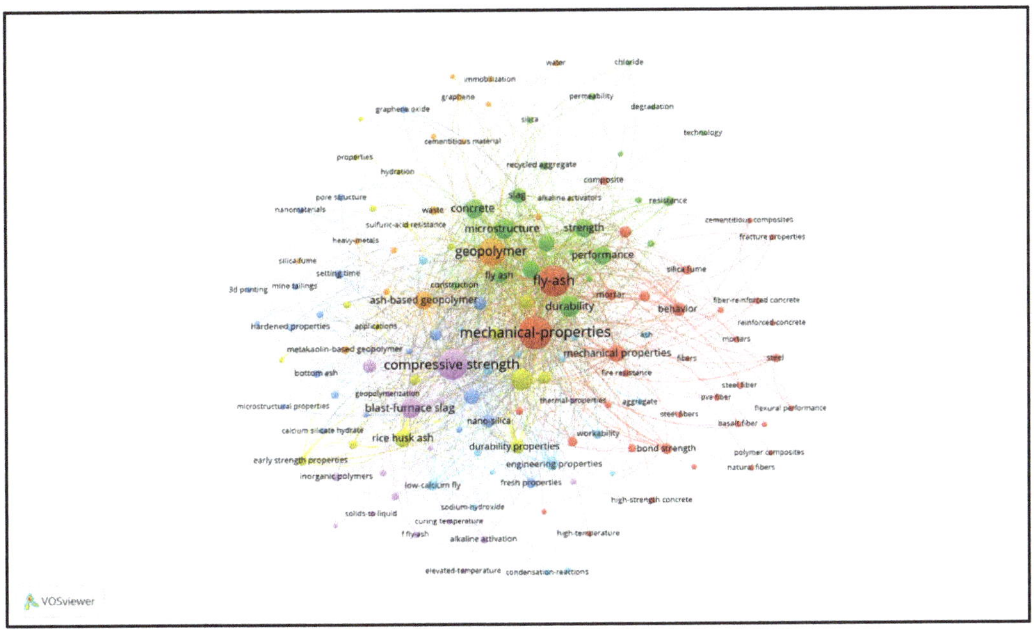

Figure 1. A keyword map of existing reviews' relevance to GCs, created using VOS viewer 1.6.18.

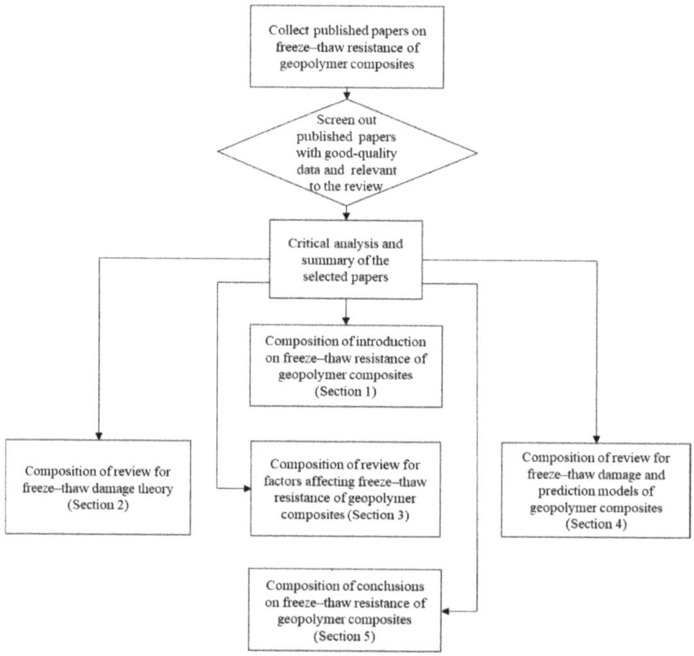

Figure 2. A process diagram for reviewing the F-T resistance of GCs.

2. Freeze–Thaw Damage Mechanism and Theory of Geopolymer Composites

2.1. Freeze–Thaw Damage Mechanism of Geopolymer Composites

Figure 3 illustrates the F-T damage process of GCs. The graph reveals that with an increase in the number of F-T cycles, the geopolymer matrix gradually undergoes deterioration. This is manifested as a reduction in the strength, RDME, and weight of the geopolymers [19,40,45]. There are numerous cracks and pores both on the surface and within the geopolymers, as shown in Figure 3a. Before the F-T cycles, water permeates into the cracks and pores of the GC due to the combined effects of capillary pressure and hydraulic pressure. When the temperature decreases, the water in the outer layer of the specimen freezes and forms ice, resulting in the volume expansion of water [46], as depicted in Figure 3b. When the ice crystals grow to fill the entire pore, they exert compressive stress on the pore wall, which is referred to as crystallization pressure. Once the crystallization pressure exceeds the tensile strength of the pore wall, microcracks will initiate in the geopolymer matrix. Additionally, during this process, the unfrozen water is forced into the interior of the matrix, and the migration of water generates a pressure known as hydrostatic pressure [13]. An overly high hydrostatic pressure can also inflict damage on the structure of the geopolymer. After multiple F-T cycles, the internal cracks in the geopolymer interconnect and propagate, forming macroscopic cracks. This leads to cracking of the geopolymer matrix, a reduction in the bonding performance, and surface detachment. After the F-T cycles, numerous cracks develop in the matrix of the GC, significantly compromising the durability and mechanical properties of the material, as illustrated in Figure 4.

The surface peeling of geopolymers is typically a destructive phenomenon under salt-freezing conditions. According to the theory of adhesive peeling [47], when the salt solution on the surface of geopolymer concrete freezes, the ice has a significantly higher expansion coefficient compared to the geopolymer concrete itself. This generates substantial tensile stress at the ice–geopolymer concrete interface, which initiates cracks and causes surface expansion of the geopolymer concrete, ultimately leading to surface detachment. Studies have indicated that salt-freezing inflicts more severe damage on geopolymers compared to water freezing [19]. In summary, whether water or a salt solution is used as the F-T medium, the main reason for the F-T damage of geopolymers is the freezing expansion of the pore solution and the pressure produced during the migration of pore water. The essence of F-T damage in GCs is a process in which the matrix transforms from a dense state to a loose state, accompanied by the initiation, growth, and propagation of microcracks. Macroscopically, this damage is manifested as a significant decrease in mass, RDME, and strength [19,33].

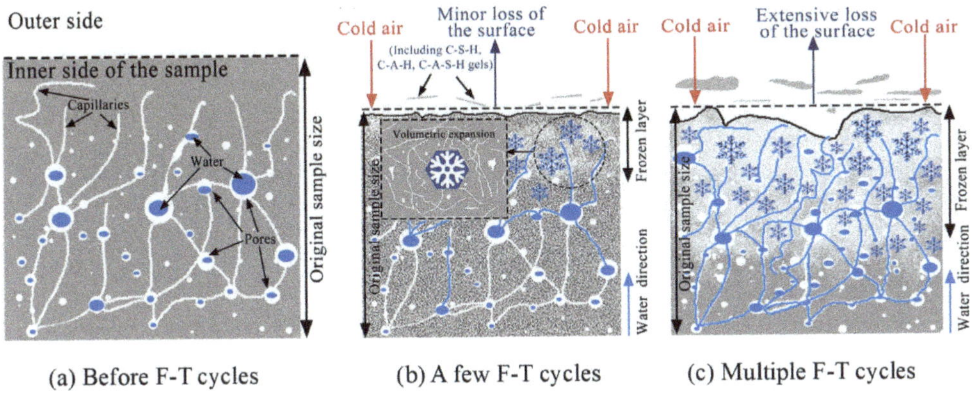

Figure 3. Schematic diagram of F-T damage mechanism of GC [21]. (Reproduced with permission from [21], Elsevier, 2022).

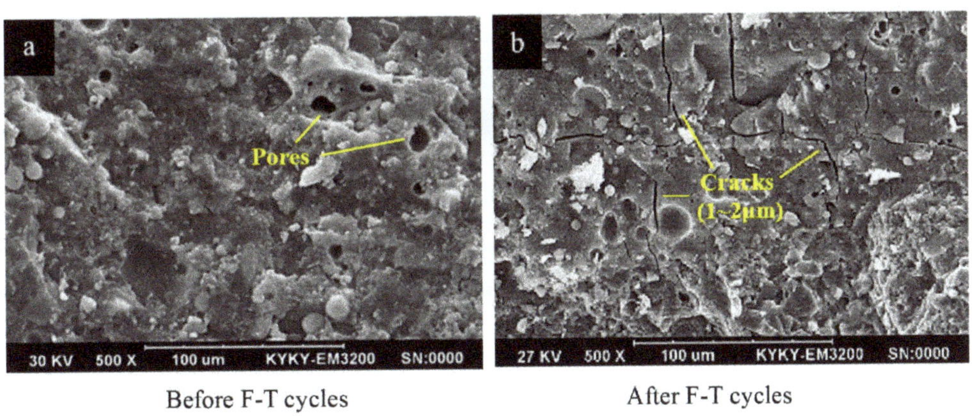

Figure 4. Scanning electron microscope (SEM) images of GC [48]. (Reproduced with permission from [48], Elsevier, 2019).

2.2. Freeze–Thaw Damage Theory

A great number of studies have investigated the mechanisms of concrete F-T failure, yielding valuable insights. Existing theoretical models of F-T damage can be categorized into two types: one is the icing pressure hypothesis [14], encompassing the crystallization pressure theory, hydrostatic pressure theory, osmotic pressure theory, etc.; the other is the temperature stress hypothesis for high-strength or high-performance concrete [14]. Although these existing mechanisms can, to a certain extent, elucidate certain aspects of the F-T damage phenomena in concrete, there is no single mechanism that can comprehensively explain all the damage phenomena that occur in concrete during the F-T process. Moreover, currently, there is relatively limited research on the F-T damage mechanism of geopolymers, which predominantly relies on the failure mechanism of cement concrete [49]. However, GCs and OPC concrete are both porous materials. As described in Section 2.1, during the F-T cycle, water will migrate and undergo phase transition in the pores of GCs, so some commonly used theories to explain F-T damage in OPC concrete also apply to GCs [50]. Building on previous research achievements, this article expounds on several commonly used theories that are applied to explain the F-T failure of GCs [49,51–54].

2.2.1. Crystallization Pressure Theory

Figure 5 presents a schematic diagram of cylindrical crystals within the pores of concrete. Due to the uniform temperature around the ice crystal, the ice undergoes simultaneous growth from both ends and the lateral sides, as depicted in Figure 5. However, the lateral growth of the ice crystal is restricted by the pore wall. When the diameter of the ice exceeds the pore size, ice crystals exert a compressive stress P_A, known as crystallization pressure [12,47]. Cracks form in the pore walls when the crystallization pressure surpasses the tensile strength of the matrix. Once the temperature around the concrete has dropped sufficiently to enable ice crystals to diffuse into most of the pores, the cumulative crystal pressure generated by the ice crystals will lead to the destruction of the concrete structure. The magnitude of the crystallization pressure is influenced by various factors, including the system temperature, the extent of ice formation, the morphology of capillary pores, and the site of initial freezing [47]. The lower the minimum temperature of the F-T cycles, the greater the loss of compressive strength and weight of the GC after F-T cycling [55,56].

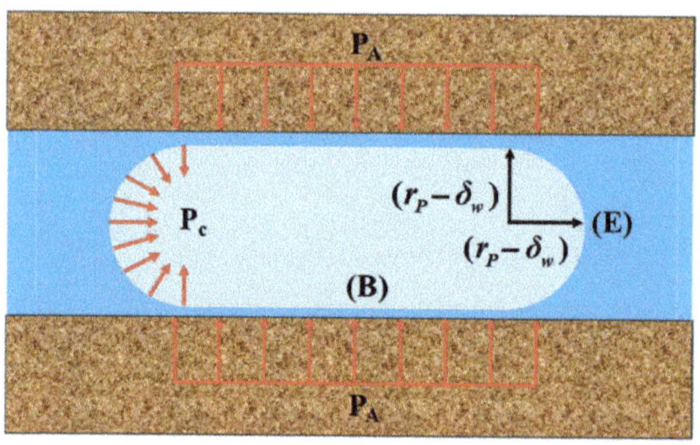

Figure 5. A schematic diagram of a cylindrical ice crystal in a pore of radius r_p [47]. The radii of the cylinder (B) and the hemispherical end (E) are both $r_p - \delta_w$. (Reproduced with permission from [47], Elsevier, 2019).

2.2.2. Hydraulic Pressure Theory

As the temperature decreases to the freezing point, ice forms on the surface of the concrete [57], as depicted in Figure 6a. The volume expansion due to the freezing of pore water causes the unfrozen water to be squeezed into the interior of the concrete, resulting in the formation of hydrostatic pressure [13]. When the hydrostatic pressure exceeds the tensile strength of the matrix, the matrix cracks, generating microcracks. Moreover, ice nucleates and grows at the junction of bubbles and pores, as shown in Figure 6b. This limits the fluidity of the unfrozen water, leading to a further increase in hydrostatic pressure. Under sustained hydrostatic pressure, microcracks within the matrix progressively propagate and coalesce, leading to cumulative damage and material degradation throughout F-T cycles [57]. The formula established by Powers [13] to estimate hydrostatic pressure P is presented in Equation (1). According to Equation (1), P decreases with a decline in the shortest distance between two bubbles L. Therefore, an AEA, which increases the number of bubbles and reduces the pore spacing coefficient, is commonly utilized to boost the F-T resistance of concrete.

$$P = a\prime(1.09 - \frac{1}{s})\frac{uR}{k}(\frac{L^3}{r_b} + \frac{3L^2}{2}) \quad (1)$$

where P represents the hydrostatic pressure, a' represents the dynamic viscosity coefficient of water, s represents the saturation coefficient of concrete, u represents the increase rate of freezing water per 1 °C temperature decrease, R represents the cooling rate, k represents the coefficient related to concrete permeability, r_b represents the average radius of the bubble, and L represents the shortest distance between two bubbles.

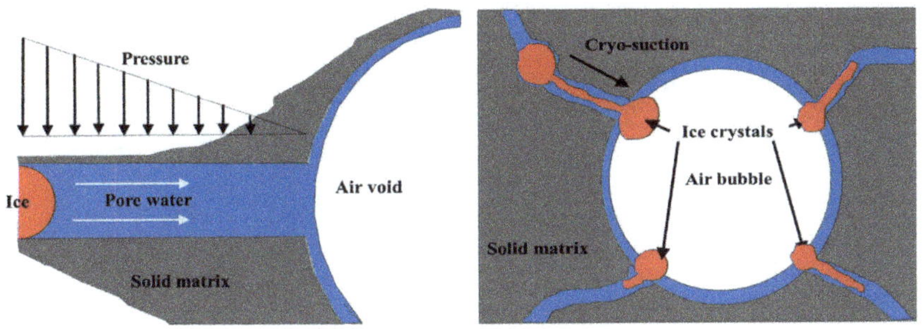

(a) Formation of hydrostatic pressure (b) Limitation of ice on flow of water

Figure 6. Schematic diagram of hydraulic pressure theory [57]. (Adapted with permission from [57], Elsevier, 2010).

2.2.3. Osmotic Pressure Theory

Concrete, being a porous material, contains numerous pores of different sizes, such as gel pores and bubble pores [58]. When the temperature decreases, a portion of the water in the large pores freezes initially, thereby increasing the salt concentration of the liquid solution inside the large pores. This creates a solution concentration difference between large and small pores. Additionally, the saturated vapor pressure of water is higher than that of ice, causing the unfrozen water to migrate to the frozen areas, as evidenced in Figure 7. Under the combined influence of the solution concentration difference and the saturated vapor pressure difference in the pores, osmotic pressure is generated inside the concrete. When the osmotic pressure surpasses the tensile strength of the concrete, microcracks will initiate and develop within the concrete structure. As the F-T cycle progresses, these microcracks gradually expand, eventually leading to the failure of the concrete structure [59]. Consequently, concrete is prone to damage caused by osmotic pressure in environments with high salt-ion concentrations, such as marine environments. The osmotic pressure theory explains why salt-freezing causes more severe damage to concrete than ordinary freezing. However, the osmotic pressure theory cannot be described by a mathematical model, making it difficult to provide a quantitative explanation of F-T failure.

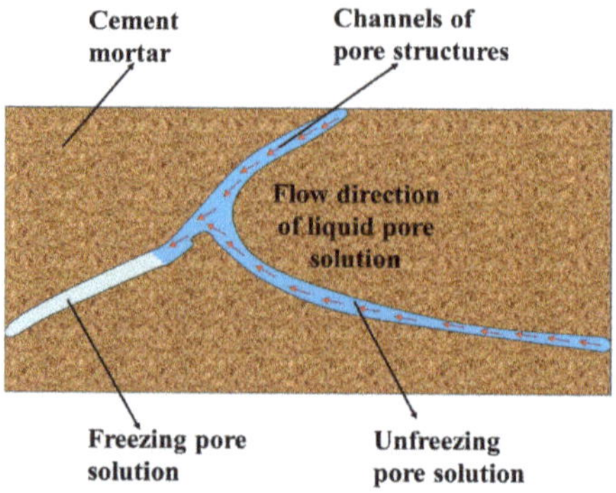

Figure 7. Schematic diagram of osmotic pressure model [60]. (Adapted with permission from [60], Elsevier, 2019).

2.2.4. Glue Spall Theory

Scherer and Valenza proposed the adhesion peeling theory [47,61,62], which is capable of effectively accounting for the surface scaling phenomenon of concrete following F-T cycles, as depicted in Figure 8. The ice on the surface of concrete forms an ice–concrete interface with the surface of the concrete. Since the shrinkage rate of ice is five times higher than that of concrete, substantial stress is generated at the interface between the ice and the concrete as the temperature drops [63]. With the temperature drops further, the ice layer cracks and forms island-shaped ice layers on the concrete surface. When the island-shaped ice shrinks, stress concentration occurs at the transition region, causing the concrete surface to crack and debond. The magnitude of the stress at the edge of the island-shaped ice layer is related to the initial concentration of the solution. Saltwater ice formed by the freezing of medium-concentration solutions (3%) causes the most severe damage to the concrete surface [61].

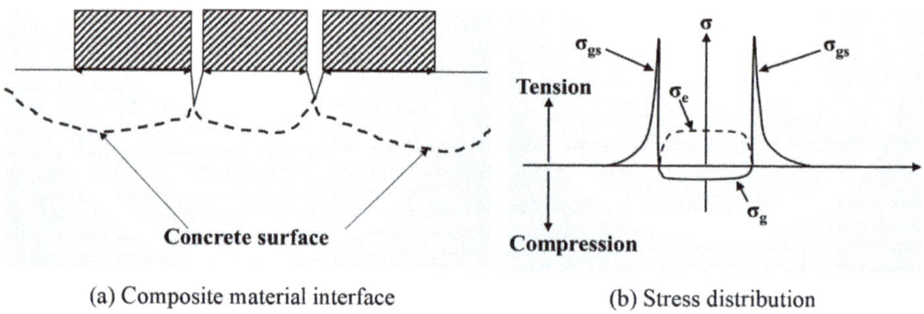

Figure 8. A schematic diagram of the glue spall mechanism [47]. σ_g, σ_e, and σ_{gs} are, respectively, the stress generated on the concrete surface, stress in the ice layer, and adhesive peeling stress around the island-shaped ice layer. (Adapted with permission from [47], Elsevier, 2007).

3. Factors Affecting the Freeze–Thaw Resistance of Geopolymer Composites

3.1. Raw Materials

3.1.1. Precursors

Unlike cement composites, GCs are fabricated from various precursors. The F-T resistance of GCs made from different precursors shows significant differences [17,19,64]. Table 1 lists the F-T durability of geopolymers fabricated with different precursors. Evidently, GCs with low-Ca precursors, such as FA and MK, exhibit poor F-T resistance.

For example, an FA-based geopolymer concrete was severely damaged after undergoing 21 F-T cycles, losing more than 28% of its mass [19]. Additionally, the results from Liang et al. [65] indicate that the compressive strength loss and weight loss of an MK-based GC were substantial after F-T cycles, reaching 63.30% and 20.24%, respectively. The explanation is that sodium aluminosilicate hydrate (N-A-S-H) gel is the primary hydration product in low-Ca systems [45], containing numerous transition pores that contribute to the poor F-T resistance of low-Ca GCs [48,66]. Moreover, due to the high water absorption of MK, water can easily enter the internal structure of the GC. According to the crystallization pressure theory and osmotic pressure theory, this increases the expansion force of ice during freezing and hydrostatic pressure, resulting in poor F-T resistance of MK-based GCs [67].

Table 1. The influence of precursors on the F-T resistance of GCs.

Precursor	Type	Sample Size (mm)	Temperature Range (°C)	F-T Cycles	Compressive Strength Loss	RDME Loss	Weight Loss	Ref.
FA	Geopolymer concrete	100 × 100 cylinder	−22~24	21	/	/	28.20%	[19]
FA/slag	Geopolymer concrete	100 × 100 × 400 prism	−18~4	125	4.30%	53.10%	0.70%	[48]
FA/slag	Geopolymer concrete	100 × 100 cylinder	−22~24	56	/	/	0.10%	[19]
Slag	Geopolymer concrete	100 × 100 × 400 prism	−18~5	300	/	8.51%	−0.48%	[17]
Slag	Geopolymer concrete	100 × 100 × 400 prism	−18~5	300	13.41%	36.33%	1.02%	[68]
FA/slag	Geopolymer mortar	100 × 100 × 400 prism	−18~5	300	/	/	0.80%	[33]
Volcanic tuff	Geopolymer mortar	50 × 50 × 50 cube	−16~3	300	19.70%	37.70%	/	[18]
MK/slag	Geopolymer mortar	50 × 50 × 50 cube	−20~20	90	34.33%	/	0.74%	[64]
MK	Geopolymer mortar	30 × 30 × 30 cube	−18~5	50	63.30%	/	20.24%	[65]

Compared to low-Ca GCs, GCs with high-Ca precursors (such as GGBFS) possess superior F-T resistance. Numerous investigations have demonstrated that GGBFS-based geopolymer concrete exhibits satisfactory F-T resistance, with a weight loss of no more than 1.1% after undergoing 300 F-T cycles [17,68]. Furthermore, compared to ordinary Portland cement concrete (OPCC), GGBFS-based geopolymer concrete has better F-T resistance [17]. This can be explained by the fact that calcium aluminosilicate hydrate (C-A-S-H) gel and calcium silicate hydrate (C-S-H) gel, which have a more compact structure compared to N-A-S-H gel, are the major hydration products in GGBFS-based GCs [48,66,69]. Additionally, the fusion of bubbles in the matrix is hindered by slag particles, reducing the average pore size and porosity of GCs [69,70]. These two reasons contribute to the high-Ca GCs having competitive F-T resistance compared to low-Ca GCs. However, Temuujin et al. [71] reported that the F-T durability of a GC prepared with class C FA was lower than that of a GC prepared with class F FA. The reason might be that the crystalline Ca component in class C FA expands when exposed to water, leading to a weakened microstructure and poor F-T resistance.

To strengthen the F-T resistance of low-Ca GCs, part of the low-Ca precursors is replaced with GGBFS to fabricate hybrid-precursor GCs [19,33,48]. Abundant research has shown that the F-T durability of FA-based geopolymer elevates with an increase in the slag proportion in the precursor. For instance, Figure 9 shows that an FA-based geopolymer with 10% slag experienced a 25% loss of compressive strength after just 5 F-T cycles, whereas increasing the slag content to 50% reduced the strength loss to only 4.3% even after 125 F-T cycles [48]. Another study found that the weight loss of a geopolymer with 70% slag was only 0.1% after F-T tests [19]. In addition, the F-T resistance of a GC is also influenced by the dosage of precursor. The geopolymer matrix gradually densifies and the cracks within the matrix decrease with an increase in precursor dosage after F-T cycles, as shown in Figure 10. This leads to a reduction in its permeability and an enhancement in F-T resistance [72]. Moreover, the Na/Al and Si/Al ratios also affect the F-T resistance of MK-based GCs. Research results have indicated that the F-T resistance of an MK-based GC was enhanced with an increase in the Na/Al ratio and decreased with the increase in the Si/Al ratio [20]. This is due to the fact that an elevation in the Na/Al ratio was capable of elevating the compressive strength of the GC.

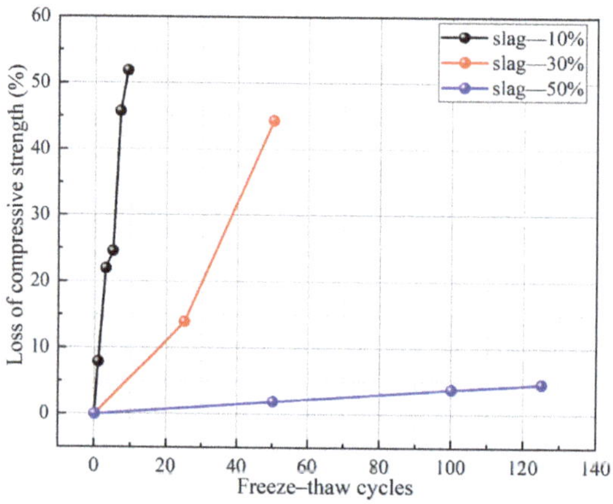

Figure 9. Loss of compressive strength of GCs with different slag contents after F-T cycles [48]. (Adapted with permission from [48], Elsevier, 2019).

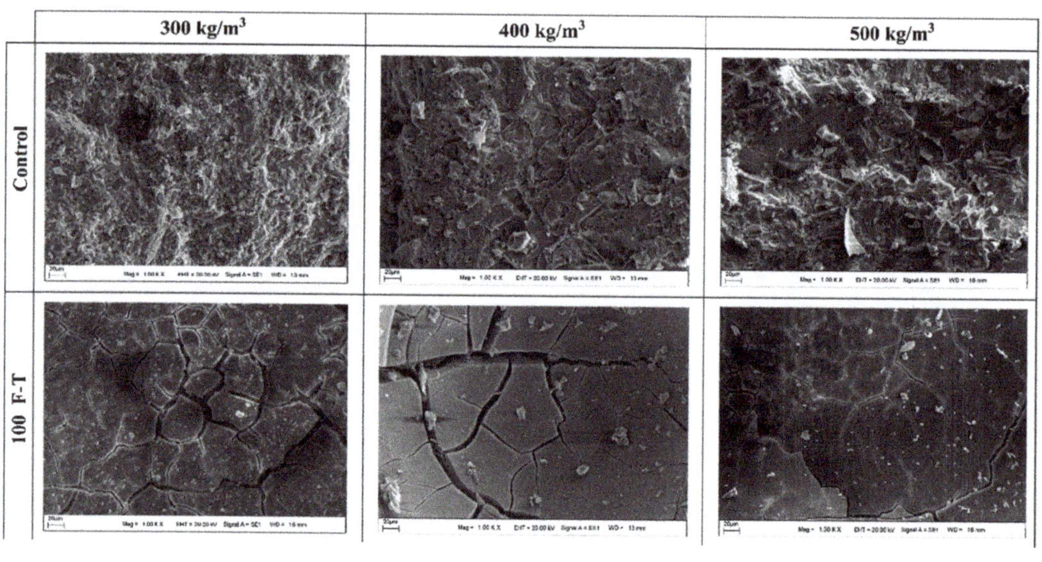

Figure 10. SEM images of GCs with different binder dosages [72]. (Reproduced with permission from [72], Elsevier, 2021).

3.1.2. Activator

Geopolymers are synthesized through the reaction of precursors with alkali activators. This indicates that the type, modulus, and dosage of alkali activators also influence the F-T resistance of GCs. Min et al. [21] revealed that geopolymers activated solely by sodium hydroxide solution exhibited poor F-T resistance. In contrast, GCs activated with a mixed solution of sodium hydroxide and sodium silicate demonstrated more favorable F-T resistance compared to those activated solely by sodium hydroxide [25], as illustrated in Figure 11. This improvement can be ascribed to the fact that the additional $[SiO_4]^{4-}$ from sodium silicate enhances the dissolution of Ca^{2+} ions, which promotes the formation of C-A-S-H gel and reduces matrix porosity [21,73]. Furthermore, the F-T resistance of GCs activated by a sodium-based activator is superior to that of GCs activated by a potassium-based activator [22]. This is because the ionic radius of Na^+ is smaller than that of K^+. This difference increases the dissolution rate of the precursor, elevates the reaction between the alkaline activator and the silicate precursor, and improves the bonding within the geopolymer structure [22]. A ternary alkali metal activator derived from carbide slag was more effective in improving the F-T resistance of geopolymer concrete based on volcanic ash than a binary alkali metal activator [16]. This is mainly because the ternary alkali activator promoted the dissolution of aluminosilicate precursors and geopolymerization, resulting in an increase in gel production.

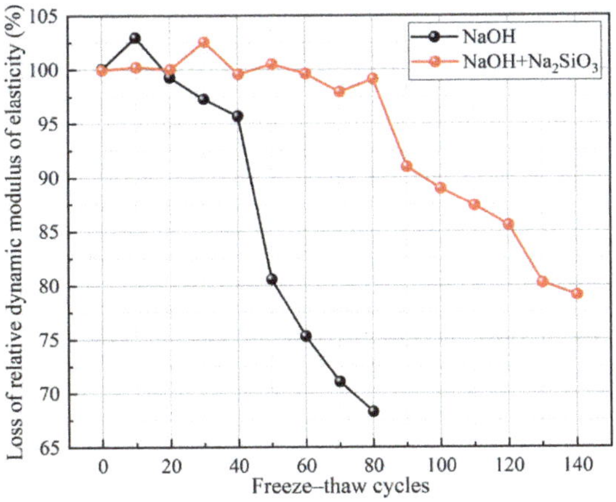

Figure 11. Influence of alkali activator type on F-T resistance of GCs [25]. (Adapted with permission from [25], Elsevier, 2021).

Moreover, the modulus of the alkali activator significantly influences the F-T durability of GCs. Zhang et al. [74] reported that the use of an alkaline activator with a modulus of 1.3 (M13) significantly enhanced the freeze–thaw resistance of GCs, as depicted in Figure 12. The reason is that appropriately increasing the modulus of the alkali activator decreases the quantity of harmful pores in the matrix. However, an excessively high modulus of the alkali activator can interfere with the geopolymerization reaction, leading to a decrease in the F-T resistance of GCs. During the curing process, some sodium silicate directly aggregated into solid particles, which reduced the compactness of the GC [67]. In addition, some researchers [24,75] have noted that GCs with higher alkali activator content exhibit better F-T resistance than those with lower activator content. Specifically, after 100 F-T cycles, a GC activated with 20% sodium metasilicate solution exhibited 31% lower compressive strength loss compared to 10% activated counterparts [75]. This is due to the fact that the increase in the content of the alkali activator facilitates the dissolution of the raw materials and the formation of gels, thereby resulting in a more compact matrix [19,23,24]. Nevertheless, Tekle et al. [76] discovered that the RDME loss of a GC with a 0.22 alkali solids-to-binder ratio (AS/B) reached 25%, while the RDME of a GC with a 0.14 AS/B ratio was almost unchanged. This is because an excessive amount of activator solution leads to an excess of water or insufficient alkali reactions in the GC, thereby weakening the adhesive forces within the matrix [77,78]. Overall, GCs activated by a mixture of sodium hydroxide and sodium silicate exhibit better F-T resistance than those activated solely by sodium hydroxide alkaline activator, with the alkaline activator modulus being most effective within the range of 1.3.

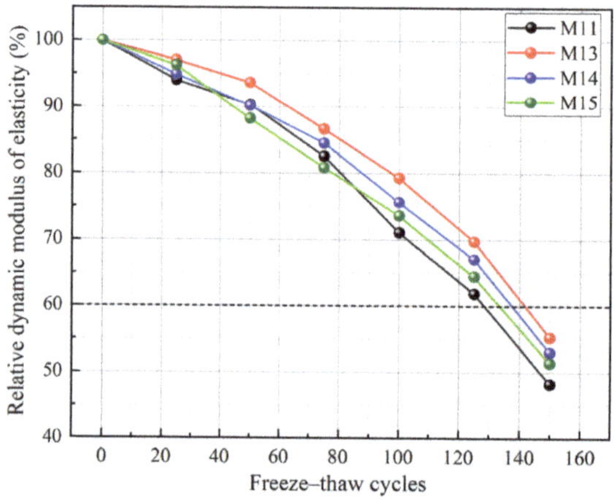

Figure 12. Influence of alkaline activator modulus on RDME [74]. (Adapted with permission from [74], Elsevier, 2023).

3.1.3. Aggregates

Aggregates are one of the crucial raw materials for preparing GCs. The F-T durability of GCs is likewise influenced by the types and properties of aggregates. Some industrial wastes, such as RPs and recycled concrete aggregate (RCA), are employed to substitute aggregates during the preparation of GCs [26–30]. Research has revealed that the relative compressive strength of GCs exhibits a pattern of initially rising and subsequently declining as the RP content increases, with an optimal RP content of 15% (Figure 13) [27]. This phenomenon is mainly due to the fact that an excessive addition of RPs will significantly increase the air content within the matrix, leading to the formation of deep and continuous cracks that propagate outward in the matrix. When the mortar on the surface of the concrete peels off, these cracks provide pathways for water to enter the interior of the matrix. Under the action of F-T cycles, these cracks further expand, allowing more water to enter the matrix and exacerbating the damage [79]. When compared with GCs without RPs, those with RPs demonstrated a substantial reduction in cracks following F-T cycles [28], as illustrated in Figure 14. The reason is that RPs absorb a portion of the stress induced by F-T cycles, resulting in a decrease in cracks [80]. Furthermore, the permeability of GCs is decreased by the addition of RPs due to their hydrophobicity. Meanwhile, RPs impede water movement in capillaries, increasing the tortuosity of water transport paths and enhancing the F-T cycle resistance of GCs [81].

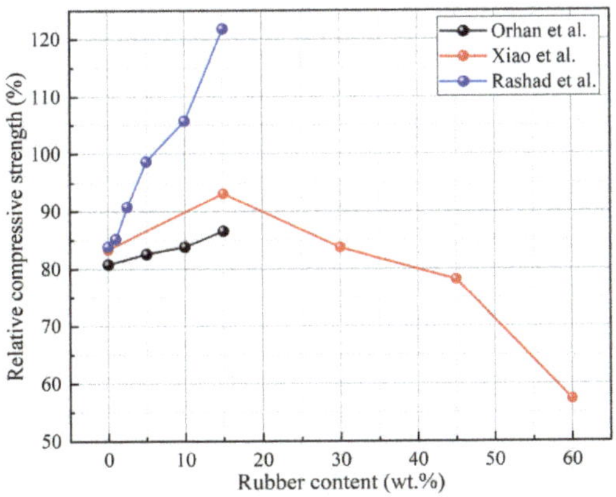

Figure 13. Effect of RPs on relative compressive strength of GCs after F-T cycles [26,27,29]. (Data from [26,27,29]).

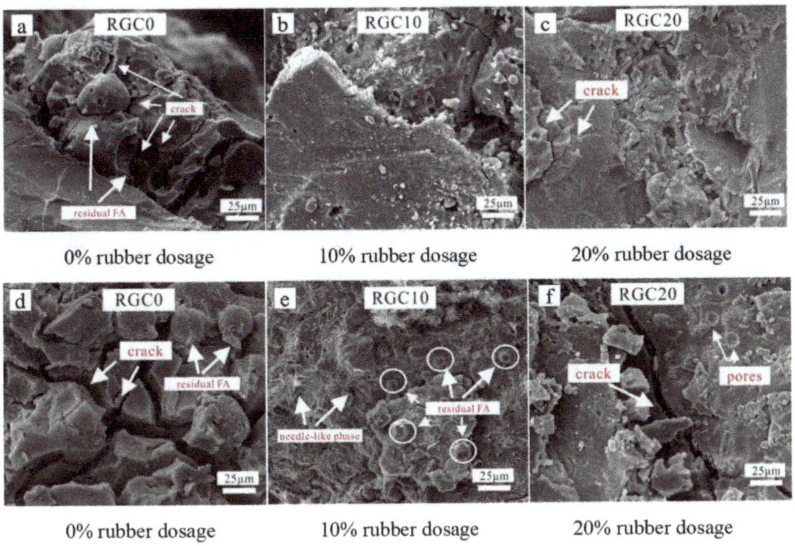

Figure 14. SEM images of rubberized geopolymer concrete before F-T cycles (**a–c**); SEM images of rubberized geopolymer concrete after 25 F-T cycles (**d–f**) [28]. (Reproduced with permission from [28], Elsevier, 2021).

The utilization of RCA effectively mitigates waste emissions, carbon emissions, and energy consumption. Nevertheless, RCA exhibits higher water absorption and weaker mechanical properties compared to natural aggregates [72]. Consequently, the incorporation of RCA leads to an increase in the amount of water infiltrating into the GC, thereby accelerating the F-T damage of the GC. Although the addition of RCA leads to an elevation in compressive strength loss and weight loss in GCs after F-T cycling, the rate of increase is not substantial, as depicted in Figure 15. Ugurlu et al. [72] reported that the loss of compressive strength of GCs without RCA was 11.8%, whereas that of samples with 100% RCA was 13.5%. This indicates that the utilization of RCA in GCs exerts a minimal impact on their F-T resistance [72,82]. Similarly, using waste glass particles instead of some natural aggregates as aggregates for geopolymer concrete also did not result in a dramatic decrease in the F-T resistance of GCs [83]. In contrast, replacing 100% of natural aggregates with coal gangue resulted in a 70% increase in weight loss after 75 F-T cycles compared to GCs without coal gangue [84]. The cause of this phenomenon is that coal gangue possesses low strength and a loose internal structure. Moreover, the adhesion between coal gangue and the gel material is weak, and there are more voids and pores in the interface transition zone [84].

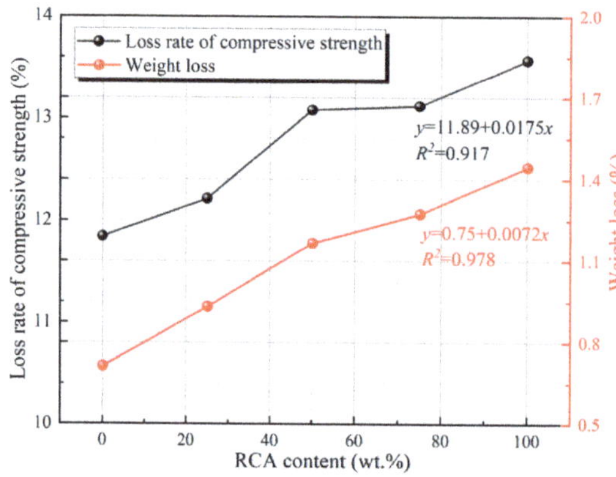

Figure 15. Influence of RCA dosage on the F-T resistance index of geopolymer [72]. (Adapted with permission from [72], Elsevier, 2021).

Apart from the aforementioned aggregates, the utilization of other aggregates can intensify the F-T resistance of GCs. Replacing part of RCA with limestone powder can enhance the F-T resistance of GCs [85]. This is mainly because limestone particles fill the pores among the hydration products, reducing the porosity [86]. Moreover, the nucleation of limestone facilitates the hydration process and the formation of hydration products [87]. Sahin et al. [88] investigated the F-T resistance of GCs prepared with six different types of sand (silica sand, river sand, sandstone, Rilem sand, RCA, and basalt sand (BS)). They discovered that GCs prepared with BS had higher compressive strength and UPV than GCs prepared with several other sands after F-T cycles. This is because the structure of geopolymer mortar filled with BS is more compact and the aggregate paste interface is strengthened. The replacement of natural aggregates with converter steel slag effectively reinforced the F-T durability of geopolymer. This is because the Ca released from the converter steel slag facilitates the formation of C-A-S-H gels. These gels fill the pores and bind the adjacent solid phases together, forming a continuous and dense matrix and a dense interface transition zone [25,89]. In summary, selecting suitable aggregates increases the density of the GC, ameliorates the interface transition zone, and thus enhances the F-T resistance of the GC. Adding 15% RP to GCs is beneficial for improving their F-T resistance, while adding RCA reduces their F-T resistance.

3.2. Curing Conditions

In addition to the raw materials used, the curing conditions employed exert a significant influence on the F-T durability of GCs. The suitable curing conditions for GCs synthesized from diverse precursors differ. Table 2 provides a compilation of the impacts that diverse curing conditions have on the F-T resistance of GCs. It can be seen that an appropriate increase in the curing temperature can elevate the F-T resistance of GCs, particularly for low-Ca GCs [65,90,91]. For instance, the F-T durability of a FA–red mud slurry (FA-RMS)-based GC solidified at a temperature of 50 °C and a relative humidity (RH) of 40–50% was determined to be optimal. The reason is that thermal curing accelerates the geopolymerization degree, thereby improving the uniformity and density of the matrix [31,92]. However, thermal curing causes rapid loss of moisture, which increases the cracking tendency in GCs [93]. Therefore, sealed curing is a suggested method, which reduces water evaporation in the structure and avoids cracking of the structure during thermal curing [72,94]. Furthermore, performing dry–wet cycles after thermal curing can reduce the compressive strength loss of geopolymer composite materials by 8.4%, as it promotes the generation of geopolymer gels and strengthens Si-O-Si bonds [95].

Table 2. Impact of solidification conditions on F-T resistance of GCs.

Precursor	Curing Condition	Temperature Range (°C)	Sample Size (mm)	F-T Cycles	Compressive Strength Loss	RDME Loss	Weight Loss	Ref.
FA-RMS	① Sealed curing under 23 °C and RH 40–50%—14 d	−10~4	50.8 × 101.6 cylinder	50	34.40%	/	3.83%	[31]
FA-RMS	① Sealed curing under 23 °C and RH 40–50%—14 d ② Standard curing-14 d	−10~4	50.8 × 101.6 cylinder	44	/	/	20.57%	[31]
FA-RMS	① Sealed curing under 50 °C—7 d ② Sealed curing under 23 °C and RH 40–50%—7 d	−10~4	50.8 × 101.6 cylinder	50	1.63%	/	−3.09%	[31]
FA-RMS	① Sealed curing under 50 °C—7 d ② Sealed curing under 23 °C and RH 40–50%—7 d ③ Ambient curing under 23 °C and RH 40–50%—14 d	−10~4	50.8 × 101.6 cylinder	50	50.2%	/	−9.49%	[31]
FA-RMS	① Sealed curing under 80 °C—24 h ② Sealed curing under 23 °C and RH 40–50%—13 d	−10~4	50.8 × 101.6 cylinder	50	3.83%	/	−8.18%	[31]
FA-RMS	① Sealed curing under 80 °C—24 h ② Sealed curing under 23 °C and RH 40–50%—13 d ③ Ambient curing under 23 °C and RH 40–50%—14 d	−10~4	50.8 × 101.6 cylinder	50	51.21%	/	−2.87%	[31]
MK	① Sealed curing under 60 °C—3 d ② Sealed curing—25 d	−20~20	100 × 100 × 100 cube	90	34.28%	/	0.74%	[64]
MK	① Sealed curing under 60 °C—3 d ② Sealed curing—25 d	−18~4	100 × 100 × 400 prism	300	28.70%	/	0.43%	[90]
MK	① Steam curing under 50 °C—28 d	−18~5	30 × 30 × 30 cube	50	63.30%	/	20.24%	[65]
Class F FA–Slag	① Standard curing—24 d	−18~5	100 × 100 × 400 prism	100	/	−2.41%	0.12%	[33]
Class F FA–Slag	① Steam curing under 60 °C—24 h ② Standard curing—23 d	−18~5	100 × 100 × 400 prism	100	/	40.12%	−0.47%	[33]
Class C FA	① Standard curing—24 d	−18~5	100 × 100 × 400 prism	100	/	3.89%	16.50%	[33]
Class C FA	① Steam curing under 60 °C—24 h ② Standard curing—23 d	−18~5	100 × 100 × 400 prism	100	/	4.51%	1.05%	[33]
Slag	① Steam curing under 85 °C—12 h ② Standard curing—27.5 d	−20~20	40 × 40 × 160 prism	150	17.05%	/	1.77%	[96]
Slag	① Standard curing—24 d	−18~5	100 × 100 × 400 prism	150	21.87%	6.74%	0.54%	[68]
Slag	① Water curing—90 d	−18~4	100 × 100 × 100 cube	300	6.14%	/	4.50%	[97]
Slag	① Sealed curing under 80 °C—24 h ② Water curing—27 d	−18~4	50 × 50 × 50 cube	100	12.04%	/	0.71%	[72]

Note: ①, ②, and ③ refer to the curing sequence.

The source of Ca in the precursor also affects the suitable curing conditions for a GC. Steam curing effectively improves the F-T resistance of GCs based on class C FA, while

GCs that are a mixture of class F FA and slag are more appropriate for standard curing conditions. This is because the steam curing method accelerates the geopolymerization process and densifies the internal structure of class C FA based GCs [33]. However, there are numerous cracks within the GC cured via steam that is based on class F FA mixed with slag. In contrast, under standard curing conditions, the hydration products of the GC based on class F FA mixed with slag are homogeneous and dense, and there is no distinct transition zone between sand and gel [33,98]. Compared with steam-cured GCs, water-cured GCs exhibit lower early-age strength, yet their gel products are more uniformly distributed within the matrix, and the matrix has a lower porosity [96].

3.3. Modified Materials

3.3.1. Fiber

GCs sustain damage during the F-T cycle as a result of the influences of expansion pressure and water pressure. Consequently, some researchers have incorporated fibers, such as SFs and basalt fibers (BFs), into GCs to mitigate F-T degradation. The influence of adding SFs and BFs on the F-T resistance of GCs is illustrated in Figure 16 [40,41,64,99–102]. Most studies indicate that adding an appropriate amount of SF and BF reduces the loss of mechanical properties in GCs after F-T cycles, such as compressive strength loss, UPV loss, and flexural strength loss [40,41,64]. For example, when compared with control specimens without SF, the compressive strength loss of GCs containing 0.8% SF decreased by approximately 50% (Figure 16a) [40]. The reason is that SFs resist the expansion pressure generated by pore-water freezing through fiber confinement, and also limit the propagation of cracks [39]. In comparison to adding SFs, the effect of adding BFs on the F-T durability of GCs is less significant [40,64]. Nazir et al. [41] observed that the weight of GCs increased, rather than decreased, as shown in Figure 16d. This is because new microcracks inside GCs are generated during F-T cycles. External water infiltrates these microcracks, leading to an increase in weight [41,100].

Adding polymer fibers to GCs can also improve their durability [41,89,101,103]. The effect of polymer fibers on the F-T resistance of GCs is exhibited in Figure 17 [41,99,101,104]. For instance, in contrast to the control group without polypropylene (PP) fibers, the compressive strength loss of GCs with 0.4% PP fibers decreased by approximately 10% after F-T cycles [89]. When compared with the control group without fiber addition, incorporating 1.0% polyethylene (PE) fibers into GCs reduced the loss of compressive strength by approximately 92.70% [41]. Incorporating polyvinyl alcohol (PVA) fibers into GCs effectively reduces weight loss of GCs following F-T cycles [101,104], as depicted in Figure 17d. The reason is that PVA fibers decrease the water absorption rate of GCs. Moreover, PVA fibers act as crack-bridging agents and restrict their propagation, thus reducing the crystallization pressure and water pressure induced by water freezing [89,101,105].

Adding 6.0% wood fibers can strengthen the F-T resistance of GCs. This is because wood fibers restrict the propagation of cracks and increase the cohesion of the matrix [106]. The incorporation of 0.1% modified multi-walled carbon nanotubes (MWCNTs) together with 2.0% PVA fibers can augment the number of F-T cycles that GCs can endure [14]. The underlying reason lies in the fact that the crack arrest effect (Figure 18b), mechanical interlocking effect, nano-filling effect (Figure 18a), and nano-nucleation effect of MWCNTs render the geopolymer mortar denser and reduce the capillary porosity of the mortar [14].

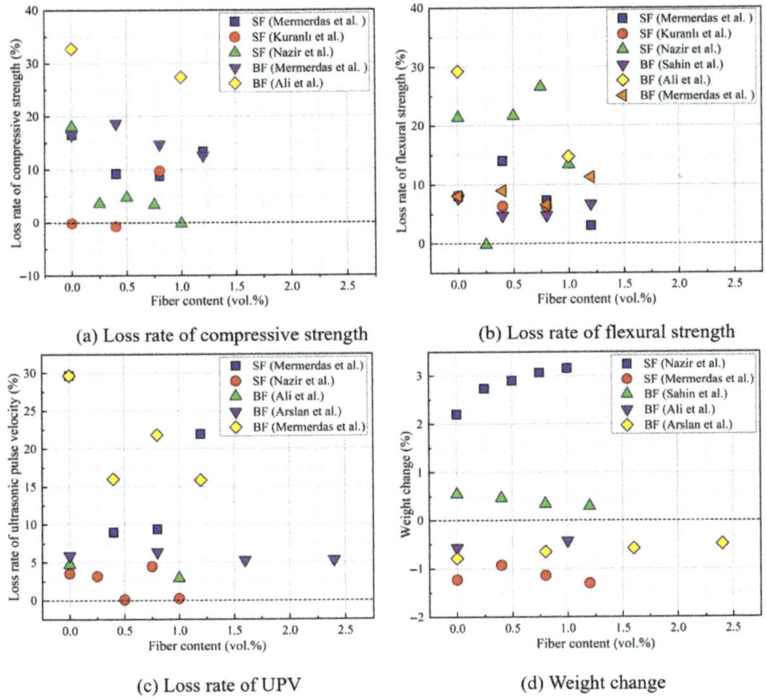

Figure 16. Influence of SF and BF on F-T resistance of GCs [40,41,64,99–102]. (The date from [40,41,64,99–102]).

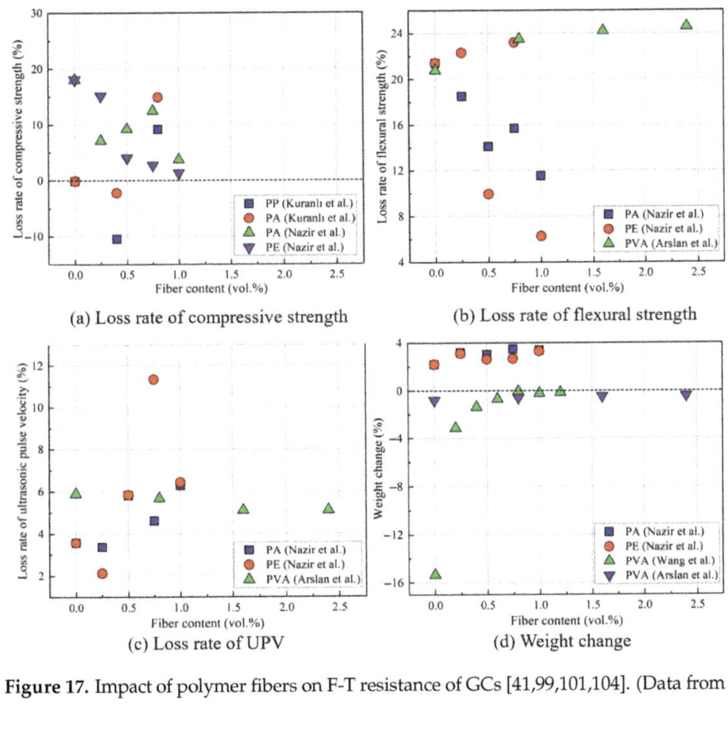

Figure 17. Impact of polymer fibers on F-T resistance of GCs [41,99,101,104]. (Data from [41,99,101,104]).

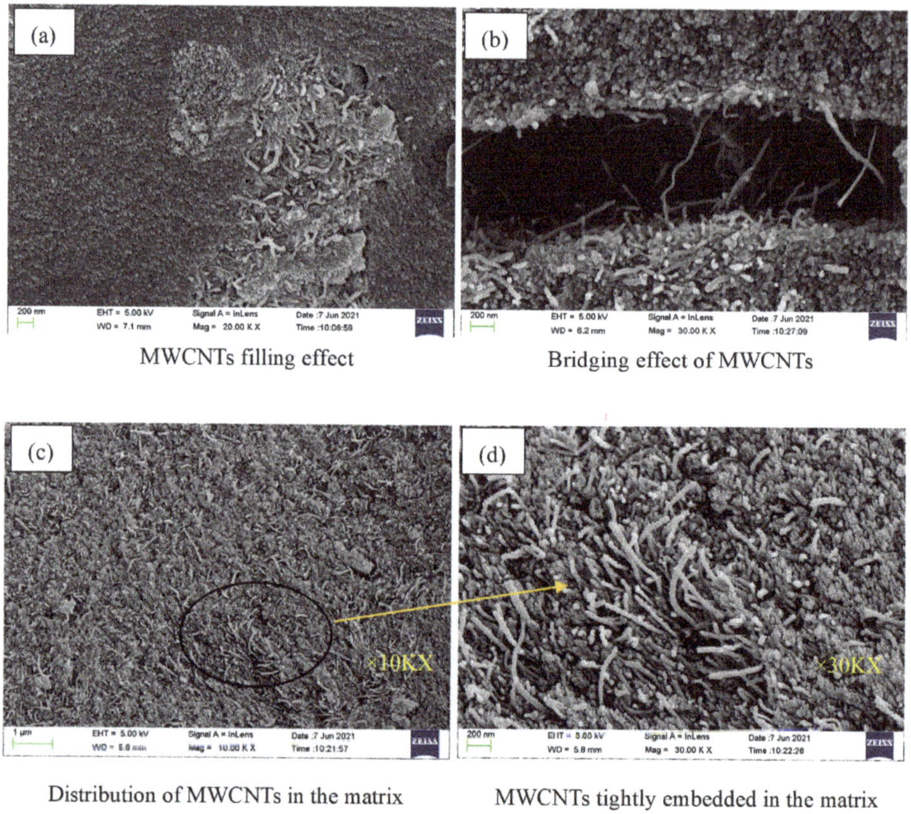

Figure 18. SEM images of GCs with modified MWCNTs incorporated after F-T cycles [14]. (Reproduced with permission from [14], Elsevier, 2022).

3.3.2. Nano-Materials

Due to the fact that nano-materials exhibit excellent volcanic ash and filling effects [107], some researchers have incorporated nano-materials into GCs to elevate their F-T properties. The incorporation of nano-materials into GCs effectively reduces the loss of compressive strength following F-T cycles, as is evident from Figure 19 [97,108–110]. For example, when compared with the control group without nano-graphite (NG), a GC containing 0.1% NG exhibited the lowest loss of compressive strength following F-T cycles, with a value amounting to merely 0.5% [108]. This is mainly because NG reduces the water absorption rate of GCs, thus reducing the formation of ice. In addition, during the F-T cycles, NG can also bridge the cracks and limit the propagation of cracks [108], as shown in Figure 20. The incorporation of GO densifies the geopolymer matrix, optimizes the pore structure, and inhibits water transport [109]. Additionally, GO promotes the generation of abundant aluminosilicate gel, such as flower-like and layered hydration products, as presented in Figure 21. When the GO content was 0.06%, the reduction in compressive strength loss reached 41.1% compared to a sample without GO [44].

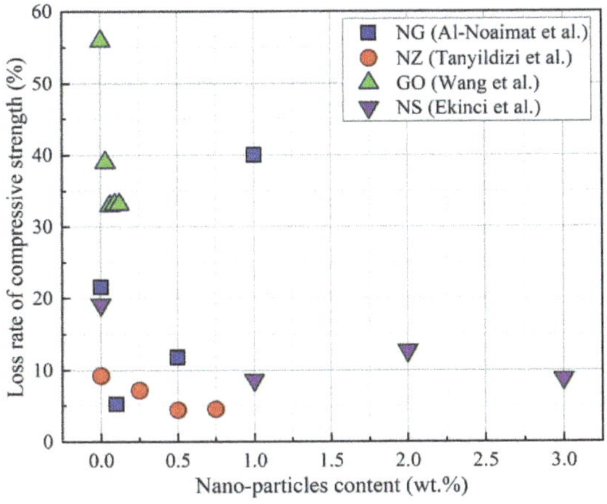

Figure 19. The influence of nano-particles on the loss rate of compressive strength [97,108–110]. (Data from [97,108–110]).

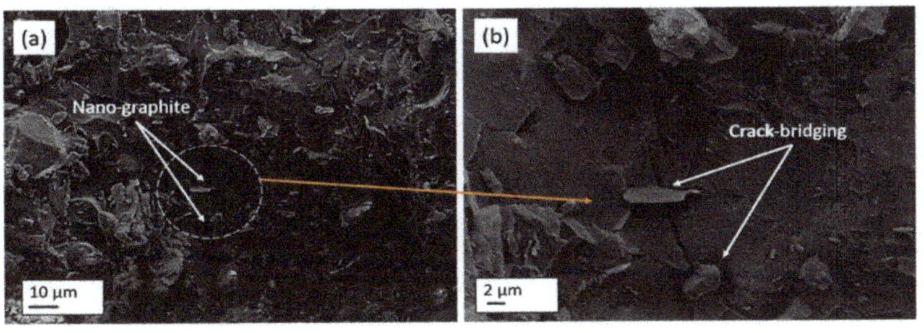

Image under 10μm

Image under 2μm

Figure 20. Schematic diagram of NG bridging function [108]. (Reproduced with permission from [108], Elsevier, 2023).

NS, nano-alumina (NA), and nano-clay (NC) promote the hydration reaction and the formation of gel products, enhancing the degree of geopolymerization. Moreover, they refine the microstructure of geopolymer and form a dense geopolymer composite slurry owing to their filling effect [34–36]. In comparison with NA and NC, NS exerts a more substantial influence on improving the F-T resistance of GCs [97]. The reason for this is that NS provides more silicon dioxide, which increases the generation of geopolymer products [42]. The majority of studies have shown that integrating 1.0% to 2.0% of NS into GCs is capable of improving the F-T resistance of GCs. [18,97,104]. Incorporating nano-zinc oxide (NZ) into geopolymer reduced the loss of compressive strength of GCs following F-T cycles, and the residual compressive strength of a GC containing 0.5% NZ was 95.72% after F-T cycles [110]. The interfacial adhesion between NZ particles and the geopolymer matrix diminishes the range of the interfacial transition zone [110]. Additionally, the existence of nano-zinc oxide (NZ) results in a more compact microstructure of GCs, as shown in Figure 22. However, an excessive incorporation of NZ leads to nano-agglomeration and weakens the F-T resistance of GCs [110]. In conclusion, considering the comprehensive economic benefits of nano-materials and their degree of improvement on F-T resistance, the addition of 1.0% NS is more conducive to enhancing the F-T resistance of GCs than other nano-materials.

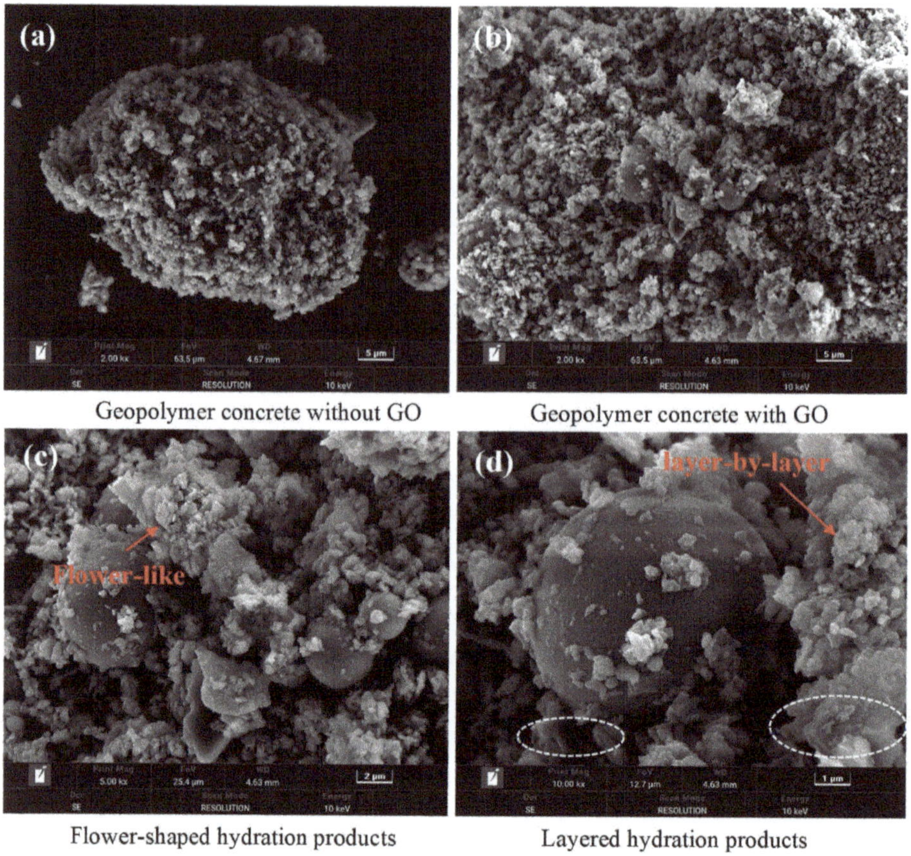

Figure 21. SEM images of geopolymer foam concrete [44]. (Reproduced with permission from [44], Elsevier, 2023).

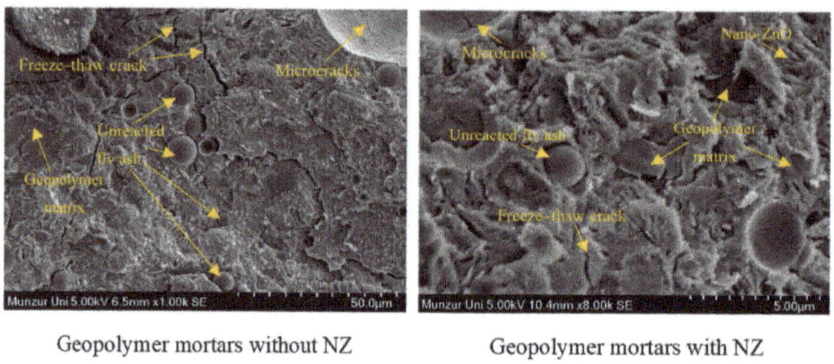

Figure 22. SEM of geopolymer mortars after F-T cycles [111]. (Reproduced with permission from [111], Elsevier, 2024).

3.3.3. Air-Entraining Agents

Numerous studies have demonstrated that AEAs effectively improve the F-T resistance of OPCC [112–115]. The reason is that AEAs incorporate tiny bubbles (20–50 μm) into concrete, thereby providing space for water expansion and reducing the internal pressure within the concrete [116]. However, the addition of AEAs to GC has not had a significant effect on improving their F-T resistance, as presented in Table 3. Sun et al. [117] discovered that there was no significant difference in the weight loss and RDME loss of FA-based geopolymer mortar with and without an AEA after 300 F-T cycles. The research findings of Aygörmez et al. [90] indicate that an AEA reduced the weight loss of MK-based geopolymer composite materials, but the effect was not substantial. Brooks et al. [118] found that FA-based geopolymers with added AEAs exhibited slight scaling after 40 F-T cycles, whereas FA-based GCs without added AEAs did not show any scaling after 40 F-T cycles. This could potentially be ascribed to the circumstance that the addition of AEA fails to form a homogeneous and stable structure within GCs [118].

Table 3. Influence of AEAs on F-T resistance of GCs.

Type	AEA Content	Sample Size (mm)	Temperature Range (°C)	F-T Cycles	Compressive Strength Loss	RDME Loss	Weight Loss	Ref.
Geopolymer mortar	0%	23.5 × 23.5 × 50.8 prism	−18~4	300	5.00%	8.40%	0.12%	[117]
Geopolymer mortar	0.20%	23.5 × 23.5 × 50.8 prism	−18~4	300	0%	6.80%	0.17%	[117]
Geopolymer mortar	0%	100 × 100 × 400 prism	−18~4	300	28.31%	/	0.43%	[90]
Geopolymer mortar	0.10%	100 × 100 × 400 prism	−18~4	300	23.73%	/	0.12%	[90]

4. Freeze–Thaw Damage and Prediction Models of Geopolymer Composites

4.1. Experience Model

By testing the degradation of GCs under F-T cycling, various F-T resistance indicators can be acquired, which can be quantified to establish a damage model for GCs under F-T cycling. These models assume a pivotal role in assessing the F-T resistance of GCs and forecasting the extent of their degradation. The RDME and compressive strength, which reflect the mechanical properties and internal structure of GCs, are generally used as damage variables to establish F-T damage models [14,84,119]. Common F-T damage models of GCs are summarized in Table 4. Most of the F-T damage models are established using exponential functions or power functions, as listed in Table 4. Compared with those using power functions, models established using exponential functions yield more accurate predictive results. Furthermore, the root mean square error (RMSE) of the nonlinear regression model put forward by Sun et al. [120] for predicting the F-T life of geopolymer concrete was 0.0299, indicating that the model had a satisfactory predictive effect. Porosity is also utilized to develop F-T damage predictive models. Wu et al. [121] developed a prediction model regarding the residual compressive strength of GCs following F-T cycles, as presented in Equations (2) and (3). The coefficient of determination (R^2) of the model was approximately 0.99, indicating that the model is capable of efficiently predicting the residual compressive strength of geopolymer concrete following F-T cycles.

$$\frac{F_N}{F_0} = \frac{1-\xi D_N}{1-\xi D_0} \tag{2}$$

$$D_i = 1-(1-\frac{\varphi_i}{\varphi_c})^{\frac{v}{2}} \cdot (1-\varphi_i)^{m+0.5} \tag{3}$$

where F_N, D_N, φ_i are the compressive strength, degree of damage, and porosity of geopolymer concrete after F-T cycles, respectively; N represents the number of F-T cycles; ξ is a correction factor; φ_c is the percolation threshold of the material; v is the scale index; and m is a parameter related to shrinkage properties.

Table 4. Empirical model of F-T damage.

F-T Evaluation Model	F-T Damage Model	Evaluating Index	Ref.
$w = 1 - ae^{bN}$	$w = 1 - E_N/E_0$	R^2: 0.910~0.986	[14]
$w = aN^b$	$w = 1 - E_N/E_0$	R^2: 0.936~0.992	[84]
$w = a(1 - e^{-bN})$	$w = 1 - E_N/E_0$	R^2: 0.974~0.996	[84]
$w = a \cdot e^{-bN}$	$w = F_N/F_0$	R^2: 0.950	[15]
$w = a \cdot N^b$	$w = F_N/F_0$	R^2: 0.790	[15]
$w = a \cdot e^{-bN}$	$w = 1 - F_N/F_0$	R^2: 0.958	[15]
$w = a \cdot N^b$	$w = 1 - F_N/F_0$	R^2: 0.998	[15]
$w = a \cdot e^{-bN}$	$w = E_N/E_0$	R^2: 0.860	[15]
$w = aN^b$	$w = E_N/E_0$	R^2: 0.600	[15]
$w = a \cdot e^{-bN}$	$w = 1 - E_N/E_0$	R^2: 0.971	[15]
$w = aN^b$	$w = 1 - E_N/E_0$	R^2: 0.897	[15]
$w = a \cdot e^{bN}$	$w = 1 \pm \frac{E_N/E_0 - 0.60}{0.40} \cdot \frac{0.25 - F_N/F_0}{0.25}$	RSME: 0.030	[120]

Note: w is the F-T damage index, E_N is the RDME under N F-T cycles, E_0 is the RDME before the F-T cycles, and a and b are constant.

4.2. Machine Learning Models

In addition to empirical models, some researchers have also established ML models to predict the F-T damage of GCs. ML is a method of extracting implicit mapping relationships from existing data through model training, aiming to achieve relatively ideal training outcomes and accurate predictions [122]. Deep learning, which is a part of machine learning, makes use of neural networks featuring three or more hidden layers. Through these networks, it is able to learn intricate patterns and acquire meaningful representations. The artificial neural network (ANN) model proposed by Abadel et al. [123] revealed acceptable precision in predicting the F-T resistance of GCs, with an R^2 value of 0.99. Three ML models, namely backpropagation neural network (BPNN), convolutional neural network (CNN), and gated recurrent unit (GRU), were employed by Yao et al. [124] to forecast the compressive strength of one-part geopolymer after F-T cycles. They used 216 sets of data, with the ratio of the training set to the validation set being 8:2. The input features included the FA/GGBF ratio, freezing temperature, and F-T cycles, while the output variable was compressive strength. Their standard deviations were 0.157, 6.251, 3.917, and 0.716, respectively. The results indicated that all models demonstrated satisfactory predictive performance, suggesting that all three models were reliable in their prediction of the F-T resistance of GCs. Among the three models, the CNN model exhibited the highest prediction accuracy, with an R^2 value of 0.9966 and an RMSE value of 0.0414, as illustrated in Figure 23a. Moreover, the innovation of metaheuristic algorithms is an approach to optimize neural networks. Algorithms like particle swarm optimization (PSO) and genetic algorithms have the capacity to enhance both the performance and the generalization capability of neural networks. Particle swarm optimization was applied by Zhang et al. [125] to optimize BPNN for the durability prediction of geopolymer mortar. They used 22 sets of data, with 16 sets for training the model and the remaining 6 sets for testing the prediction. The input layer included MK dosage, FA dosage, NS dosage, and PVA fiber dosage, while the output layer was the compressive strength loss rate. Their standard deviations were 3.671, 3.377, 0.807, 0.394, and 3.592, respectively. The predicted results of PSO-BPNN were closer to the actual values than those of BPNN [125], as depicted in Figure 23b. Therefore, it is feasible to predict the F-T durability of GCs accurately and scientifically using PSO-BPNN.

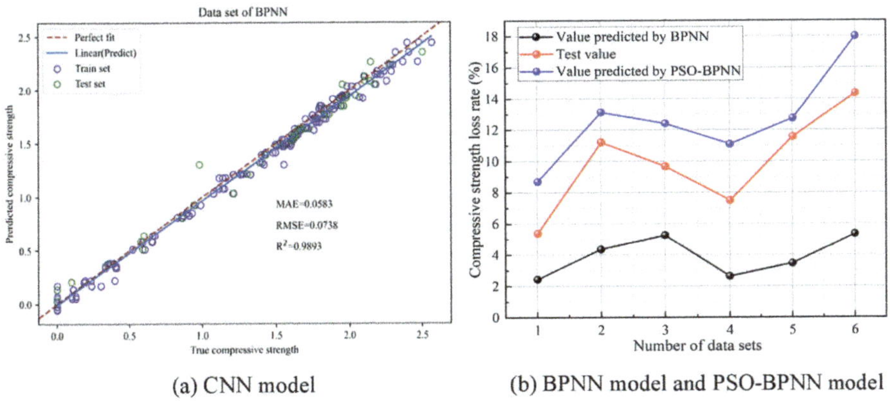

Figure 23. Prediction results of different ML models [124,125]. (Reproduced with permission from [124,125], Elsevier, 2024).

5. Conclusions

This review article offers a comprehensive overview of the F-T damage process of GCs, along with some common theories pertaining to F-T damage. It also provides an in-depth and comprehensive summary of the factors that influence the F-T resistance of GCs. By doing so, this review contributes to a more profound understanding of the elements influencing the F-T resistance of GCs and their underlying mechanisms, thereby laying a solid foundation for both engineering applications and academic research. The influencing factors encompass raw materials, curing conditions, and modified materials. Moreover, this review summarizes the models developed through regression analysis and machine learning techniques for the evaluation and prediction of the F-T damage of GCs. The main conclusions of this article are as follows:

(1) The degree of F-T damage of GCs is influenced by pore water pressure and crystallization pressure. The F-T failure process of GCs is predominantly categorized into three distinct stages: water absorption and saturation, ice crystallization during the freezing phase, and microstructural damage leading to macroscopic failure. As the quantity of F-T cycles rises, the surface layer of the geopolymer will start to flake off, and fissures will develop within its internal structure. Three commonly used F-T damage theories are introduced, namely the crystallization pressure theory, hydrostatic pressure theory, and osmotic pressure theory. The theory of crystallization pressure elucidates the process of crystal failure in porous materials.

(2) The Ca content in the precursor can affect the F-T resistance of the geopolymer. GCs with a high Ca content exhibit better F-T resistance than those with a low Ca content. Multiple studies have shown that GCs activated by a mixture of sodium hydroxide and sodium silicate possess better F-T resistance compared to those activated using sodium hydroxide alkaline activator alone. The modulus of the alkaline activator is most effective within the range of 1.3. Replacing natural aggregates with recycled aggregates weakens the F-T resistance of GCs, although this effect is not pronounced. When the proportion of RPs replacing fine aggregates is in the range of approximately 15%, it can augment the F-T resistance of GCs.

(3) The suitable curing conditions for GCs are influenced by the source and amount of Ca contained in the precursor. The F-T resistance of GCs can be enhanced by appropriately increasing the curing temperature to the range of approximately 50 °C

to 80 °C, particularly for low-Ca GCs. Desirable results can be obtained when the curing temperature is set within the range of 50 °C to 70 °C.

(4) Fibers, nano-particles, and AEAs are modified materials that influence the F-T resistance of GCs. Extensive experimental studies have demonstrated that fibers can strengthen the F-T resistance of GCs. However, an excessive amount of fibers can form aggregates and cause defects within the matrix. Incorporating an appropriate amount of nano-particles (ranging from 0.45% to 2%) into GCs can improve their F-T resistance. The impact of AEAs on the F-T resistance of GCs is relatively limited, and the findings reported in the literature are still highly controversial.

(5) In this review, the assessment and prediction models of F-T damage were summarized, and the coefficient of determination R^2 values of these models were all above 0.9. Most of the empirical models for F-T damage were established based on exponential and power functions. When compared with traditional empirical models, most of the prediction models of geopolymer F-T damage established using neural network algorithms possess higher accuracy and broader applicability. Among these models, the prediction results of the CNN model and the ANN model are relatively accurate. Their coefficient of determination R^2 values are all above 0.99.

Funding: This research was funded by [Program for Leading Talents in Central Plains Science and Technology Innovation] grant number [254000510027].

Institutional Review Board Statement: Not applicable.

Informed Consent Statement: Not applicable.

Data Availability Statement: No new data were created or analyzed in this study.

Acknowledgments: The authors would like to acknowledge the financial support received from the Program for Leading Talents in Central Plains Science and Technology Innovation (Grant No. 254000510027).

Conflicts of Interest: The authors declare no conflicts of interest.

Abbreviations

OPC	ordinary Portland cement
GC	geopolymer composite
FA	fly ash
GGBFS	ground granulated blast furnace slag
MK	metakaolin
F-T	freeze–thaw
RDME	relative dynamic modulus of elasticity
UPV	ultrasonic pulse velocity
Ca	calcium
AEA	air-entraining agent
SF	steel fiber
PE	polyethylene
GO	graphene oxide
RP	rubber particle
NS	nano-silica
ML	machine learning
SEM	scanning electron microscopy
N-A-S-H	sodium aluminosilicate hydrate
OPCC	ordinary Portland cement concrete
C-S-H	calcium silicate hydrate

C-A-S-H	calcium aluminosilicate hydrate
RCA	recycled concrete aggregate
BS	basalt sand
FA-RMS	fly ash–red mud slurry
RH	relative humidity
BF	basalt fiber
PP	polypropylene
PVA	polyvinyl alcohol
MWCNTs	multi-walled carbon nanotubes
NG	nano-graphite
NA	nano-alumina
NC	nano-clay
NZ	nano-zinc oxide
RMSE	root mean square error
ANN	artificial neural network
BPNN	backpropagation neural network
CNN	convolutional neural network
GRU	gated recurrent unit
PSO	particle swarm optimization

References

1. Wang, A.; Zheng, Y.; Zhang, Z.; Liu, K.; Li, Y.; Shi, L.; Sun, D. The durability of alkali-activated materials in comparison with Ordinary Portland Cements and concretes: A review. *Engineering* **2020**, *6*, 695–706. [CrossRef]
2. Singh, N.B.; Middendorf, B. Geopolymers as an alternative to Portland cement: An overview. *Constr. Build. Mater.* **2020**, *237*, 117455. [CrossRef]
3. Li, V.C. High-Performance and multifunctional cement-based composite material. *Engineering* **2019**, *5*, 250–260. [CrossRef]
4. Monteiro, P.J.M.; Miller, S.A.; Horvath, A. Towards sustainable concrete. *Nat. Mater.* **2017**, *16*, 698–699. [CrossRef]
5. Amran, Y.H.M.; Alyousef, R.; Alabduljabbar, H.; El-Zeadani, M. Clean production and properties of geopolymer concrete; A review. *J. Clean. Prod.* **2020**, *251*, 119679. [CrossRef]
6. Wang, W.S.; Zhang, P.; Guo, J.J.; Wang, F. Abrasion resistance assessment of geopolymer concrete reinforced with nano-SiO_2 and steel-polyvinyl alcohol hybrid fiber. *Constr. Build. Mater.* **2025**, *487*, 15. [CrossRef]
7. Zhang, P.; Zhang, X.; Guo, J.J.; Zheng, Y.X.; Gao, Z. Mechanical Properties of Cement-Based Gel Composites Reinforced by Plant Fiber: A Review. *Gels* **2025**, *11*, 33. [CrossRef]
8. Davidovits, J. Synthesis of New High-Temperature Geo-Polymers for Reinforced Plastics/Composites. 1979; pp. 151–154. Available online: https://www.scopus.com/pages/publications/0024630792?inward= (accessed on 6 July 2025).
9. Provis, J.L. Alkali-activated materials. *Cem. Concr. Res.* **2018**, *114*, 40–48. [CrossRef]
10. Xie, C.; Cao, M.; Yin, H.; Guan, J.; Wang, L. Effects of freeze-thaw damage on fracture properties and microstructure of hybrid fibers reinforced cementitious composites containing calcium carbonate whisker. *Constr. Build. Mater.* **2021**, *300*, 123872. [CrossRef]
11. Wang, R.; Zhang, Q.; Li, Y. Deterioration of concrete under the coupling effects of freeze-thaw cycles and other actions: A review. *Constr. Build. Mater.* **2022**, *319*, 126045. [CrossRef]
12. Scherer, G.W. Crystallization in pores. *Cem. Concr. Res.* **1999**, *29*, 1347–1358. [CrossRef]
13. Powers, T.C. A working hypothesis for further studies of frost resistance of concrete. *J. ACI* **1945**, *14*, 245–272.
14. Li, F.; Chen, D.; Lu, Y.; Zhang, H.; Li, S. Influence of mixed fibers on fly ash based geopolymer resistance against freeze-thaw cycles. *J. Non-Cryst. Solids* **2022**, *584*, 121517. [CrossRef]
15. Bao, W.X.; Yin, Y.; Mi, W.J.; Chen, R.; Lin, X.H. Durability and microstructural evolution of high-performance ecological geopolymer concrete under low-pressure-salt-erosion-freeze-thaw cycling conditions. *Constr. Build. Mater.* **2024**, *426*, 136197. [CrossRef]
16. Zheng, Y.; Rao, F.; Yang, L.; Zhong, S. Comparison of ternary and dual combined waste-derived alkali activators on the durability of volcanic ash-based geopolymers. *Cem. Concr. Compos.* **2023**, *136*, 104886. [CrossRef]
17. Fu, Y.; Cai, L.; Wu, Y. Freeze-thaw cycle test and damage mechanics models of alkali-activated slag concrete. *Constr. Build. Mater.* **2011**, *25*, 3144–3148. [CrossRef]

18. Ekinci, E.; Türkmen, İ.; Kantarci, F.; Karakoç, M.B. The improvement of mechanical, physical and durability characteristics of volcanic tuff based geopolymer concrete by using nano silica, micro silica and Styrene-Butadiene Latex additives at different ratios. *Constr. Build. Mater.* **2019**, *201*, 257–267. [CrossRef]
19. Aiken, T.A.; Kwasny, J.; Sha, W.; Tong, K.T. Mechanical and durability properties of alkali-activated fly ash concrete with increasing slag content. *Constr. Build. Mater.* **2021**, *124330*, 124330. [CrossRef]
20. Yan, D.M.; Xie, L.J.; Qian, X.Q.; Ruan, S.Q.; Zeng, Q. Compositional dependence of pore structure, strengthand freezing-thawing resistance of metakaolin-based geopolymers. *Materials* **2020**, *13*, 2973. [CrossRef]
21. Min, Y.F.; Wu, J.; Li, B.; Zhang, M.Y.; Zhang, J.J. Experimental study of freeze-thaw resistance of a one-part geopolymer paste. *Case Stud. Constr. Mater.* **2022**, *17*, e01269. [CrossRef]
22. Bilir, T.; Aygörmez, Y.; Bastan, Z.; Uysal, M.; Aygun, B.F. Unraveling the characteristics of geopolymer mortars: A deep dive into the impact of marble powder as fine aggregate and varied activators. *Constr. Build. Mater.* **2024**, *422*, 135767. [CrossRef]
23. Xue, L.; Zhang, Z.; Wang, H. Early hydration kinetics and microstructure development of hybrid alkali activated cements (HAACs) at room temperature. *Cem. Concr. Compos.* **2021**, *123*, 104200. [CrossRef]
24. Mazaheri, A.; Bayat, A.; Hosinzadeh, F. Investigating the effect of alkali-activated slag on the strength of clay soil. *Arab. J. Geosci.* **2021**, *14*, 2662. [CrossRef]
25. Sun, K.K.; Peng, X.Q.; Chu, S.H.; Wang, S.P.; Zeng, L.; Ji, G.X. Utilization of BOF steel slag aggregate in metakaolin-based geopolymer. *Constr. Build. Mater.* **2021**, *300*, 124024. [CrossRef]
26. Rashad, A.M.; Sadek, D.M. Behavior of alkali-activated slag pastes blended with waste rubber powder under the effect of freeze/thaw cycles and severe sulfate attack. *Constr. Build. Mater.* **2020**, *265*, 120716. [CrossRef]
27. Xiao, R.; Shen, Z.; Si, R.; Polaczyk, P.; Li, Y.; Zhou, H.; Huang, B. Alkali-activated slag (AAS) and OPC-based composites containing crumb rubber aggregate: Physico-mechanical properties, durability and oxidation of rubber upon NaOH treatment. *J. Clean. Prod.* **2022**, *367*, 132896. [CrossRef]
28. Zhang, B.; Feng, Y.; Xie, J.; Lai, D.; Yu, T.; Huang, D. Rubberized geopolymer concrete: Dependence of mechanical properties and freeze-thaw resistance on replacement ratio of crumb rubber. *Constr. Build. Mater.* **2021**, *310*, 125248. [CrossRef]
29. Orhan, T.Y.; Karakoç, M.B.; Özcan, A. Durability characteristics of slag based geopolymer concrete modified with crumb rubber. *Constr. Build. Mater.* **2023**, *404*, 132851. [CrossRef]
30. Bayraktar, O.Y.; Benli, A.; Bodur, B.; Öz, A.; Kaplan, G. Performance assessment and cost analysis of slag/metakaolin based rubberized semi-lightweight geopolymers with perlite aggregate: Sustainable reuse of waste tires. *Constr. Build. Mater.* **2024**, *411*, 134655. [CrossRef]
31. Zhao, M.; Zhang, G.; Htet, K.W.; Kwon, M.; Liu, C.; Xu, Y.; Tao, M. Freeze-thaw durability of red mud slurry-class F fly ash-based geopolymer: Effect of curing conditions. *Constr. Build. Mater.* **2019**, *215*, 381–390. [CrossRef]
32. Yılmaz, A.; Degirmenci, F.N.; Aygörmez, Y. Effect of initial curing conditions on the durability performance of low-calcium fly ash-based geopolymer mortars. *Bol. Soc. Esp. Cerám. Vidr.* **2023**, *63*, 238–254. [CrossRef]
33. Jiao, Z.; Li, X.; Yu, Q. Effect of curing conditions on freeze-thaw resistance of geopolymer mortars containing various calcium resources. *Constr. Build. Mater.* **2021**, *313*, 125507. [CrossRef]
34. Malik, M.A.; Sarkar, M.; Xu, S.L.; Li, Q.H. Effect of PVA/SiO_2 NPs additive on the structural, durability, and fire resistance properties of geopolymers. *Appl. Sci.* **2019**, *9*, 1953. [CrossRef]
35. Deb, P.S.; Sarker, P.K.; Barbhuiya, S. Sorptivity and acid resistance of ambient-cured geopolymer mortars containing nano-silica. *Cem. Concr. Compos.* **2016**, *72*, 235–245. [CrossRef]
36. Mustakim, S.M.; Das, S.K.; Mishra, J.; Aftab, A.; Alomayri, T.S.; Assaedi, H.S.; Kaze, C.R. Improvement in fresh, mechanical and microstructural properties of fly ash- blast furnace slag based geopolymer concrete by addition of nano and micro silica. *Silicon* **2021**, *13*, 2415–2428. [CrossRef]
37. Gao, Z.; Zhang, P.; Dai, X.B.; Zheng, Y.X.; Feng, H. Assessment of bonding behavior of hybrid fiber alkali-activated concrete for tunnel lining concrete restoration. *J. Clean. Prod.* **2025**, *514*, 14. [CrossRef]
38. Feng, Z.; Zhang, P.; Guo, J.J.; Zheng, Y.X.; Hu, S.W. Single and synergistic effects of nano-SiO2 and hybrid fiber on rheological property and compressive strength of geopolymer concrete. *Constr. Build. Mater.* **2025**, *472*, 15. [CrossRef]
39. Zada Farhan, K.; Azmi Megat Johari, M.; Demirboğa, R. Evaluation of properties of steel fiber reinforced GGBFS-based geopolymer composites in aggressive environments. *Constr. Build. Mater.* **2022**, *345*, 128339. [CrossRef]
40. Mermerdas, K.; Ipek, S.; Mahmood, Z. Visual inspection and mechanical testing of fly ash-based fibrous geopolymer composites under freeze-thaw cycles. *Constr. Build. Mater.* **2021**, *283*, 122756. [CrossRef]
41. Nazir, K.; Canpolat, O.; Uysal, M. Durability properties of steel, polyamide, and polyethylene fiber-reinforced geopolymer mortar made with recycled concrete aggregate and glass powder as fillers. *J. Build. Eng.* **2023**, *76*, 107313. [CrossRef]
42. Adak, D.; Sarkar, M.; Mandal, S. Structural performance of nano-silica modified fly-ash based geopolymer concrete. *Constr. Build. Mater.* **2017**, *135*, 430–439. [CrossRef]

43. Wang, W.S.; Zhang, P.; Dai, X.B.; Zheng, Y.X.; Hu, S.W. Workability of self-compacting geopolymer concrete: The effect of nano-SiO_2 and steel-polyvinyl alcohol hybrid fiber. *Constr. Build. Mater.* **2025**, *460*, 12. [CrossRef]
44. Wang, W.J.; Zhong, Z.W.; Kang, X.; Ma, X.Y. Physico-mechanical properties and micromorphological characteristics of graphene oxide reinforced geopolymer foam concrete. *J. Build. Eng.* **2023**, *72*, 106732. [CrossRef]
45. Miyan, N.; Omur, T.; Amed, B.; Özkan, H.; Aydin, R.; Kabay, N. Recycled waste concrete and metakaolin based alkali-activated paste: Characterization, optimization, and life cycle assessment. *Constr. Build. Mater.* **2024**, *416*, 16. [CrossRef]
46. Pilehvar, S.; Szczotok, A.M.; Rodríguez, J.F.; Valentini, L.; Lanzón, M.; Pamies, R.; Kjoniksen, A.L. Effect of freeze-thaw cycles on the mechanical behavior of geopolymer concrete and Portland cement concrete containing micro-encapsulated phase change materials. *Constr. Build. Mater.* **2019**, *200*, 94–103. [CrossRef]
47. Valenza, J.J.; Scherer, G.W. A review of salt scaling: II. Mechanisms. *Cem. Concr. Res.* **2007**, *37*, 1022–1034. [CrossRef]
48. Zhao, R.; Yuan, Y.; Cheng, Z.; Wen, T.; Li, J.; Li, F.; Ma, Z.J. Freeze-thaw resistance of class F fly ash-based geopolymer concrete. *Constr. Build. Mater.* **2019**, *222*, 474–483. [CrossRef]
49. Tian, L.Y.; He, D.P.; Zhao, J.N.; Wang, H.G. Durability of geopolymers and geopolymer concretes: A review. *Rev. Adv. Mater. Sci.* **2021**, *60*, 1–14. [CrossRef]
50. Zhang, P.; Wen, Z.; Han, X.; Guo, J.; Hu, S. A state-of-the-art review on frost resistance of fiber-reinforced geopolymer composites. *Sustain. Chem. Pharm.* **2025**, *45*, 102006. [CrossRef]
51. Li, J.; Yang, L.; Rao, F.; Tian, X. Gel Evolution of Copper Tailing-Based Green Geopolymers in Marine Related Environments. *Materials* **2022**, *15*, 4599. [CrossRef]
52. Chen, J.; Bai, B.; Du, Q. Durability evaluation of a high-performance red mud-based composite material. *Mater. Today Commun.* **2024**, *39*, 108684. [CrossRef]
53. Bahafid, S.; Hendriks, M.; Jacobsen, S.; Geiker, M. Revisiting concrete frost salt scaling: On the role of the frozen salt solution micro-structure. *Cem. Concr. Res.* **2022**, *157*, 106803. [CrossRef]
54. Zhang, H.E.; Sarker, P.K.; Xiao, L.; Ai, J.H.; He, B.; Ren, Q.; Zhu, X.P.; Zhang, Y. Durability of low-carbon geopolymer mortar: Different responses to cryogenic attack caused by water content and freeze-thaw mediums. *Cem. Concr. Compos.* **2023**, *139*, 105065. [CrossRef]
55. Fan, L.F.; Zhong, W.L.; Wang, G.; Xi, Y. Optimal slag content for geopolymer composites under freeze-thaw cycles with different freezing temperatures. *J. Zhejiang Univ.-SCI A* **2023**, *24*, 366–376. [CrossRef]
56. Zhong, W.L.; Wang, G.; Xi, Y.; Fan, L.F. Damage evaluation of geopolymer under three freezing-thawing treatments with different freezing temperatures based on ultrasonic technique. *J. Build. Eng.* **2023**, *69*, 106268. [CrossRef]
57. Zeng, Q.; Li, K.; Fen-Chong, T.; Dangla, P. A study of the behaviors of cement-based materials subject to freezing. In Proceedings of the 2010 International Conference on Mechanic Automation and Control Engineering, MACE 2010, Wuhan, China, 26–28 June 2010; pp. 1611–1616. [CrossRef]
58. Das, S.; Yang, P.; Singh, S.S.; Mertens, J.C.E.; Xiao, X.; Chawla, N.; Neithalath, N. Effective properties of a fly ash geopolymer: Synergistic application of X-ray synchrotron tomography, nanoindentation, and homogenization models. *Cem. Concr. Res.* **2015**, *78*, 252–262. [CrossRef]
59. Powers, T.C.; Helmuth, R.A. Theory of Volume Changes in Hardened Portland Cement Paste During Freezing. In Proceedings of the Highway Research Board Proceedings, Washington, DC, USA, 13–16 January 1953.
60. Sun, M.; Xin, D.; Zou, C. Damage evolution and plasticity development of concrete materials subjected to freeze-thaw during the load process. *Mech. Mater.* **2019**, *139*, 103192. [CrossRef]
61. Valenza II, J.J.; Scherer, G.W. Mechanism for Salt Scaling. *J. Am. Ceram. Soc.* **2006**, *89*, 1161–1179. [CrossRef]
62. Valenza, J.J.; Scherer, G.W. Mechanism for salt scaling of a cementitious surface. *Mater. Struct.* **2007**, *40*, 259–268. [CrossRef]
63. Scherer, G.W. Characterization of saturated porous bodies. *Mater. Struct.* **2004**, *37*, 21–30. [CrossRef]
64. Ali, N.; Canpolat, O.; Aygörmez, Y.; Al-Mashhadani, M.M. Evaluation of the 12-24 mm basalt fibers and boron waste on reinforced metakaolin-based geopolymer. *Constr. Build. Mater.* **2020**, *251*, 118976. [CrossRef]
65. Liang, G.W.; Zhu, H.J.; Li, H.X.; Liu, T.J.; Guo, H.H. Comparative study on the effects of rice husk ash and silica fume on the freezing resistance of metakaolin-based geopolymer. *Constr. Build. Mater.* **2021**, *293*, 123486. [CrossRef]
66. Nemecek, J.; Smilauer, V.; Kopecky, L. Nanoindentation characteristics of alkali-activated aluminosilicate materials. *Cem. Concr. Compos.* **2011**, *33*, 163–170. [CrossRef]
67. Feng, B.W.; Liu, J.S. Durability of repair metakaolin geopolymeric cement under different factors. *Processes* **2022**, *10*, 1818. [CrossRef]
68. Chen, B.; Wang, J. Experimental study on the durability of alkali-activated slag concrete after freeze-thaw cycle. *Adv. Mater. Sci. Eng.* **2021**, *2021*, 9915639. [CrossRef]
69. Provis, J.L.; Myers, R.J.; White, C.E.; Rose, V.; van Deventer, J.S.J. X-ray microtomography shows pore structure and tortuosity in alkali-activated binders. *Cem. Concr. Res.* **2012**, *42*, 855–864. [CrossRef]

70. Ravikumar, D.; Peethamparan, S.; Neithalath, N. Structure and strength of NaOH activated concretes containing fly ash or GGBFS as the sole binder. *Cem. Concr. Compos.* **2010**, *32*, 399–410. [CrossRef]
71. Temuujin, J.; Minjigmaa, A.; Davaabal, B.; Bayarzul, U.; Ankhtuya, A.; Jadambaa, T.; MacKenzie, K.J.D. Utilization of radioactive high-calcium Mongolian flyash for the preparation of alkali-activated geopolymers for safe use as construction materials. *Ceram. Int.* **2014**, *40*, 16475–16483. [CrossRef]
72. Ugurlu, A.I.; Karakoc, M.B.; Ozcan, A. Effect of binder content and recycled concrete aggregate on freeze-thaw and sulfate resistance of GGBFS based geopolymer concretes. *Constr. Build. Mater.* **2021**, *301*, 124246. [CrossRef]
73. Melo Neto, A.A.; Cincotto, M.A.; Repette, W. Drying and autogenous shrinkage of pastes and mortars with activated slag cement. *Cem. Concr. Res.* **2008**, *38*, 565–574. [CrossRef]
74. Zhang, B.; Yan, B.; Li, Y. Study on mechanical properties, freeze–thaw and chlorides penetration resistance of alkali activated granulated blast furnace slag-coal gangue concrete and its mechanism. *Constr. Build. Mater.* **2023**, *366*, 130218. [CrossRef]
75. Turkoglu, M.; Bayraktar, O.Y.; Benli, A.; Kaplan, G. Effect of cement clinker type, curing regime and activator dosage on the performance of one-part alkali-activated hybrid slag/clinker composites. *J. Build. Eng.* **2023**, *68*, 106164. [CrossRef]
76. Tekle, B.H.; Ly, T.V.; Hertwig, L.; Holschemacher, K. Freeze-thaw resistance and sorptivity of fine-grained alkali-activated cement concrete. *Struct. Concr.* **2023**, *24*, 4286–4296. [CrossRef]
77. Ling, Y.F.; Wang, K.J.; Wang, X.H.; Hua, S.D. Effects of mix design parameters on heat of geopolymerization, set time, and compressive strength of high calcium fly ash geopolymer. *Constr. Build. Mater.* **2019**, *228*, 116763. [CrossRef]
78. Ruiz-Santaquiteria, C.; Skibsted, J.; Fernández-Jiménez, A.; Palomo, A. Alkaline solution/binder ratio as a determining factor in the alkaline activation of aluminosilicates. *Cem. Concr. Res.* **2012**, *42*, 1242–1251. [CrossRef]
79. Han, X.Y.; Ding, N.; Chen, A.J.; Wang, Z.H.; Xu, Y.; Feng, L.Y.; Ji, Y.T.; Li, K.L.; Jing, J.L.; Sun, S.; et al. Experimental study on freeze-thaw failure of concrete incorporating waste tire crumb rubber and analytical evaluation of frost resistance. *Constr. Build. Mater.* **2024**, *439*, 137356. [CrossRef]
80. Coussy, O.; Monteiro, P.J.M. Poroelastic model for concrete exposed to freezing temperatures. *Cem. Concr. Res.* **2008**, *38*, 40–48. [CrossRef]
81. Ma, C.; Zhao, B.; He, Y.Z.; Li, F.; Long, G.C.; Du, Y.F. Preparation and properties of sustainable magnesium phosphate cement composites with recycled tire rubber particles. *J. Clean. Prod.* **2020**, *262*, 121253. [CrossRef]
82. Nazarpour, H.; Jamali, M. Mechanical and freezing cycles properties of geopolymer concrete with recycled aggregate. *Struct. Concr.* **2020**, *21*, 1004–1012. [CrossRef]
83. Saccani, A.; Manzi, S.; Lancellotti, I.; Barbieri, L. Manufacturing and durability of alkali activated mortars containing different types of glass waste as aggregates valorisation. *Constr. Build. Mater.* **2020**, *237*, 117733. [CrossRef]
84. Zhu, H.G.; Yang, S.; Li, W.J.; Li, Z.H.; Fan, J.C.; Shen, Z.Y. Study of mechanical properties and durability of alkali-activated coal gangue-slag concrete. *Materials* **2020**, *13*, 5576. [CrossRef]
85. Tammam, Y.; Uysal, M.; Canpolat, O.; Kuranli, Ö. Effect of waste filler materials and recycled waste aggregates on the production of geopolymer composites. *Arab. J. Sci. Eng.* **2023**, *48*, 4823–4840. [CrossRef]
86. Wang, D.H.; Shi, C.J.; Farzadnia, N.; Shi, Z.G.; Jia, H.F.; Ou, Z.H. A review on use of limestone powder in cement-based materials: Mechanism, hydration and microstructures. *Constr. Build. Mater.* **2018**, *181*, 659–672. [CrossRef]
87. Tammam, Y.; Uysal, M.; Canpolat, O. Effects of alternative ecological fillers on the mechanical, durability, and microstructure of fly ash-based geopolymer mortar. *Eur. J. Environ. Civ. Eng.* **2022**, *26*, 5877–5900. [CrossRef]
88. Sahin, F.; Uysal, M.; Canpolat, O. Systematic evaluation of the aggregate types and properties on metakaolin based geopolymer composites. *Constr. Build. Mater.* **2021**, *278*, 122414. [CrossRef]
89. Ahiskali, A.; Ahiskali, M.; Bayraktar, O.Y.; Kaplan, G.; Assaad, J. Mechanical and durability properties of polymer fiber reinforced one-part foam geopolymer concrete: A sustainable strategy for the recycling of waste steel slag aggregate and fly ash. *Constr. Build. Mater.* **2024**, *440*, 137492. [CrossRef]
90. Aygörmez, Y.; Canpolat, O.; Al-mashhadani, M.M.; Uysal, M. Elevated temperature, freezing-thawing and wetting-drying effects on polypropylene fiber reinforced metakaolin based geopolymer composites. *Constr. Build. Mater.* **2020**, *235*, 117502. [CrossRef]
91. Sahin, F.; Uysal, M.; Canpolat, O.; Cosgun, T.; Dehghanpour, H. The effect of polyvinyl fibers on metakaolin-based geopolymer mortars with different aggregate filling. *Constr. Build. Mater.* **2021**, *300*, 124257. [CrossRef]
92. Moghadam, A.S.; Roshan, A.M.G.; Omidinasab, F. Utilization of agricultural wastes as fiber, binder and aggregates of geopolymer mortars: Application of taguchi method for strength and durability optimization. *J. Build. Eng.* **2023**, *75*, 106906. [CrossRef]
93. Perera, D.S.; Uchida, O.; Vance, E.R.; Finnie, K.S. Influence of curing schedule on the integrity of geopolymers. *J. Mater. Sci.* **2007**, *42*, 3099–3106. [CrossRef]
94. van Jaarsveld, J.G.S.; van Deventer, J.S.J.; Lukey, G.C. The effect of composition and temperature on the properties of fly ash- and kaolinite-based geopolymers. *Chem. Eng. J.* **2002**, *89*, 63–73. [CrossRef]
95. Aygörmez, Y.; Canpolat, O.; Al-mashhadani, M.M. Assessment of geopolymer composites durability at one year age. *J. Build. Eng.* **2020**, *32*, 101453. [CrossRef]

96. Alnkaa, A.A.; Danish, A.; Yaprak, H.; Memis, S.; Gencel, O.; Amran, M.; Ozbakkaloglu, T. Performance evaluation and cost analysis of ternary blended geopolymers for sustainable built environment under different curing regimes. *Constr. Build. Mater.* **2023**, *409*, 133842. [CrossRef]
97. Shahrajabian, F.; Behfarnia, K. The effects of nano particles on freeze and thaw resistance of alkali-activated slag concrete. *Constr. Build. Mater.* **2018**, *176*, 172–178. [CrossRef]
98. Ismail, I.; Bernal, S.A.; Provis, J.L.; Nicolas, R.S.; Hamdan, S.; van Deventer, J.S.J. Modification of phase evolution in alkali-activated blast furnace slag by the incorporation of fly ash. *Cem. Concr. Compos.* **2014**, *45*, 125–135. [CrossRef]
99. Kuranlı, Ö.F.; Uysal, M.; Abbas, M.T.; Cosgun, T.; Niş, A.; Aygörmez, Y.; Canpolat, O.; Al-mashhadani, M.M. Evaluation of slag/fly ash based geopolymer concrete with steel, polypropylene and polyamide fibers. *Constr. Build. Mater.* **2022**, *325*, 126747. [CrossRef]
100. Şahin, F.; Uysal, M.; Canpolat, O.; Aygörmez, Y.; Cosgun, T.; Dehghanpour, H. Effect of basalt fiber on metakaolin-based geopolymer mortars containing rilem, basalt and recycled waste concrete aggregates. *Constr. Build. Mater.* **2021**, *301*, 124113. [CrossRef]
101. Arslan, A.A.; Uysal, M.; Yilmaz, A.; Al-mashhadani, M.M.; Canpolat, O.; Sahin, F.; Aygörmez, Y. Influence of wetting-drying curing system on the performance of fiber reinforced metakaolin-based geopolymer composites. *Constr. Build. Mater.* **2019**, *225*, 909–926. [CrossRef]
102. Abdollahnejad, Z.; Mastali, M.; Falah, M.; Shaad, K.M.; Luukkonen, T.; Illikainen, M. Durability of the reinforced one-part alkali-activated slag mortars with different fibers. *Waste Biomass Valorization* **2021**, *12*, 487–501. [CrossRef]
103. Ranjbar, N.; Zhang, M. Fiber-reinforced geopolymer composites: A review. *Cem. Concr. Compos.* **2020**, *107*, 103498. [CrossRef]
104. Wang, K.; Zhang, P.; Guo, J.; Gao, Z. Single and synergistic enhancement on durability of geopolymer mortar by polyvinyl alcohol fiber and nano-SiO_2. *J. Mater. Res. Technol.-JMRT* **2021**, *15*, 1801–1814. [CrossRef]
105. Zhang, P.; Feng, Z.; Guo, J.J.; Zheng, Y.X.; Yuan, P. Mechanical behavior and microscopic damage mechanism of hybrid fiber-reinforced geopolymer concrete at elevated temperature. *Ceram. Int.* **2024**, *50*, 53851–53866. [CrossRef]
106. Ozcelikci, E.; Ozdogru, E.; Tugluca, M.S.; Ilcan, H.; Sahmaran, M. Comprehensive investigation of performance of construction and demolition waste based wood fiber reinforced geopolymer composites. *J. Build. Eng.* **2024**, *84*, 108682. [CrossRef]
107. Sumesh, M.; Alengaram, U.J.; Jumaat, M.Z.; Mo, K.H.; Alnahhal, M.F. Incorporation of nano-materials in cement composite and geopolymer based paste and mortar—A review. *Constr. Build. Mater.* **2017**, *148*, 62–84. [CrossRef]
108. Al-Noaimat, Y.A.; Chougan, M.; Al-kheetan, M.J.; Yio, M.H.N.; Wong, H.S.; Ghaffar, S.H. Upcycling end-of-life bricks in high-performance one-part alkali-activated materials. *Dev. Built Environ.* **2023**, *16*, 100231. [CrossRef]
109. Zeng, H.Y.; Lai, Y.M.; Qu, S.; Yu, F. Exploring the effect of graphene oxide on freeze-thaw durability of air-entrained mortars. *Constr. Build. Mater.* **2022**, *324*, 126708. [CrossRef]
110. Zidi, Z.; Ltifi, M.; Ben Ayadi, Z.; El Mir, L.; Nóvoa, X.R. Effect of nano-ZnO on mechanical and thermal properties of geopolymer. *J. Asian Ceram. Soc.* **2020**, *8*, 1–9. [CrossRef]
111. Tanyildizi, H.; Seloglu, M.; Coskun, A. The effect of nano zinc oxide on freeze-thaw resistance of 3D-printed geopolymer mortars. *J. Build. Eng.* **2024**, *96*, 110431. [CrossRef]
112. Farooq, M.A.; Sato, Y.; Niitani, K. Experimental investigation of monotonic behavior and stress-strain models of AE and non-AE high strength concrete with BFS fine aggregates under freezing and thawing. *Constr. Build. Mater.* **2020**, *249*, 118679. [CrossRef]
113. Shang, H. Triaxial T-C-C behavior of air-entrained concrete after freeze–thaw cycles. *Cold Reg. Sci. Technol.* **2013**, *89*, 1–6. [CrossRef]
114. Liu, K.; Yan, J.; Hu, Q.; Sun, Y.; Zou, C. Effects of parent concrete and mixing method on the resistance to freezing and thawing of air-entrained recycled aggregate concrete. *Constr. Build. Mater.* **2016**, *106*, 264–273. [CrossRef]
115. Wu, Z.; Libre, N.A.; Khayat, K.H. Factors affecting air-entrainment and performance of roller compacted concrete. *Constr. Build. Mater.* **2020**, *259*, 120413. [CrossRef]
116. Li, X.; Sun, G.X. Optimal freeze-thaw resistance air-entrained concrete with designed nanoparticle stabilised bubble system. *Constr. Build. Mater.* **2024**, *435*, 136769. [CrossRef]
117. Sun, P.; Wu, H.-C. Chemical and freeze-thaw resistance of fly ash-based inorganic mortars. *Fuel* **2013**, *111*, 740–745. [CrossRef]
118. Brooks, R.M.; Bahadory, M.; Tovia, F.; Rostami, H. Properties of alkali-activated fly ash: High performance to lightweight. *Int. J. Sustain. Eng.* **2010**, *3*, 211–218. [CrossRef]
119. Zahedi, A.; Komar, A.; Sanchez, L.F.M.; Boyd, A.J. Global assessment of concrete specimens subjected to freeze-thaw damage. *Cem. Concr. Compos.* **2022**, *133*, 104716. [CrossRef]
120. Sun, Q.; Li, B.T.; Wang, H.; Wang, Y.T. Degradation mechanism and life prediction of tailings and waste rock aggregate geopolymer concrete under freeze-thaw corrosion (vol 9, 015506, 2022). *Mater. Res. Express* **2022**, *9*, 049502. [CrossRef]
121. Wu, T.Y.; Wu, J.; Zheng, C.J.; Wang, J. Evaluation of freeze-thaw resistance of geopolymer concrete incorporating GFRP waste powder. *J. Build. Eng.* **2024**, *90*, 109465. [CrossRef]

122. Moein, M.M.; Saradar, A.; Rahmati, K.; Mousavinejad, S.H.G.; Bristow, J.; Aramali, V.; Karakouzian, M. Predictive models for concrete properties using machine learning and deep learning approaches: A review. *J. Build. Eng.* **2023**, *63*, 41. [CrossRef]
123. Abadel, A.A.; Alghamdi, H. Effect of high volume tile ceramic wastes on resistance of geopolymer mortars to abrasion and freezing-thawing cycles: Experimental and deep learning modelling. *Ceram. Int.* **2023**, *49*, 15065–15081. [CrossRef]
124. Yao, C.Q.; Hu, G.; Chen, Q.Y.; Wu, J. Prediction on the freeze-thaw resistance of a one-part geopolymer stabilized soil by using deep learning method. *Case Stud. Constr. Mater.* **2024**, *21*, e03530. [CrossRef]
125. Zhang, X.M.; Zhang, P.; Yuan, W.S.; Hu, S.W. Durability prediction of geopolymer mortar reinforced with nanoparticles and PVA fiber using particle swarm optimized BP neural network. *Nanotechnol. Rev.* **2024**, *13*, 20230214. [CrossRef]

gels

MDPI

Review

Valorization of River Sediments in Sustainable Cementitious Gel Materials: A Review of Characteristics, Activation, and Performance

Yuanxun Zheng [1,2], Yuxiao Xie [1,2], Yu Zhang [1,2,3,*], Cong Wan [1,2], Li Miao [1,2,*] and Peng Zhang [1,2]

1 School of Water Conservancy and Transportation, Zhengzhou University, Zhengzhou 450001, China; yxzheng@zzu.edu.cn (Y.Z.); yuxiaoxie2023@163.com (Y.X.); wancong0518@163.com (C.W.); zhangpeng@zzu.edu.cn (P.Z.)
2 State Key Laboratory of Tunnel Boring Machine and Intelligent Operations, Zhengzhou 450001, China
3 School of Civil Engineering, Harbin Institute of Technology, Harbin 150090, China
* Correspondence: 24b933029@stu.hit.edu.cn (Y.Z.); mlcjm@zzu.edu.cn (L.M.)

Abstract: River sediments have attracted increasing attention as alternative raw materials for sustainable cementitious materials due to their abundant availability and silica–alumina-rich composition. In this study, a systematic literature search was conducted in Web of Science and Google Scholar using combinations of the keywords "river sediment," "cementitious materials," "activation," and "pozzolanic activity," covering publications up to July 2025. In addition, a citation network tool (Connected Papers) was employed to trace related works and ensure comprehensive coverage of emerging studies. This review systematically examines the properties of river sediments from diverse regions, along with activation and modification techniques such as alkali/acid activation, thermal calcination, and mechanical milling. Their applications in various cementitious systems are analyzed, with mix design models compared to elucidate the effects of replacing fine aggregates, coarse aggregates, and cement on workability, strength, and durability. Multi-scale characterization via XRD, FTIR, and TG-DSC reveals the mechanisms of C–S–H and C–A–S–H gel formation, pore refinement, and interfacial transition zone densification. The review highlights three key findings: (1) moderate sediment replacement (20–30%) improves strength without compromising flowability; (2) alkali–water glass activation and calcination at 600–850 °C effectively enhance pozzolanic activity; and (3) combining the minimum paste thickness theory with additives such as water reducers, fibers, or biochar enables high-performance and low-carbon concrete design. This review provides a comprehensive theoretical foundation and technical pathway for the high-value utilization of river sediments, carbon reduction in concrete, and sustainable resource recycling.

Keywords: river sediments; activation techniques; optimization of concrete properties; low-carbon building materials; proportion design methods

1. Introduction

1.1. Research Background

Amid growing global concerns over resource scarcity and environmental sustainability, the construction materials industry is undergoing a significant green transformation. As the most widely used human-made material, concrete is under scrutiny for its high consumption of natural resources and associated carbon emissions during production and use [1,2]. Over time, large-scale extraction of natural sand, gravel, and cement has led to resource depletion and ecological degradation. Moreover, cement production is energy-intensive and emission-heavy, making it a key target for carbon peaking and neutrality

 https://doi.org/10.3390/gels11090755

efforts [3,4]. Consequently, developing low-carbon, high-performance, and sustainable alternative raw materials has become a global research focus [5].

River sediment, generated in large volumes through dredging during urban and natural river management, often exceeds hundreds of millions of tons annually. However, most of it remains unused, occupying land and posing environmental risks such as heavy metal leaching [6–8]. Compositionally, river sediments contain fine particles, clay minerals, and reactive silica–alumina components, showing similarities with traditional concrete materials in terms of gradation and mineralogy [9–11]. This has prompted interest in their use as fine aggregates, partial cement replacements, or auxiliary admixtures, offering a pathway for transforming waste into a resource and aligning environmental governance with material recycling goals [11,12]. The existing literature confirms that using sediments in ternary cementitious systems is a mature and promising research direction. Several studies have successfully applied sediments in ternary blends, showing improved mechanical properties and refined microstructures [13,14]. To date, various applications of river sediments have yielded promising results: modification into flood control materials [15]; use as pavement base and sub-base layers [16]; soil remediation and land reconstruction in low- and medium-yield sandy areas along the Yellow River, where optimized filling strategies have been developed [17–19]; and production of recycled bricks [20,21], lightweight aggregates [22], and ceramic granules [23] (Figure 1).

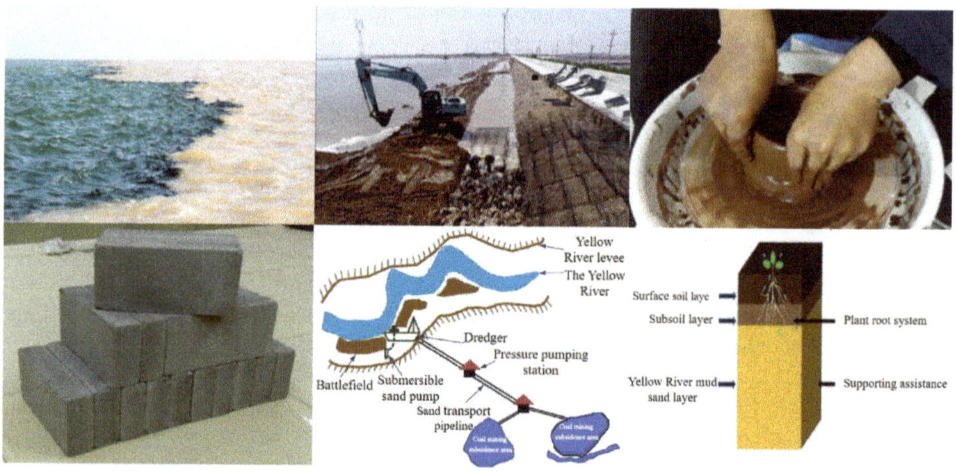

Figure 1. Yellow River sediment resource utilization.

Based on sediment characteristics and engineering requirements, researchers have developed sediment-based concrete for a wide range of applications. These include pervious concrete, lightweight concrete, foam concrete, self-compacting mortar, polymer mortar, autoclaved aerated concrete (AAC), ultra-high-performance concrete (UHPC), and engineered cementitious composites (ECCs), as shown in Figure 2. In these applications, sediments function either as a replacement for sand or as a substitute for cementitious components.

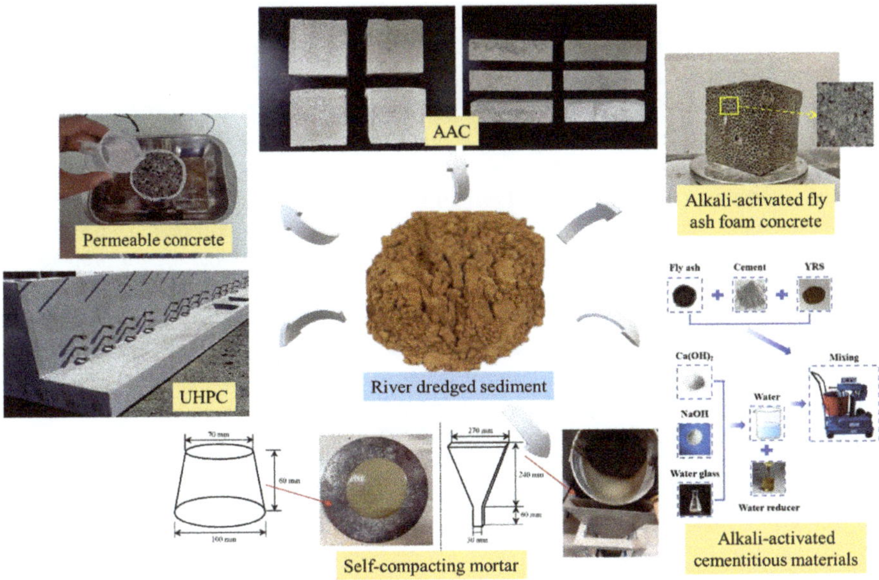

Figure 2. Application of river sediment in concrete (Permeable concrete [24], AAC [25], UHPC [26], Alkali-activated fly ash foam concrete [27]; Self-compacting mortar [28]; Alkali-activated cementitious materials [29]).

Although river sediments have promising application potential, their use in concrete still faces multiple challenges due to variability in physicochemical properties, high impurity content, and low pozzolanic activity [26]. Sediments formed under different geographical and hydrological conditions exhibit significant differences in particle size distribution, mineral composition, and organic content, which directly influence their suitability for concrete applications [30,31]. Moreover, high moisture content, low reactivity, and the presence of humus or heavy metals can adversely affect workability, strength, and durability if not properly treated [32]. Therefore, identifying key physical properties, establishing applicability evaluation criteria, and enhancing reactivity through targeted techniques are essential to advancing sediment-based engineering applications. Recent studies have explored activation strategies to address these issues. Thermal treatment disrupts crystal structures and releases active phases [33,34]; alkali activation promotes reconstruction of the silica–alumina skeleton and formation of binding gels [35]; and mechanical milling increases surface area and exposes reactive sites [36,37]. These methods help overcome the limitations of weak cementitious activity.

However, current research in this field lacks a systematic and multi-scale framework, which limits the efficient, value-added utilization of river sediments in concrete. The main research gaps are (1) a reliance on isolated case studies rather than comparative analyses to establish general principles; (2) an insufficient understanding of microstructural evolution and interface interactions; (3) low substitution levels that hinder practical application; and (4) a shortage of life cycle assessments validating environmental and economic benefits. And, current research still faces several limitations: (1) most studies focus on single sediment types, lacking systematic comparisons to support universal mix design systems; (2) emphasis is placed on mechanical performance, while microstructural evolution and interfacial transition mechanisms remain insufficiently explored; (3) substitution levels are typically low and fail to meet performance thresholds required for real-world application; and (4) life cycle-based environmental and economic assessments are scarce, limiting large-scale adoption. In this context, systematically evaluating multi-path utilization strategies is essential. Such efforts can reveal the fundamental interactions between sediment particle characteristics, mineral composition, and cementitious systems, offering theoretical and technical support for the development of green building materials. A comprehensive analysis of sediment-based composites—from rheology and hydration to microstructure and durability—can enable performance optimization and functional material design. Furthermore, integrating life cycle and carbon footprint assessments will support the transformation of sediments from low-value alternatives to high-performance green resources. This review focuses on the use of river sediments in concrete, summarizing their properties, activation and modification methods, substitution strategies, and performance enhancement mechanisms. It also examines their role in hydration, microstructure evolution, and durability, while proposing future research directions aligned with engineering demands and low-carbon goals. The findings aim to provide a systematic theoretical basis and technical framework for the high-value utilization of river sediments and contribute to the sustainable transformation of the concrete industry.

1.2. Methodology

This systematic review was conducted using a structured and reproducible protocol to identify and analyze relevant studies on the use of river sediments in cementitious materials, with a focus on activation mechanisms and pozzolanic activity. The search was carried out primarily using the Web of Science Core Collection and Google Scholar. To ensure comprehensive coverage, an extensive set of keywords and Boolean combinations was employed. The search strings included the following: ("river sediment" OR "dredged sediment" OR "silt") AND ("cementitious material" OR "alkali-activated" OR "geopolymer" OR "supplementary cementitious material") AND ("activator" OR "mechanochemical" OR "thermal treatment") AND ("volcanic" OR "pozzolan" OR "ash"). The search covered all publications in these databases up to July 2025.

The study selection followed predefined criteria. Publications were included if they (1) focused on river/dredged sediments as raw materials; (2) examined their use in cementitious or alkali-activated binders; (3) detailed activation methods (mechanical, thermal, or chemical); and (4) discussed pozzolanic/volcanic activity or reaction mechanisms. Exclusion criteria included conference abstracts, editorials, and book chapters without original experimental data. Screening was conducted in two phases. First, all retrieved articles were screened by title and abstract. Then, the full texts of potentially relevant articles were assessed for eligibility. To capture emerging studies not yet indexed, the Connected Papers tool was used to trace backward and forward citations of key articles, ensuring comprehensive coverage. A standardized data extraction form was used to collect information from the included studies. The initial search retrieved 369 records. After title and abstract screening, 188 documents proceeded to full-text evaluation. Ultimately, 149 studies met the criteria and were included for data extraction and analysis. Key data included (1) sediment characteristics (e.g., origin and chemical/mineralogical composition); (2) activation process details (e.g., method and parameters); (3) composite mix designs (e.g., binder composition and replacement ratios); (4) curing conditions; and (5) measured properties (e.g., strength, reaction products, and microstructure). Given methodological heterogeneity, a narrative synthesis was adopted. Findings were thematically organized to compare the effects of different activation techniques on sediment pozzolanic activity and to discuss reaction mechanisms.

While every effort was made to ensure comprehensiveness, this review has limitations. Differences in activation and testing protocols restricted the possibility of quantitative meta-analysis. Despite multiple search strategies, some recent or unpublished work may not have been captured.

2. Physical Characteristics and Activation Measures of River Sediments

2.1. Fundamental Characteristics

2.1.1. Physical Characteristics

Before dredging and utilizing river sediments, the sediments can be characterized based on the contaminant content, organic matter content and particle size distribution of the deposits, and statistical analysis of the resulting database can help to categorize these sediments, which can then be used to experimentally quantify the impact of the various sediments on concrete in a more efficient manner [38]. In some areas, the newly dredged sediments inevitably contain pollutants such as waste metals, and the total pollutant content can be detected by Inductive Coupled Plasma [39].

The sediments were classified into deposited fine sand and fine-grained sediments according to the particle size, and the appearance comparison with ordinary river sand as well as mechanism sand as shown in Figure 3, which has a big difference in morphology and color. In terms of particle size distribution, the particle size of fine sand is similar to that of small quartz sand, and the particle size of micro-powder is slightly larger than that of cement and other auxiliary cementitious materials, as shown in Figure 4a,b. Additionally, a few studies have examined larger sediment particles used as coarse aggregates in cementitious materials [24,39]. Since aggregate properties—such as moisture content, water absorption, and density—strongly affect cementitious performance, Table 1 summarizes their physical properties. Sedimentary micropowders are widely used as cement substitutes, and analyzing their chemical and mineralogical composition is essential for understanding macro- and micro-scale behavior. This topic is discussed in the next section. According to Table 1, sediment moisture content ranges from 0.065% to 10.69%, which directly influences the effective water-cement ratio. Water absorption also strongly affects slump and other physical properties. Highly absorbent aggregates often have high porosity and low strength, creating weaknesses in concrete. When absorption exceeds 2.5%, rapid uptake of mixing water leads to slump loss. In addition, highly absorbent materials usually have low density, which reduces hardened concrete strength and durability. Therefore, when such sediments are used, pretreatment or water-cement ratio adjustment is required.

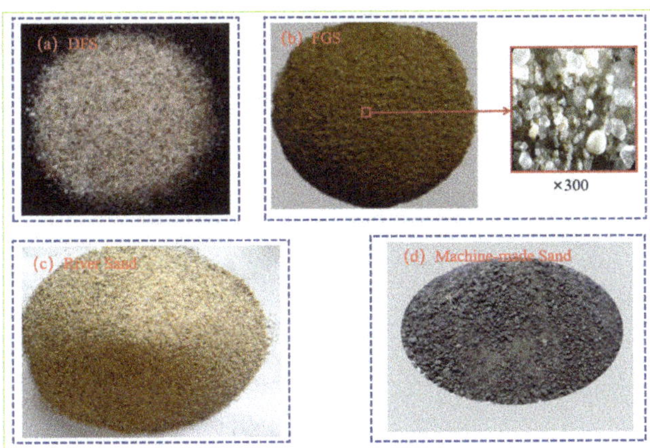

Figure 3. Comparison of material morphology of different sands. (**a**) Deposited fine sand (DFS) [40], (**b**) fine-grained sediments (FGS) [41], and its 300× micrograph [29]; (**c**) river sand; and (**d**) machine-made sand.

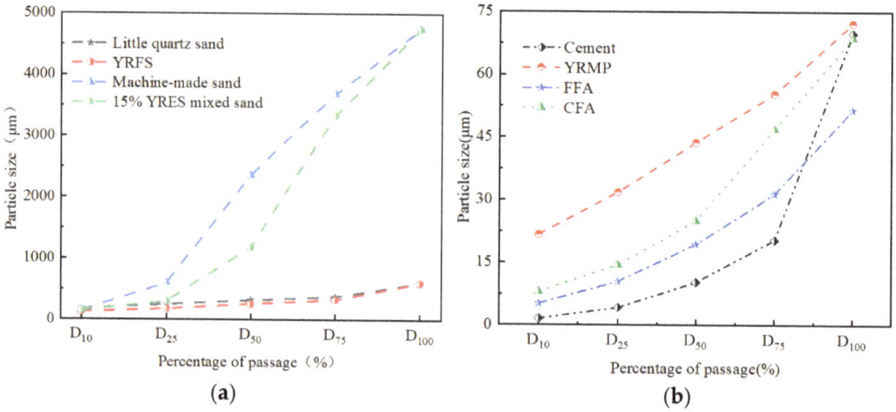

Figure 4. Particle size distribution of different types of sand/particles. (**a**) Particle size distribution of small quartz sand, deposited fine sand, mechanism sand, and a blend of 15% dosed Yellow River Fine Sand(YRFS) and mechanism sand; (**b**) particle size distribution of ordinary silicate cement [42], low calcium fly ash (FFA) [43], high calcium fly ash [44] (CFA), and Yellow River Micro-Powder (YRMP) [40].

Table 1. Moisture content, water absorption, and density of river sediments.

		Water Content (%)	Absorption (%)	Density (g/cm^3)
Conventional aggregates [39]	Sand	0.081	4.7	2.41
	Gravel	0.065	2.3	2.53
Neuilly raw sediment [39]	Sand	N.D.	3.0	2.45
	Gravel	10.69	1.8	2.53
Puteaux raw sediment [39]	Sand	N.D.	3.6	2.46
	Gravel	6.43	2.6	2.47
Preparation of lightweight aggregates [22]	Gravel	N.D.	5.5–9.5	1.01–1.38
Preparation of ceramic granules [23]	Gravel	N.D.	5.9	0.879
Seine Basin [24]	Sand	N.D.	N.D.	2.24–2.41
	Gravel	N.D.	3.7–17.2	2.05–2.41
Yangtze River ultra-fine dredged sand [45]	Sand	N.D.	4.5	2.69

Note: N.D. (Not determined).

2.1.2. Chemical Composition

X-ray fluorescence analysis (Table 2) shows that the chemical composition of river sediments differs significantly from that of cement. Unlike cement, which is CaO-rich, sediments contain higher SiO_2 and moderate Al_2O_3, resembling fly ash in composition [18,46]. As illustrated in Figure 5, sediments exhibit intermediate characteristics: their SiO_2 and Al_2O_3 contents are higher than those of cement but lower than those of fly ash, while CaO content is lower than cement but higher than fly ash. Comparison of aggregate composition in Table 2 with ASTM C618 shows that the total SiO_2, Al_2O_3, and Fe_2O_3 in most sediments exceeds 70%, meeting the minimum requirement for type N pozzolan in ASTM C618. This "medium silica–alumina with moderate calcium" profile indicates potential pozzolanic activity and Ca-supplement capacity, making sediments suitable as supplementary cementitious materials, especially for partial cement replacement or use with activators in low-carbon concrete.

Table 2. Chemical composition of river sediment and cement.

Sports Event	SiO_2 (%)	Al_2O_3 (%)	CaO (%)	Fe_2O_3 (%)	Na_2O (%)	K_2O (%)	MgO	LOI
Cement 1 [29]	21.49	5.24	64.16	2.89	0.76	0.42	2.12	1.0
Cement 2 [5]	18.093	5.882	64.394	3.904	N.D.	1.219	1.944	N.D.
Yellow River sediment 1 [29]	68.73	11.08	7.56	3.64	1.76	3.21	2.11	2.85
Yellow River sediment 2 [23]	60.5	15.9	9.96	4.77	1.56	2.81	3.18	N.D.
Yangtze River sediment 1 [47]	68.2	11.4	5.66	3.22	1.88	2.31	2.46	N.D.
Yangtze River sediment 2 [45]	68.74	11.4	5.56	3.20	1.84	2.3	2.42	N.D.
Mud and sand sediment 1 [46]	47.50	15.60	10.20	6.70	0.30	1.90	2.40	15.1
Mud and sand sediment 2 [47]	75.717	11.988	1.59	4.971	0.029	1.857	0.951	N.D.
Mud and sand sediment 3 [48]	33.25	8.65	13.1	3.89	0.45	149	0.75	N.D.
Mud and sand sediment 3 calcined at 750 °C [48]	43.45	10.30	15.4	4.95	0.63	1.84	0.91	N.D.
Mud and sand sediment 4 [25]	56.93	18.98	2.14	12.05	0.70	4.07	2.07	4.13
Fly ash 1 [18]	50.6	27.2	2.8	7.0	0.5	2.6	0.97	1.14
Fly ash 2 [25]	53.7	27.3	7.7	5.70	0.7	0.12	1.8	0.40

Note: LOI is short for loss on ignition at 1000 °C; N.D. = not determined.

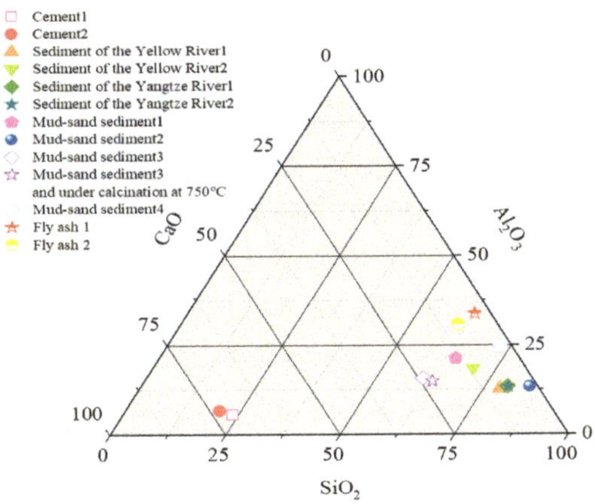

Figure 5. Comparison of chemical composition of different materials [5,18,23,25,29,45–48].

Given these characteristics, deposited fine sand can feasibly replace or blend with river sand, manufactured sand, or quartz sand as a fine aggregate. This is particularly advantageous, as manufactured and quartz sands often suffer from high porosity, poor gradation, low workability, and high angularity [49,50]. Sedimentary sand, being finer and comparable to quartz sand, is environmentally favorable for partial substitution in concrete [51–54]. Currently, most studies treat deposited fine sand as inert aggregate, optimizing mix designs with limited dosages. However, due to its low reactivity, performance improvement remains restricted [55,56], and low replacement levels reduce economic feasibility [57,58]. In contrast, finer sedimentary powders show greater reuse potential. As shown in Table 2, sediments are primarily composed of SiO_2 and Al_2O_3, with lower levels of CaO, Fe_2O_3, K_2O, MgO, and Na_2O. As aluminosilicate-rich materials, they possess theoretical potential for geopolymerization under suitable conditions. Activating this reactivity could enable cement substitution and offer a new pathway for sediment resource utilization.

2.1.3. Mineral Composition

Given the growing focus on ternary cement and the synergistic effects of calcined clay and other cementitious materials, it is important to discuss the mineralogical composition of sediments to demonstrate their potential in producing alternative cement.

Subramanian et al. [59] investigated sediments from the Yamuna River, a Himalayan tributary of the Ganges, and found that quartz and feldspar were the most abundant minerals. The clay mineral assemblage was mainly illite and chlorite, with minor kaolinite and montmorillonite. Hamdy et al. [60] studied the entire Ganges system and reported that the clay fraction was dominated by illite, followed by smectite and kaolinite/chlorite. Li et al. [61] studied rivers in Taiwan, China, and found that sediments mainly consisted of illite, smectite (montmorillonite-group), chlorite, and kaolinite, with smectite reaching 40–80% in some rivers. Singh et al. [62] studied the Kaveri River in southern India and found the main clay minerals to be montmorillonite, kaolinite, and illite.

These studies show that quartz and feldspar are the dominant light minerals in sand and silt fractions, typical products of continental crust weathering. Analysis of sediment composition shows high silica and alumina, indicating quartz (SiO_2), clay minerals such as illite and kaolinite, and possibly feldspathic phases [63,64]. These aluminosilicates are critical for pozzolanic behavior, as they react with $Ca(OH)_2$ in cementitious systems to form C–S–H phases [65]. The moderate calcium content supports self-cementing potential under activation, bridging traditional pozzolans and latent hydraulic materials such as GGBS [66]. The fine particle size distribution enhances reactivity by providing nucleation sites for hydration and promoting microstructural densification [67]. Low contents of K_2O, Na_2O, and MgO reduce risks of expansion and ASR cracking, supporting safe use as a construction material [68].

In summary, river sediments rich in reactive silica and alumina, with supplementary calcium, show pozzolanic potential and alkali activation compatibility, supporting their use as sustainable SCMs in modern concrete.

2.2. *Activation Measures for Fine-Grained River Sediments*

Li et al. [69] demonstrated that Pisha sandstone—the dominant mineral resource within Yellow River sediments—constitutes a distinctive clay-rich formation. This lithology comprises non-crystalline clay minerals (montmorillonite, illite, mica, etc.) and crystalline phases (feldspar, quartz, calcite, etc.), thereby providing evidence for the low pozzolanic activity inherent to fine-grained river sediments. To enable its use as a cement substitute, activation is necessary to enhance its reactivity. Properly activated sediment powder—via calcination or mechanical treatment—transforms kaolinite and other clays into amorphous metakaolin, which, in the presence of $Ca(OH)_2$ and water, forms C–S–H and C–A–H gels. This process effectively regenerates micro-scale cementitious phases and improves matrix strength and densification [70].

2.2.1. Chemical Excitation Activation

(1) Categories of chemical excitants

Alkali activators enhance reactivity by disrupting mineral structures and releasing active components [29]. Among these, NaOH and water glass are the most common. Li et al. [69] demonstrated that using NaOH and water glass (modulus 3) significantly increased the compressive strength of Pisha sandstone. Water glass alone can also activate sediments [71]. Jiang et al. [27] and Jing et al. [72] found that mono-doping with 10–15% $Ca(OH)_2$ optimized pozzolanic reactivity. Ze et al. [29] conducted a study on the preparation of Yellow River sediment/fly ash/cement-based alkali-activated cementitious materials for coal mine filling. The study compared different activators, including $Ca(OH)_2$, NaOH, sodium silicate (water glass), and their combinations. All these activators promoted more complete reactions of cement, fly ash, and Yellow River sediment, which led to the formation of additional C–S–H and C–A–S–H gels. Among them, the combination of NaOH and sodium silicate proved most effective in refining pores and improving the microstructure. However, Junakova et al. [73] argued that NaOH alone is ineffective for activating sediments. Regarding this contradictory phenomenon, research by Palomo et al. [74] revealed that excessive NaOH use, due to its high alkalinity, increases the alkalinity of the hydration solution and reduces the hydration of anhydrous silicates, thereby decreasing compressive strength.

Salt activators also show promise. Hai et al. [57] used a 6% mixture of $CaCl_2$ and water glass (1:1) to activate sediments. Ca^{2+} exchanged with ions in clay minerals, releasing soluble Si and Al, while reacting with C_3A to form hydrated calcium chloroaluminate, thus enhancing strength. $CaCl_2$ also accelerates feldspar hydrolysis, while water glass fills pores with silica and calcium silicate gels. However, the chloride ions in $CaCl_2$ may induce long-term durability issues. Liu et al. [21] proposed sodium bisulfite as an activator, though its mechanism requires further clarification.

In addition, acidic activation has gained attention. Wang [75] studied Yellow River sediment and used acidic activators to replace cement in cement–sand specimens of the same particle size. The results showed that acid activation provided stable strength, improved energy efficiency, and offered environmental benefits while avoiding durability problems related to alkali. Phosphoric acid, acetic acid, and hydrochloric acid corroded particle surfaces, increased surface area, and promoted gel formation. Acid–base synergistic activation further accelerated ion release and hydration, enhanced density, inhibited salt migration, and effectively mitigated alkali–silica reaction.

(2) Activation reaction mechanisms

As shown in Figure 6a–c [29], under alkaline excitation, the matrix incorporating activators exhibited a denser structure than the blank matrix, with fly ash and YRS particles encapsulated by C–S–H and C–A–S–H gels. Similarly, in Figure 6d [27], the addition of $Ca(OH)_2$ led to the formation of abundant honeycomb and fibrous C–S–H gels, enhancing matrix densification and reducing average pore size. In the Na_2CO_3 and Na_2SO_4 systems (Figure 6e,f), hydration between sediment and activator was limited. The resulting structure was loose, with flocculated geopolymer gels coexisting with unreacted matrix and feldspar clasts wrapped in gels. In the acidic systems (Figure 6g–i [75]), the 1.5% phosphoric acid group produced abundant needle-like and flocculent hydration products, forming a dense and continuous gel skeleton. These products included C–S–H gels, $Ca(OH)_2$ crystals, and $Ca_3(PO_4)_2$, effectively filling pores and increasing strength. In contrast, the 1% acetic acid and 1.5% hydrochloric acid groups also generated C–S–H gels and calcite, but with lower product content and poor connectivity, resulting in weaker excitation effects than the phosphoric acid group.

The hydration products and microstructures of the fillers changed significantly under different activators. XRD results showed that doping with $Ca(OH)_2$, NaOH, water glass, or $CaCl_2$ increased C–S–H and C–A–S–H gel formation. Co-doping with NaOH and water glass depleted $Ca(OH)_2$, while excitation with $CaCl_2$ eliminated natrium feldspar peaks and introduced kaolinite peaks, indicating ion exchange and mineral transformation (Figure 7a,d). TG analysis confirmed that activators enhanced hydration reactions. Dehydration of products increased with $Ca(OH)_2$ depletion, $CaCO_3$ content decreased, and gel production rose significantly (Figure 7b). FTIR results showed that doping eliminated $Ca(OH)_2$ characteristic peaks, caused shifts in Si–O peaks, and $CaCl_2$ enhanced O–H absorption peaks, indicating increased hydroxyl content that promoted particle bonding. Overall, excitants significantly improved hydration and microstructural densification (Figure 7c,e) [29,75].

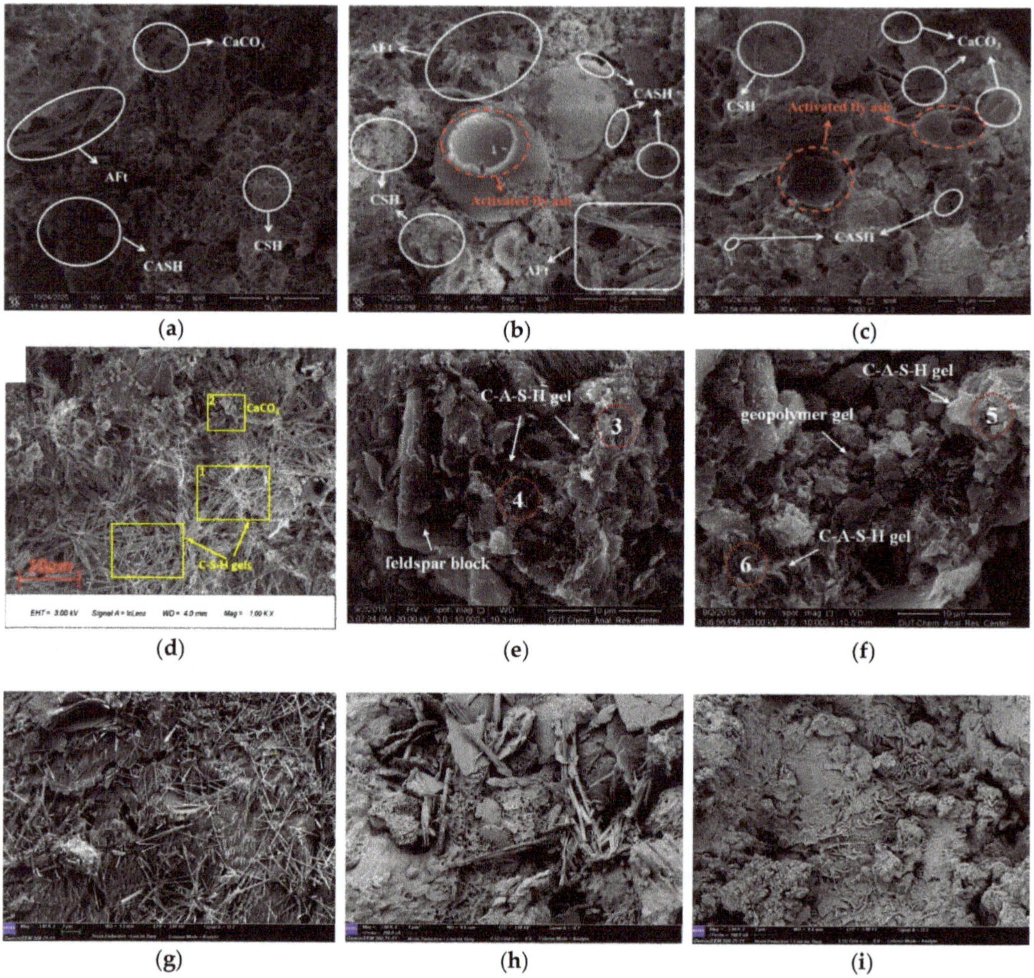

Figure 6. Microscopic morphology of cementitious materials after adding different chemical excitants. (**a**) NaOH [29]; (**b**) water glass [29]; (**c**) water glass + NaOH [29]; (**d**) $Ca(OH)_2$ [27]; (**e**) Na_2CO_3 [71]; (**f**) Na_2SO_4 [71]; (**g**) 1.5% sodium pyrophosphate [75]; (**h**) 1% acetic acid [75]; and (**i**) 1.5% hydrochloric acid [75]. (The scale bar length in (**g**,**h**) is 2 μm.)

The above results indicate significant differences in the efficacy of chemical activators. The choice of the optimal activator depends on its overall performance in the chain of "destroying the original structure, providing reactive components, and forming stable products." NaOH–water glass enhances gel formation and structure through synergistic effects in alkaline environments. Phosphoric acid, in contrast, produces a strong and durable microstructure through corrosion and stable precipitation in acidic conditions. However, the Cl^- introduced by $CaCl_2$ induces steel corrosion, posing a serious threat to long-term durability and greatly limiting its practical application.

In summary, the microstructure and activity of river sediments were improved to a great extent under the action of chemical exciters, in which the activation principles of acidic and alkaline exciters differed. Currently, there is a lack of systematic research on the selection of river sediments activating agents, optimal modulus, optimal dosage, and their relationship with hydration characteristics and macro-microstructure, and the future should focus on exploring these aspects.

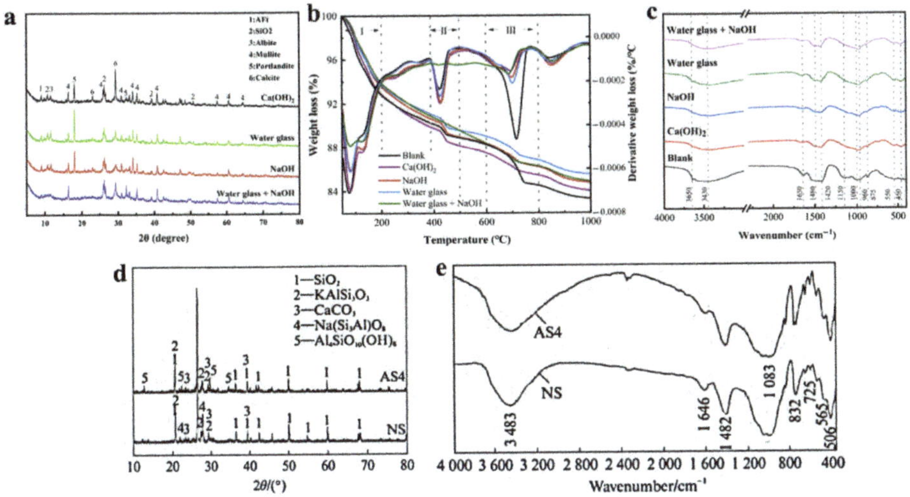

Figure 7. XRD, TG and FTIR patterns of the prepared filling materials from Yellow River sediments under different excitants. (**a–c**) $Ca(OH)_2$, NaOH, water glass, water glass + NaOH [29]; (**d**,**e**) $CaCl_2$ + water glass [75].

2.2.2. Thermal Activation

Thermal activation enhances the pozzolanic activity of sediments by converting crystalline clay phases into an amorphous state [48,76]. For instance, Ferone et al. [46] calcined clay sediments from two reservoirs in southern Italy at 400 °C and 750 °C for 2 h at 10 °C/min. Li et al. [77] studied Pisha sandstone decomposition at 600 °C and 800 °C. Wang et al. [23] investigated the effect of calcination temperature on Yellow River sediment-based ceramic grains. To reduce energy use, Snellings et al. and Duc Chinh Chu et al. [78,79] applied flash calcination to treat sediments. Post-treatment, visible color differences between 650 °C and 850 °C (Figure 8a,b) suggested compositional changes. SEM images (Figure 8c–f) showed granular structures with surface recrystallization, indicating localized melting. Samples treated at 650 °C contained fine particles, while those at 850 °C showed melted and recrystallized fines [80].

Figure 9 presents XRD patterns at various calcination temperatures. Quartz remained thermally stable between 550 and 1000 °C. Feldspar showed peak shifts but incomplete decomposition at 1000 °C. Clay minerals, especially kaolinite, underwent major changes—its (001) peak disappeared above 550 °C, confirming dehydroxylation and the formation of amorphous metakaolinite ($Al_2O_3{\cdot}2SiO_2$), which improved pozzolanic activity [81,82]. Although reactivity increased up to 800 °C, temperatures above 950 °C reduced activity due to mullite crystallization. Chlorite began dehydroxylation at 650 °C and completed by 800 °C, indicating a narrow activation window [83]. Cook [84]. noted its recrystallization near 850 °C. Illite and muscovite were more thermally stable, with peaks present even at 950 °C, where they became most reactive [85,86]. Hematite was the only recrystallized mineral detected, with peaks appearing from 600 °C and intensifying at higher temperatures, indicating progressive crystallization. Thus, thermal treatment at 550–950 °C effectively activates clay-rich dredged sludge, with careful temperature control key to optimizing amorphous phase formation [46].

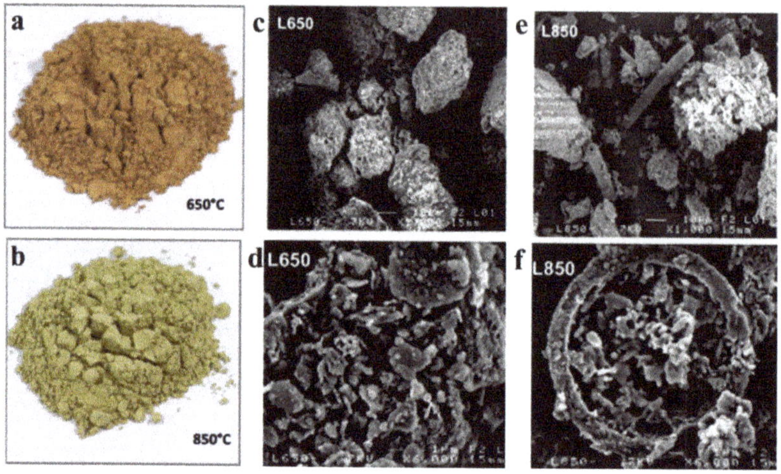

Figure 8. **(a,b) Visual aspect of sediment heated at 650 °C and 850 °C**; (**c**,**d**) SEM images at 650 °C with magnifications of 1kx and 6kx; (**e**,**f**) SEM images at 850 °C with magnifications of 1kx and 6kx [80].

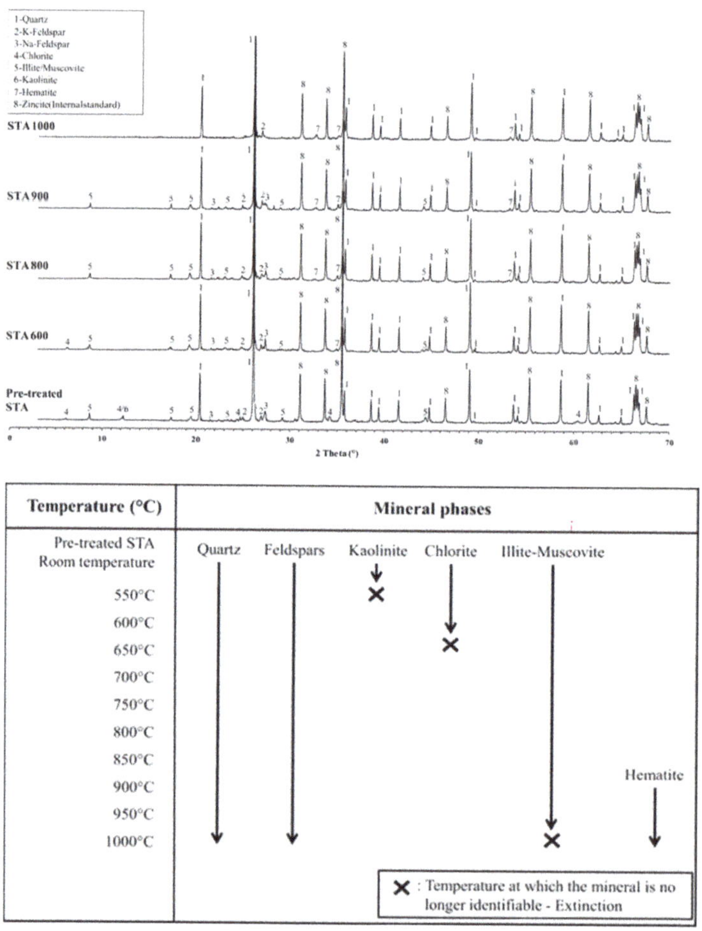

Figure 9. XRD patterns and identification of crystalline phases at different calcination temperatures [87].

Figure 10a shows greater mass loss between 105 and 400 °C in mixtures with treated sediments than in Portland cement, indicating sediment involvement in hydration. In Figure 10b, 650 °C-treated samples fell below the dashed line, showing pozzolanic behavior [88]; 850 °C-treated samples were above the line due to calcite decarbonization forming reactive CaO. Figure 10c confirms lower $CaCO_3$ in 850 °C samples, supporting $Ca(OH)_2$ formation [80]. Figure 10d shows that at high substitution rates, 650 °C-treated samples exhibited higher compressive strength than limestone.

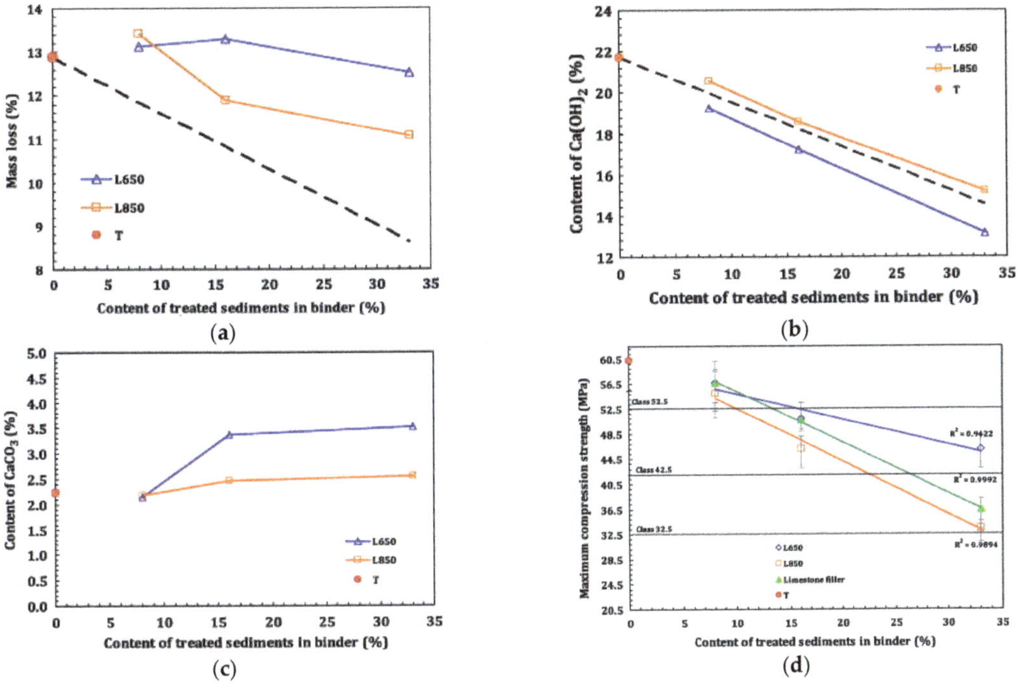

Figure 10. (**a**) Amount of bound water (between 105 °C and 400 °C) versus the amount of treated sediment in the slurry (The dashed line presents the amount of bound water corresponding to the part of Portland cement in the blended paste); (**b**) Amount of $Ca(OH)_2$ in the slurry (by mass) versus the substitution ratio (The dashed line presents the amount of calcium hydroxide corresponding to the part of Portland cement in the blended paste); (**c**) Amount of $CaCO_3$ in the slurry (by mass) versus the substitution ratio; and (**d**) 28-day compressive strength of the slurry versus the treated sediment and limestone filler substitution rates [80].

In summary, thermal activation alters sediment mineral structures, greatly enhancing activity without introducing external substances. For clay-rich minerals, the optimal calcination temperature is 550–950 °C, where amorphous transformation is highest and reactivity is strongest. This enhances early strength and long-term durability of the cementitious system. Samples treated at 850 °C produced highly active CaO, which promoted secondary hydration and generated more C-S-H gel, significantly improving matrix density and strength. Samples treated at 650 °C showed higher compressive resistance than limestone. Optimizing the calcination process achieves a balance between strength and durability, providing key technical support for high-performance cementitious materials. However, it requires high energy, large equipment, and may burn off active components. Chemical activation operates at room temperature, is simpler and adjustable, but may introduce impurities and environmental risks. Each method has advantages and limitations and should be selected based on application needs. A combined approach may also be considered [46].

2.2.3. Mechanical Milling

Mechanical milling, as a physical activation method, effectively improves the sediment's cementitious activity for partial cement replacement. Grinding increases specific surface area and exposes reactive sites, accelerating interactions with hydration products [89,90]. Kou et al. [5] and Beddaa et al. [24,39] found that grinding sediments can enhance hydration reactions by providing nucleation sites and promoting micro-flocculation. This improves packing density, pore structure, and durability. Junakova and Junak [73] further compared pure dry milling, co-milling with NaOH, with fly ash, and with both. NaOH alone had a limited effect, while composite treatments, especially those with fly ash, significantly enhanced sediment reactivity.

In summary, chemical activation operates at room temperature, is simple and adjustable, but may introduce impurities and environmental risks. Thermal activation fundamentally alters the crystalline structure, creating a stable amorphous phase with consistent reactivity, ideal for high-performance applications. Mechanical milling with additives such as biochar and fibers forms a "micro-cement + filler" composite, improving 28-day compressive strength by 10–20%. Mechanical milling enhances sediment reactivity and improves structure and performance through refinement and surface activation, providing strong support for sustainable construction. Each method has advantages and limitations, and selection should depend on application needs. A combined approach may also be considered.

2.2.4. Pozzolanic Reactivity Assessment Methods

Activated dredged sediments are expected to exhibit pozzolanic activity and must be evaluated to confirm activation. Four evaluation methods are outlined below:

(1) A rapid evaluation method for the activity of pozzolanic materials was used, and the activity rate (K_α) of pozzolanic materials was defined as the ratio of the total reactive SiO_2 and Al_2O_3 (reacted with saturated limewater) to the total amount of SiO_2 and Al_2O_3, as shown in Equation (1) [91].

$$K_\alpha = \frac{\text{Active}(SiO_2+Al_2O_3)}{\text{Total}(SiO_2+Al_2O_3)} \tag{1}$$

(2) The Fratini test assesses pozzolanic reactivity by monitoring changes in OH^- and Ca^{2+} concentrations in a system comprising 20% mineral admixture and 80% CEM I cement. After sealing at 40 °C for 8–15 days, ion concentrations are compared with the Ca^{2+} solubility curve to determine activity [92].
(3) The strength activity index method evaluates mechanical performance by comparing the compressive strength of cement paste containing supplementary cementitious material with that of control paste made from ordinary Portland cement [87].
(4) Calorimetry is used to assess the effect of activated sedimentary pozzolanic material on cement hydration rate, thereby indirectly evaluating pozzolanic activity [87].

3. Performance-Enhancement Design for Sediment-Based Concrete

3.1. Mix Proportioning Methodology

River sediments typically have high water absorption and broad particle size distribution, making traditional mix design methods unsuitable [93]. Current approaches mainly rely on empirical or trial-and-error methods [20,94], which are inefficient and lack precision. Therefore, developing a scientific and efficient mix design method is essential for effective sediment utilization. This section reviews several mix design theories used for fine sand and ultrafine powder concrete and explores their applicability to river sediment concrete. The main methods are listed in Table 3:

Table 3. The design method of the concrete mix proportion.

Method	Name	Principle	Features
Aggregate-based method	Compressive Packing Model (CPM) [95]	This approach uses virtual packing density to model particle combinations and improve packing efficiency.	It requires full particle size distribution data.
	Andreasen and Andersen model [26,96,97]	This method determines component ratios by optimizing a continuous particle size distribution curve.	It provides more precise control than the traditional residual fitting method.
	Absolute Volume Method [98–100]	This theory derives component ratios from aggregate volume.	It is complex and requires separate volume data for each material.
	Packing Density Modeling (PDM) [101]	This model predicts mixture density using energy input, material densities, and particle sizes.	It avoids the separate calculation of packing parameters and achieves relatively high accuracy.
Slurry-based method	The minimum paste theory [102].	This theory considers concrete as an aggregate skeleton coated with the minimum paste.	Reducing paste volume improves volumetric stability and crack resistance while maintaining workability and strength.

Current mix design models fall into two categories: aggregate-based and slurry-based. Aggregate-based models optimize particle packing but often fail to address the high paste demand caused by fine sediments' large surface area and high water absorption, limiting effectiveness. For example, Maherzi et al. [101] and Ennahal et al. [103] applied the PDM method to combine particle grades and minimize porosity. Jun et al. [26] optimized solid sizes with an improved Andreasen and Andersen model to design UHPC containing Yellow River ultrafine sand. However, these methods mainly focus on aggregate structure while neglecting paste dosage and distribution. This makes it difficult to resolve poor workability and low durability caused by high fines, large surface area, and high-water demand in river sediments. Slurry-based methods involve determining powder proportions, calculating aggregate voids, setting the average paste thickness (APT), and deriving component dosages. Studies show that adjusting parameters such as fine-to-coarse ratio, sand rate, water-cement ratio, fly ash/slag content, and water-reducer dosage reduces paste content, lowering cost and carbon emissions [104,105]. For instance, Luan et al. [105] applied this theory to design dredged sand concrete mixes by adjusting target strength, APT, and sand content. They found that increasing APT first enhances compressive strength before it declines, while workability keeps improving. This demonstrates the feasibility and effectiveness of the minimum paste theory for dredged ultrafine sand concrete. In contrast, paste-based methods directly regulate paste dosage and distribution. They offer tailored solutions for improving workability and durability in high-fines, high-absorption sediment concretes by minimizing excess paste while maintaining performance.

3.2. Performance Enhancement in Sediment-Functionalized Concrete

Although the fine-grained sediments are used as a high silica–alumina material, their activity is low and cannot directly participate in the hydration reaction. Although a series of activation measures have been taken, with the gradual increase in the dosage of its replacement cementitious material, the generation efficiency of hydration products such as C–S–H and C–A–S–H will still be affected, resulting in a gradual decrease in the macro-mechanical properties of the specimen. Deposited fine sand also introduces excessive defects, leading to the loss of properties when the substitution rate is too high [106].

Therefore, there is an urgent need to continue to investigate the performance enhancement mechanism of sediment-deposited concrete on this basis.

3.2.1. Sediment as Partial Aggregate Replacement

The incorporation of river sediments as aggregates in concrete compensates for the lack of fines in washed mechanical sand, improves particle gradation, and enhances mechanical properties [45,107,108]. After particle size sorting, sediment can partially or fully replace natural coarse and fine aggregates [38]. Beddaa et al. [39] achieved C30 concrete by fully replacing aggregates with sediment, requiring only 5% more cement to meet the target strength; the dynamic modulus was comparable to the control. Junakova et al. [109] reported that substituting 20 wt% coarse sediment yields similar compressive strength to conventional concrete.

Sediment-based aggregates are now used in various cement systems to study the effects of different replacement rates. In alkali-activated systems, a 25% substitution of Yangtze dredged sand showed the best performance, improving compressive strength by about 5%, maintaining workability, and producing a denser interfacial zone [45,106]. Similarly, concrete designed with ultrafine dredged sand using the minimum slurry theory achieved the lowest porosity and highest strength at 25% substitution, confirming the feasibility of ultrafine sediment incorporation [105]. Sediment is also used as a polymer mortar aggregate. Maherzi et al. [101] optimized particle packing to reduce porosity, while Ennahal et al. [103] showed that polyester encapsulation stabilizes sediment ions and improves durability. Lightweight aggregates made from roasted sediments have low density and moderate water absorption, making them suitable for lightweight and self-compacting concrete with technical, ecological, and social benefits [22,26,110].

In summary, with proper particle size control and the use of admixtures or polymers, river sediments can replace fine, coarse, or full aggregates to improve performance and durability. The optimal replacement rate is typically 20–30%. For higher rates, adjustments such as modifying the water-cement ratio, adding superplasticizers, or using sintered lightweight aggregates are necessary, providing a practical approach for sediment resource utilization.

3.2.2. Sediment as Partial Cementitious Material Replacement

(1) Chemical activation

As discussed in Section 2.2, various activation methods have been explored to induce pozzolanic activity in river sediments. Incorporating pozzolanic materials prolongs setting time, enhances Al and Si reactions to form (N,C)–A–S–H gels, improves hydration and mechanical properties, lowers cost, and reduces carbon emissions [77,111,112]. Activation is thus an effective way to enhance sediment concrete performance and will not be elaborated here.

(2) Performance-enhancing additives

To enhance the performance of dredged sediments as partial cement replacements, composite modification via external additives has gained attention. Functional additives can regulate hydration, microstructure, and mechanical properties across scales, improving applicability and durability.

Zhang et al. [113] showed that adding 0–2% biochar to sediment-based lightweight concrete promoted hydration and carbonation, improving microstructure and increasing 28-day compressive strength from 3.92 to 4.61 MPa. This effect was due to biochar's porous structure and carbon content, which enhance nucleation and carbonation. Lang's team explored the synergistic reinforcement of sediments with fibers and nanomaterials. Polypropylene, rice straw, and wheat straw fibers improved crack resistance and ductility via bridging effects [114,115]. Specifically, 3 mm polypropylene fibers enhanced interfacial bonding and provided strain-hardening behavior [114], while straw fiber doses above 0.5% reduced performance due to poor dispersion [115]. Nanomaterials such as nano-SiO_2 and nano-MgO refined the pore structure and accelerated hydration, boosting strength by up to 40% [116]. Nano-MgO also improved volume stability due to its slight expansion [107]. Lang's team proposed a fiber-nanomaterial synergy strategy: combining rice straw fiber and nano-SiO_2 increased compressive and tensile strengths by 35% and 28%, respectively—better than using either alone [116]. Polypropylene fibers with nano-MgO further achieved both high strength and ductility [117]. This synergy arises from nanomaterials optimizing the matrix, fibers enhancing macro-properties, and improved interfacial transition zones.

In addition, moderate use of superplasticizers in blended cement systems slightly delays peak hydration but improves particle packing and workability. Especially at high sediment replacement rates (30–40%), superplasticizers help ensure compatibility and control air content [78].

In summary, external modification using functional additives significantly enhances the reactivity, strength, and durability of sediment-based cementitious materials through multiscale mechanisms, offering a critical path for their high-value application.

4. Comprehensive Performance Analysis of River-Sediment Concrete

4.1. Hydration Heat Release

Deposited fine sand does not slow down hydration and slightly increases total heat release, as shown in Figure 11a [24]. In contrast, fine-grained sediments significantly slow down hydration and reduce heat release due to their high soluble humus content. Humus is complex organic matter formed by the decomposition of animal and plant remains in river ecosystems. Beddaa et al. [24] reported that organic compounds in fine sediments—especially humic and fulvic acids—adsorb onto cement surfaces and hydration nucleation sites. This process delays the dissolution of cement clinker minerals and the growth of C–S–H gel. It slows hydration and reduces cumulative heat release. Its role is primarily physical filling rather than chemical participation, see Figure 11b [24]. Similarly, Hamideh et al. [28] found that increasing amounts of fine-grained sediments delayed the main exothermic peak, confirming its hydration-delaying effect, see Figure 11c. However, previous thermal analyses did not explain the change in intensity of the small shoulder peak after the main exothermic peak, which is generally attributed to continued C_3A hydration. The influence of sediments on C_3A hydration thus warrants further investigation.

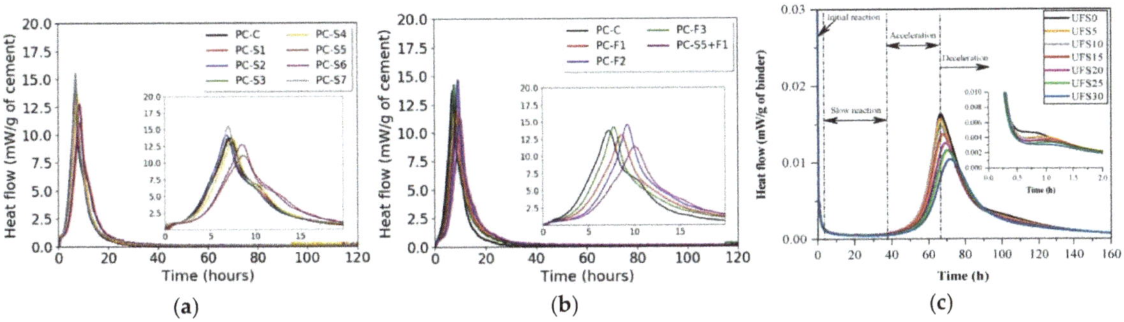

Figure 11. Hydration kinetics of concretes based on sediments: (**a**) sand sediment [24]; (**b**,**c**) fine sediment [24,28] (S1–S7: dredged sands from different areas of the same watershed; F1–F3: different dredged material powders pulverized at 105 °C and sieved through an 80 μm sieve; UFS: ultra-fine sediment).

4.2. Rheological Behavior

As shown in Figure 12a,c, ultrafine dredged sand particles are smaller and more rounded than the angular and irregularly shaped mechanism sand (Figure 12b) or the larger river sand (Figure 12d), both of which increase interparticle friction and reduce concrete fluidity [118]. According to the minimum paste thickness theory, even with increased dredged sand content, maintaining average paste thickness ensures improved slump, demonstrating the theory's effectiveness. However, without controlling paste thickness, increasing the dredged sand lowers the slump [119].

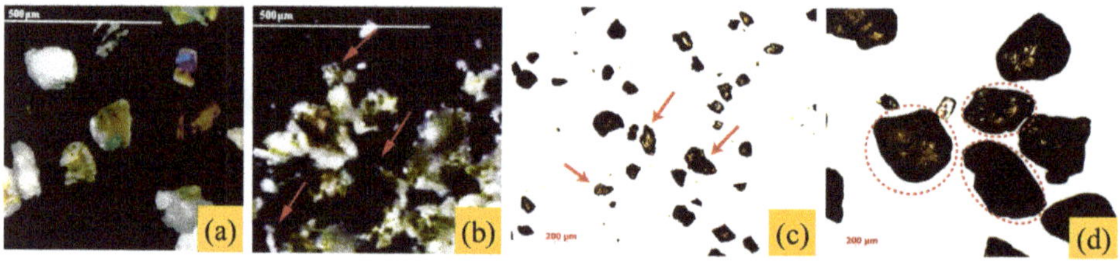

Figure 12. (**a**) Morphology of ultrafine dredged sand 1 and (**b**) mechanism sand [105]; (**c**) ultrafine dredged sand 2 and (**d**) river sand [45].

Pervious concrete using deposited fine sand or micronized powder exhibits similar zero-slump behavior [24]. Hamideh et al. [28] showed that increasing fine-grained sediments raises porosity and reduces free water, significantly decreasing slurry fluidity (Figure 13a). The type and dosage of activators also strongly affect workability [29] (Figure 13b). For example, 1 wt% $Ca(OH)_2$ improves the slump, which slightly drops at 2 wt%. NaOH has a limited impact, while increased water glass sharply reduces fluidity due to coagulation and viscosity, reaching a slump as low as 230 mm with NaOH addition. These results underscore the sensitivity of sediment-based systems to activator selection and dosage.

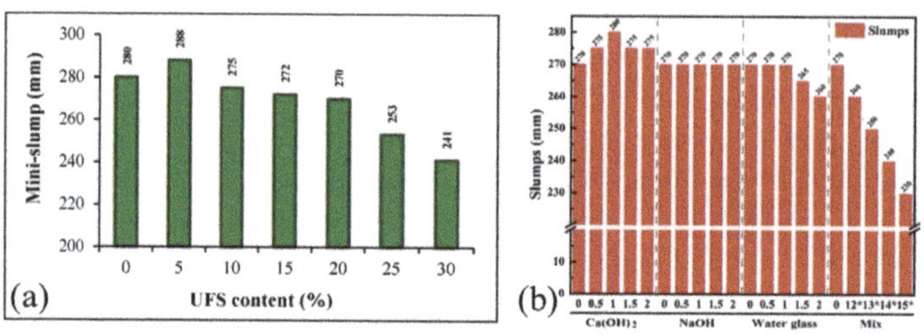

Figure 13. (**a**) Effect of fine-grained sediments substitution on the slump of cement paste [28]. (**b**) The slumps of filling cementitious materials (* indicates 0.5 wt% NaOH-doped) [29].

4.3. Shrinkage Behavior

Mechanically ground river sediments exert a dual effect of heterogeneous nucleation and microaggregate filling, which promotes hydration, refines pores, and densifies the matrix [90]. Their pozzolanic activity accelerates C–S–H formation, but reduced internal humidity and pore size lead to increased early self-shrinkage (Figure 14). In alkali-activated systems, ultrafine dredged sand affects drying shrinkage based on dosage: at 25%, 90-day shrinkage drops by 27%, but increases by up to 80% when the dosage exceeds 50% [45] (Figure 15a). Additionally, high clay content, water absorption, and low stiffness in fine sediments raise water demand and aggravate shrinkage [38,120] (Figure 15b). Thus, optimizing micronized powder dosage and precursor type is essential to control shrinkage while leveraging filling and activation benefits.

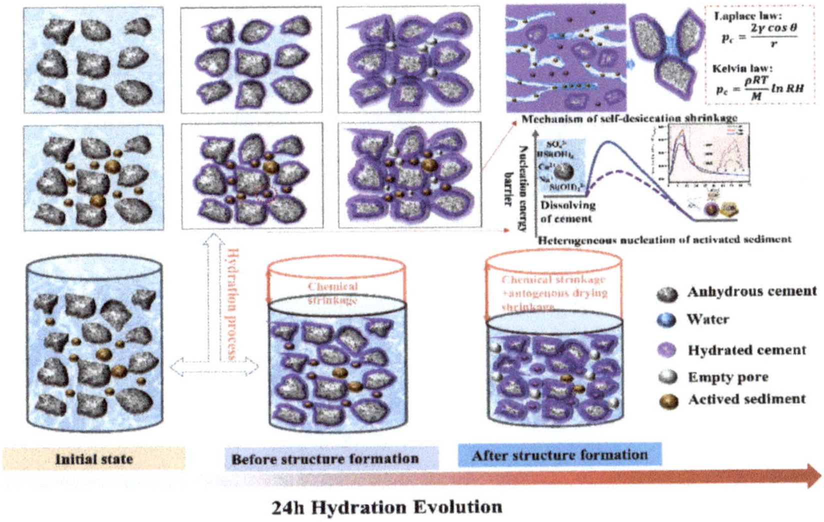

Figure 14. Schematic representation of the hydration process and early shrinkage changes in cement partially replaced by fine-grained sediments in the evolution of 24 h hydration [90].

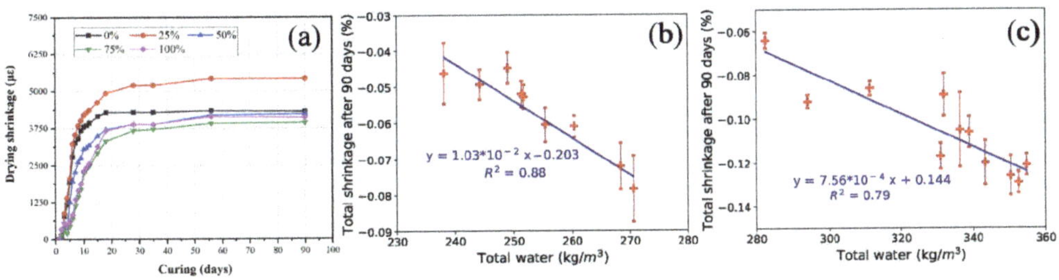

Figure 15. (**a**) Drying shrinkage of alkali-excited slag/fly ash mortar with different ultrafine dredged sand contents [45]. (**b**) Total shrinkage of sediment-sand concrete after 90 days versus total water in the mixture [38]. (**c**) Total shrinkage of deposited fine sand concrete after 90 days versus total water in the mixture [38].

4.4. Fundamental Mechanical Properties

In this section, we summarize recent experimental data in Table 4 on the effects of three sediment utilization pathways—substitution of fine aggregates, substitution of cementitious materials, and synergistic modification with admixtures—on the basic mechanical properties of concrete (compressive and flexural/splitting strength), and extract the following key insights:

(1) Fine aggregate substitution: Ultrafine dredged sand can increase strength by 3–10% at a 20–50% replacement ratio; above 60%, insufficient paste coating causes a sharp strength reduction.

(2) Cementitious material substitution: Flash-calcined or alkali-activated sediments exhibit significantly enhanced pozzolanic activity, and at a 10–20% replacement of OPC or GGBS, compressive strength can increase by up to 17%, showing a "low dosage, high efficiency" effect.

(3) Synergistic additives: Sediments combined with red mud, slag, or similar materials can achieve strength gains through "activation and densification" mechanisms; some systems (e.g., YRS-GGBS-RM ground polymer) show strength improvements over 20%.

Table 4. Comprehensive comparison of the mechanical properties of concrete/mortar by river sediment under different replacement strategies.

	Setup and Level	Sediment Sources/Treatment	Range of Replacement Rates (%)	Optimal Substitution Rate (%)	Change in Compressive Strength	Change in Bending/ Splitting Strength	Remarks/Key Conditions
Sediment as Fine Aggregate Replacement Systems							
[28]	Self-compacting mortar	Ultrafine sediments (unactivated) in the Yangtze River Estuary	5–30	5	45.88 → 43.51 MPa ↓ 5%	8.02 → 8.84 MPa ↑ 10%	Rapid decrease in strength after >15%
[45]	Alkali-inspired system mortar	Ultrafine sediments in the Yangtze River + Ground Granulated Blastfurnace Slag: Fly Ash = 3:7	25–100	25	25.67 → 26.36 MPa ↑ 3%	4.50 → 5.08 MPa ↑ 13%	Activation system, >50% significant decrease
[45]	Alkali-inspired system mortar	Ultrafine sediments in the Yangtze River + Ground Granulated Blastfurnace Slag: Fly Ash = 7:3	0–100	25	59.18 → 61.2 4 MPa ↑ 3%	9.09 → 9.34 MPa ↑ 3%	—
[26]	Ultra high-performance concrete	Ultrafine sediments of the Yellow River + Fine sand	0–100	80	100.3 → 104.3 MPa ↑ 4%	15.5 → 16.9 MPa ↑ 9%	Optimum 80% sand mixing ratio
[106]	Alkali-inspired concrete	Ultrafine sediments in the Yangtze River	0–100	50	49.89 → 54.60 MPa ↑ 9%	—	—
[39]	Ordinary concrete	Seine River sediments (completely replacing coarse and fine aggregates)	100	—	Requires ↑ 5% cement to reach C30 grade strength	—	Technical feasibility, economic assessment
[47]	Ordinary concrete	Yangtze River dredged sand and machine-made sand concrete	0–50	25	41.48 → 65.50 MPa ↑ 57.9%	—	—

Table 4. *Cont.*

	Setup and Level	Sediment Sources/Treatment	Range of Replacement Rates (%)	Optimal Substitution Rate (%)	Change in Compressive Strength	Change in Bending/ Splitting Strength	Remarks/Key Conditions
			Sediment–Cement Binder Systems				
[107]	OPC mortar	(Flash calcination) calcined dredging sediments	20–40	20	64.74 → 71.46 MPa ↑ 10%	—	Flash calcination activation is significant
[27]	Foam Concrete	Yellow River sludge ($Ca(OH)_2$ activation)	5–20	5	4.32 → 3.82 MPa ↓ 11%	—	High substitution rate intensity falls
[112]	Ground polymer mortar	Yellow River Silt Replacement Ground Granulated Blastfurnace Slag + Red mud	10–40	Standard maintenance: 10; High temperature water bath maintenance: 20	68.10 → 80.00 MPa ↑ 17% (Standard maintenance); 22.06 → 65.43 MPa ↑ 17.47 (High temperature water bath maintenance)	—	Standard maintenance; High temperature water bath maintenance, same trend
[112]	Porous ground-polymerized concrete	Yellow River Silt Replacement Ground Granulated Blastfurnace Slag + Red mud	10–40	10	24.35 → 26.25 MPa ↑ 8%	—	—
[111]	Alkali-inspired system mortar	Yellow River sediment + Red mud	20–80	40	16.80 → 26.52 MPa ↑ 57.86 (Natural Curing); 39.87 → 48.67 MPa ↑ 22.07% (Standard Curing)	—	The compressive strength of 28 d under standard curing can be increased by 82~132% to that under natural curing

Overall, the mechanical contribution of sediments is nonlinear, and the optimal dosage depends on particle gradation, activation method, and matrix type. Research is shifting from basic feasibility studies toward multi-scale synergistic mechanisms and engineering applications, laying the foundation for standardization and durability assessments.

Engineering concrete structures (e.g., locks, dams, long-span bridges) are exposed to complex triaxial stresses and cyclic loads [121–123], making it critical to assess the stability of sediment-admixed systems. Luan et al. [119] used CT reconstruction to study the triaxial monotonic and cyclic loading behavior of dredged sand concrete (Figure 16a). As confining pressure decreases, fracture volume and damage increase significantly (Figure 16b); cyclic loading under the same pressure causes larger fracture zones than monotonic loading, indicating that both confining pressure and loading path influence microcrack evolution and strength degradation (Figure 16c). Additionally, inert inclusions such as shell fragments, wood chips, and slag in sediments form weak interfaces and local porosity, offsetting some strength gains [39,124,125]; however, overall porosity and carbonation depth remain comparable to control concrete [20]. Particle size also plays a key role: sandy sediments have limited impact, whereas fine sedimentary sand enhances pervious concrete strength via combined filling and activation effects [24]. In conclusion, ensuring strength and durability under complex loading requires optimized sediment activation, impurity control, and tailored particle gradation.

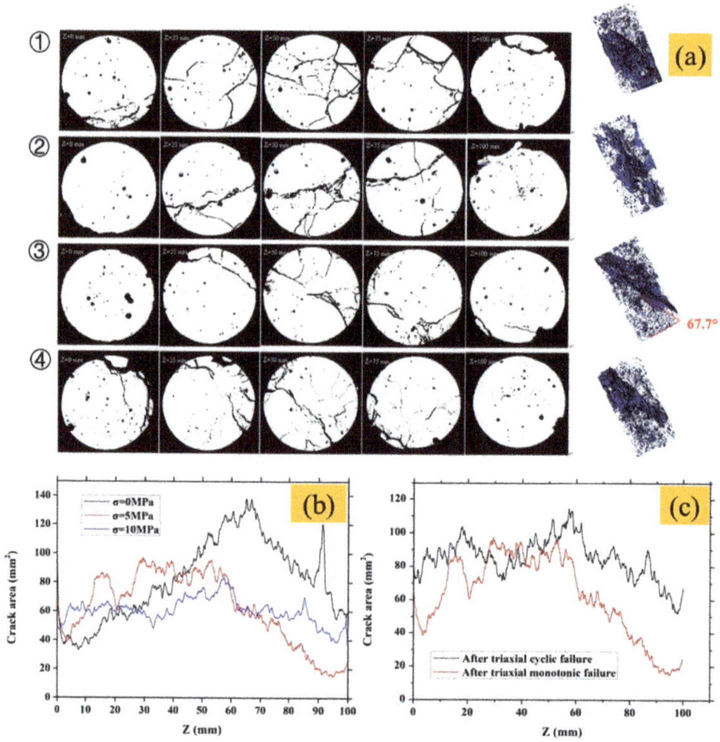

Figure 16. (**a**) Three-dimensional structure of CT binarized images of dredged sand concrete specimens at different heights z under triaxial monotonic loading (① σ_3 = 0 MPa; ② σ_3 = 5 MPa); ③ σ_3 = 10 MPa; ④ Triaxial cyclic load test σ_3 = 10 MPa); (**b**) Dredged sand concrete specimens loaded monotonically in three axes (σ = 0 MPa, 5 MPa and 10 MPa); (**c**) Evolution of cracks and pore areas along different heights z after damage by triaxial monotonic and cyclic loading of dredged sand concrete specimens (σ = 5 MPa) [119].

4.5. Durability Performance

Existing studies generally indicate that moderate activation or graded utilization of river sediments can enhance the durability of cementitious materials through various mechanisms.

(1) Early-stage water absorption/pore structure regulation

Deposited fine sand with high specific surface area and hydrophilicity absorbs over 50% of its final water content within 0–0.2 h, followed by dominant water retention [25] (Figure 17). This "fast-absorbing-slow-releasing" behavior reduces hydration heat and optimizes pore structure, offering new potential for durability design.

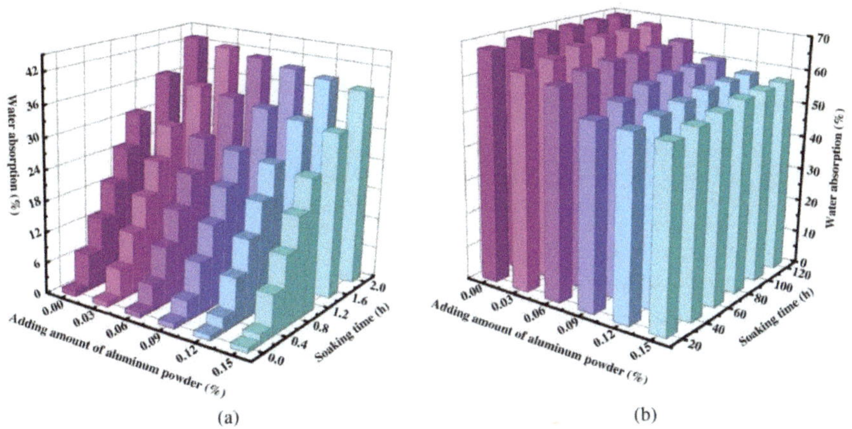

Figure 17. Effect of Aluminum Powder Addition on Moisture Content of AAC Blocks (**a**) 0–2 h; (**b**) 5–120 h [25].

(2) Sulfate attack resistance

Mortar (M1) with 15% calcined fine-grained sediments replacing cement showed the lowest mass loss in 5% $MgSO_4$ solution, the most stable potential, and strength gain within 90 days due to caliche/gypsum filling; degradation appeared only after 360 days, still outperforming higher substitution ratios [48] (Figure 18a–c). Calcined sediments containing 17% CaO continue to form C–S–H/C–A–H through pozzolanic reactions, enhancing matrix densification and inhibiting sulfate attack [70,126,127].

(3) Freeze–thaw durability

The compressive strength of sediment-based AAC with antifreeze remained $\geq$3 MPa after 15 freeze–thaw cycles [25]; concrete with 20 wt% coarse sediment substitution met XF2 requirements, with only 1.33–2.5% mass loss after 50 cycles [109].

(4) Chloride ingress resistance

High chloride permeability compromises long-term durability [128]; however, self-compacting lightweight aggregate concrete with dredged sediment and 28-day resistivity >20 kΩ·cm shows strong chloride resistance. A lower water-cement ratio further reduces cracking and mass loss [110]. Fine sand concrete from the Yellow and Liaohe Rivers also exhibited good impermeability [47].

Overall, sediment mineralogy, activation method, and particle gradation determine its durability performance. Proper calcination or mechanical activation and optimized dosage can significantly improve impermeability, erosion resistance, and freeze–thaw stability. In contrast, excessive replacement or untreated impurities may cause long-term strength loss. Future work should target durability under coupled degradation conditions to better define the limits of sediment use in high-performance concrete.

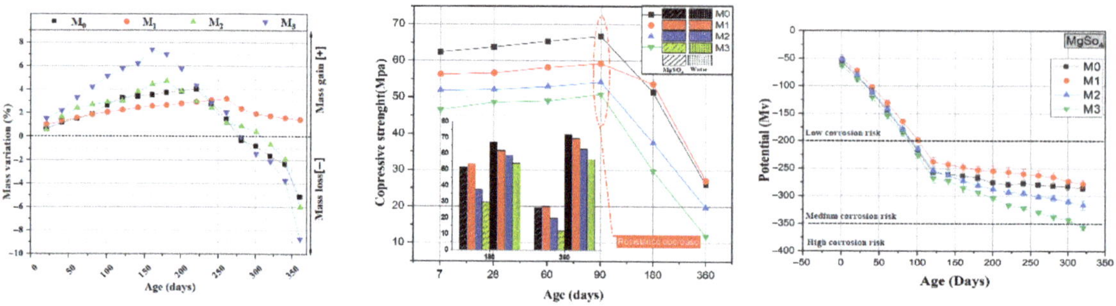

(a) (b) (c)

Figure 18. (**a**) Mass change in concrete in 5% $MgSO_4$ solution; (**b**) Compressive strength of concrete in 5% $MgSO_4$ solution and strength difference between mortar in $MgSO_4$ and water; (**c**) Potential change in 5% $MgSO_4$ solution (M0: control; M1: 15% fine-grained sediments; M2: 20%; M3: 30%) [48].

4.6. Hydration Kinetics and Microstructural Evolution

4.6.1. Thermogravimetric Analysis

Thermogravimetric analysis (TG) and derivative thermogravimetric analysis (DTG) are used to assess the thermal stability of sediment-replaced cementitious materials and the decomposition behavior of their components, with results shown in Figure 19. As the temperature rises, cement components gradually dehydrate and lose mass (Figure 19a). The DTG curve reflects decomposition rates, with each peak indicating a specific hydration product's breakdown (Figure 19b). Corresponding mass loss events and their causes are summarized in Table 5.

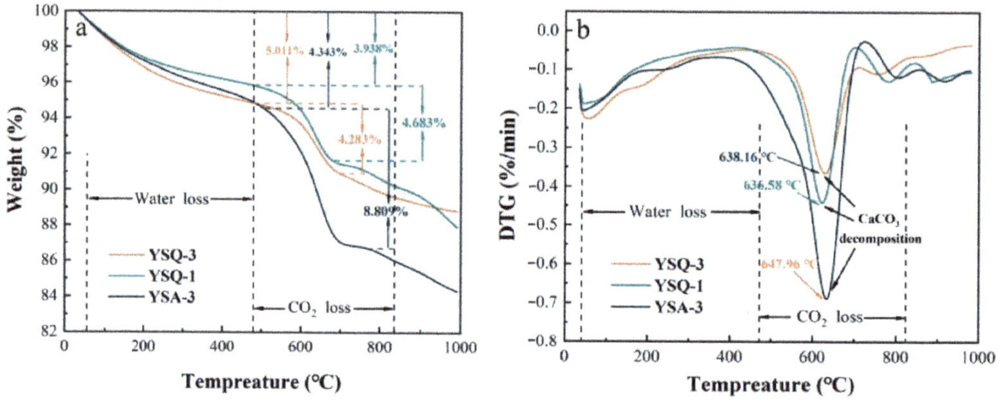

Figure 19. TG (**a**) and DTG (**b**) curves of 28-day YSQ–1, YSQ–3 and YSA–3 specimens. (YSQ-1: control, 100 wt% FA and 10 wt% $Ca(OH)_2$; YSQ-3: 90 wt% FA, 10 wt% YRS and 10 wt% $Ca(OH)_2$; YSA-3: 90 wt% FA, 10 wt% YRS and 15 wt% $Ca(OH)_2$) [27].

Table 5. Analysis of causes of mass loss at different temperatures.

Temperature Range(°C)	Main Causes of Quality Loss	Note
50–100	Free water evaporation	Corresponds to the weight loss peak at ~100 °C in the DTG curve, initial physical weight loss, which is present in all samples [129].
100–200	C–S–H and C–A–S–H initial dewatering; AFt, AFm dewatering	The appearance of a distinct weight loss peak indicates the formation of reaction products that enhance structural strength [130,131].
200–500	C–S–H and C–A–S–H continuous dewatering	The process continues and affects the mechanical strength of the samples. From this stage, it is possible to determine the promotion or inhibition of gel generation by the addition of river sediments [27].
400–500	$Ca(OH)_2$ dehydroxylation reaction (chemistry)	$Ca(OH)_2$ is involved in the reaction or consumed by carbonation [29]. It is possible to determine whether river sediments promote CH production based on the amount of CH consumed at this stage of the process. Furthermore, this densification inhibits penetration of aggressive agents, directly enhancing concrete durability.
~630	$CaCO_3$ decomposition	Related to the carbonation reaction, increased carbonation products enhance strength and densification [132–134].
500–850	Decomposition of heat-stabilized components such as calcium carbonate	The degree of overall mass loss indicates the extent to which sediment affects cement hydration.

4.6.2. Microscopic Properties

(1) Scanning electron microscope

When sediment replaces natural or manufactured sand, its effect on the matrix depends on both physical filling and hydration reactivity. From a hydrochemical perspective, Hamideh et al. [28] reported that a 15% replacement ratio increased internal microcracking due to low sediment reactivity, limited hydration product formation, and weak interfacial bonding (Figure 20). This defect can damage mechanical integrity and reduce durability, especially under complex stresses. Conversely, Huang et al. [47] found that replacing 25% of manufactured sand with dredged sediment improved the interfacial transition zone by increasing concrete density, reducing porosity, and refining pore size distribution. These microstructural enhancements improve mechanical performance and durability, including resistance to chloride penetration, freeze–thaw cycles, and chemical erosion. These findings are not contradictory but reflect the dual nature of sediment substitution: it is influenced by both physical effects (filling and grading) and chemical limitations (reactivity and bonding), which are closely tied to the sediment's source and mineralogy. Therefore, sediment replacement assessment should include pore structure and hydration chemistry analyses, correlated with macro-scale mechanical and durability indicators.

To evaluate the feasibility of partially replacing cementitious materials with sediment, it is essential to examine changes in hydration product morphology and chemistry. At low dosages, slender needle-like hydrates form (Figure 21a); at higher dosages, coarser needles form a denser skeleton (Figure 21b) [135], enhancing load-bearing capacity and fracture resistance. These coarser crystals enhance erosion resistance and can maintain or improve compressive strength [25]. EDS surface scans further show that high Ca content in raw sediment promotes extensive C–A–S–H gel formation, indicating that elemental migration and curing conditions reshape the gel structure (Figure 21c) [111]. The resulting gels improve both early and long-term strength and enhance resistance to ionic diffusion and carbonation. Standard curing activates low-reactivity components, forming Si, O-rich (N,C)–A–S–H gels that densify the matrix (Figure 21d), reduce permeability, and improve durability in harsh environments. In summary, the advantages of using sediment to replace cementitious materials arise from both morphological densification and chemical activation, and their synergy governs the enhancement of mechanical and durability performance. Optimized substitution ratios refine microstructure and produce more durable, mechanically robust concrete.

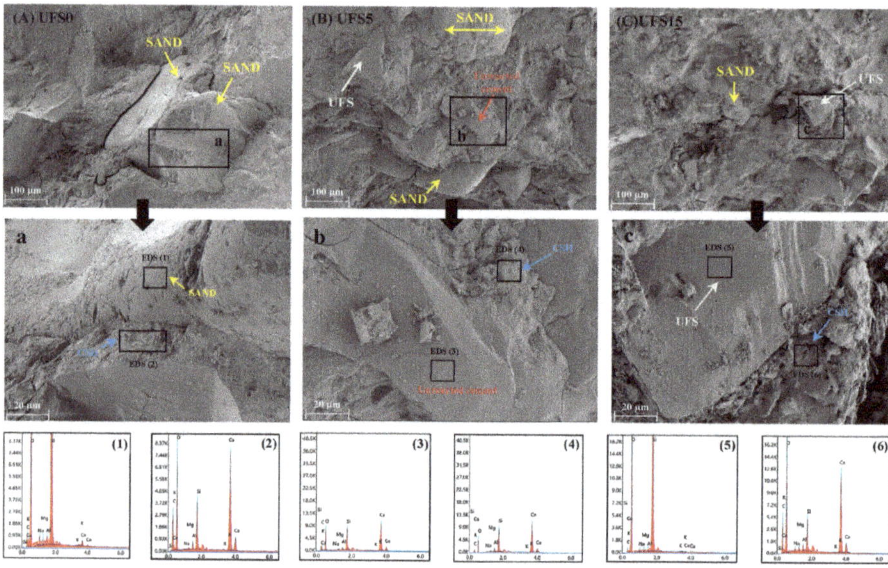

Figure 20. SEM-EDS images of 28-day self-compacting mortar samples: (**A**) control; (**B**) 5% deposit replacement cement; (**C**) 15% deposit replacement cement [28].

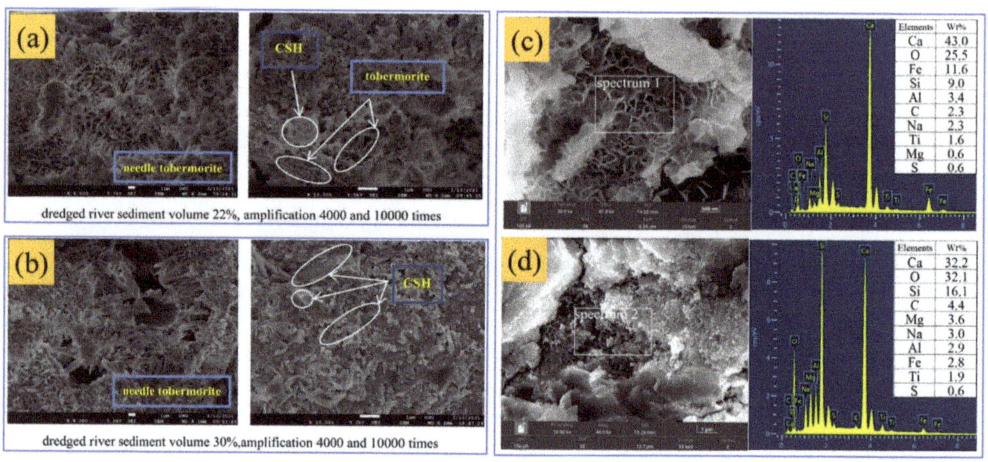

Figure 21. (**a**) Mortar with 22% dredged river mud content [25]; (**b**) mortar with 30% dredged river mud content [25]; and (**c**,**d**) dredging mud content is 40% and 60% of red mud geopolymer cement base material: natural curing (**c**) [111] and (**d**) the standard maintenance [111].

(2) Pore structure characterization

Ali Benkabouche [48] systematically analyzed the pore evolution of mortars with 0–30% sediment replacing cement using mercury intrusion porosimetry (Figure 22a–d). While sediments as mineral admixtures can enhance matrix density and mechanical strength [136,137], their effect on pore size distribution is relatively limited. Even moderate pore refinement improves mechanical consistency and reduces permeability, enhancing durability against freeze–thaw and chemical attack. In contrast, Jun [26] found that using Yellow River sedimentary sand to replace fine aggregate in UHPC significantly reduces the proportion of harmful and multi-harmful pores, transforming the pore structure toward less harmful types. This refinement mitigates strength loss and enhances fracture resistance, improving reliability and extending service life under harsh conditions (Figure 22e,f). However, when sediments are used as micronized powder, they compete with cement for filling space, and their lower filling capacity leads to increased porosity (Figure 22g), as confirmed by Hamideh et al. [28]. Increased porosity reduces compressive and flexural strength and durability by allowing fluid ingress and accelerating corrosion and degradation. Overall, the effect of sediments on pore structure depends on particle size, shape, and replacement mode. Achieving a balance between pore optimization and performance improvement requires fine-grading or synergistic blending strategies.

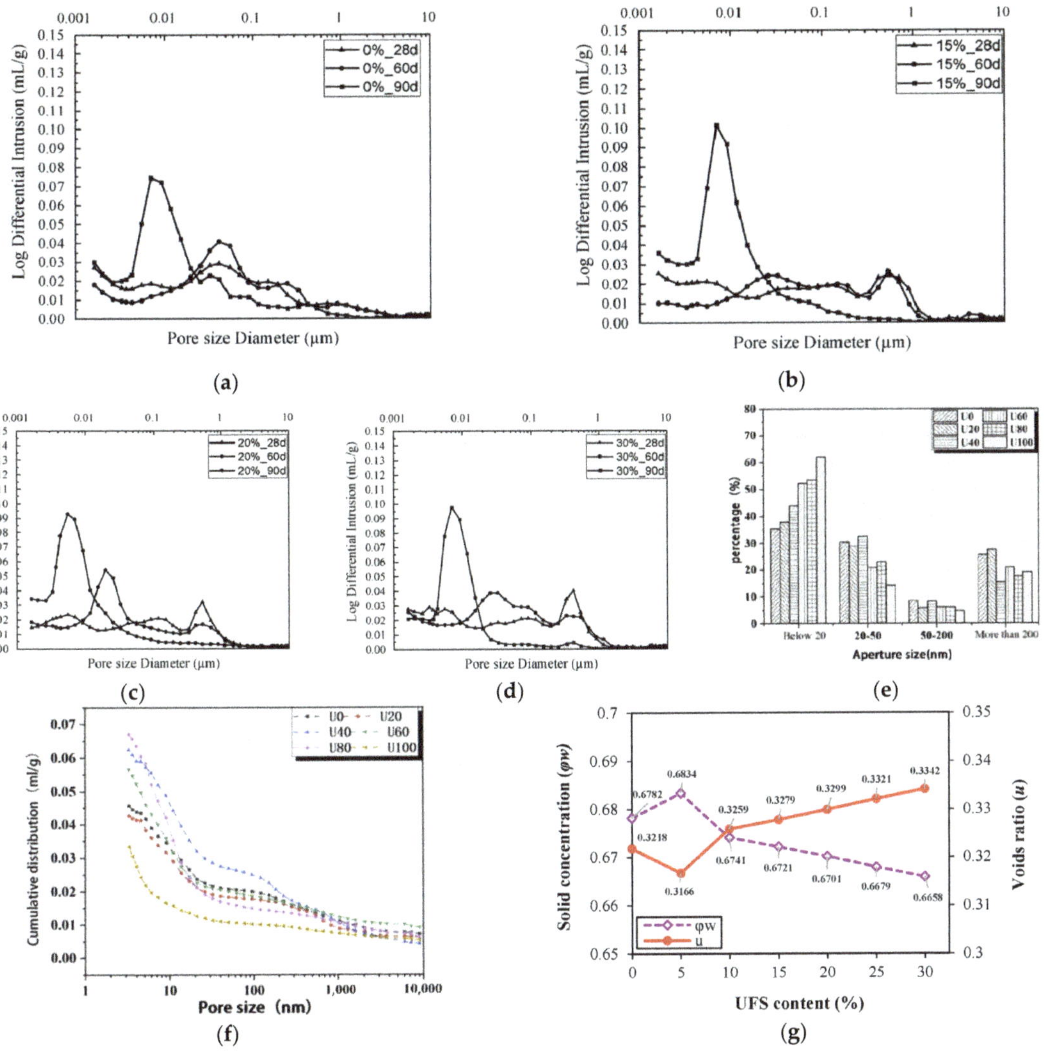

Figure 22. Porosity of mortar at different maintenance ages and at different sediment substitution rates: (**a–d**) substitution of cementitious materials [48]; (**e**,**f**) substitution of fine sand [26]; (**g**) the effect

of UFS content on the packing density (φ_w) and voids ratio (u). UFS: ultra-fine sediment [28]. The impact of activated sediment replacing cement manifests in several aspects. Initially, alite hydration increases, but the difference in reaction degree narrows after 3 days. The CH content decreases due to the pozzolanic reaction triggered by activation [26]. Activated alumina in the sediment reacts with $Ca(OH)_2$ and $CaSO_4$ to form additional ettringite in early hydration [138]. During later stages, the content of mono- and hemicarbonate AFm phases increases, and Al released from activated sediments slightly raises AFm levels [78].

5. Taxonomy and Application Scenarios of Sediment-Tailored Multifunctional Concrete

According to sediment characteristics and engineering demands, researchers have developed sediment-based concrete for diverse applications, including pervious concrete, lightweight concrete, foam concrete, self-compacting mortar, polymer mortar, autoclaved aerated concrete (AAC), ultra-high-performance concrete (UHPC), and engineered cementitious composites (ECC), as shown in Figure 22. These materials function either by replacing sand or cementitious components with sediment.

5.1. Deposited Fine Sand as Partial Sand Replacement

(1) Pervious concrete: Compared to conventional concrete, pervious concrete has lower thermal conductivity and heat capacity, helping to mitigate urban heat island effects [24]. Beddaa et al. [39] found that finer dredged sediments, used to fully replace sand, produced denser concrete with reduced porosity and permeability and improved compressive strength.

(2) Lightweight and thermal-insulating concrete: A porous ceramic masonry mortar using Yellow River sediment and coal dust fully replaced standard sand and offered lightweight properties [23]. Zhang et al. [113] further improved the performance by incorporating biochar, enhancing water retention, water resistance, and insulation, making it suitable for green building applications.

(3) Polymer-based mortar: Maherzi et al. [101] developed a polymer mortar by replacing traditional sand with sediment. The resulting material showed enhanced chemical resistance and thermal stability, with superior durability under corrosive and thermal conditions.

(4) Autoclaved aerated concrete (AAC) and non-AAC blocks: AAC blocks made with 30–34% dredged silt, 24% cement, 10% quicklime, 30% fly ash, 2% gypsum, 0.09% aluminum powder, and a 0.5 water-to-material ratio, cured under 2.2 MPa for 6 h, achieved 4.5 MPa strength and 716.56 kg/m^3 dry density [25]. Non-AAC blocks using 15% sediment, 48% cement, 20% lime, and the same water ratio reached 3.1 MPa and 924.19 kg/m^3. Both met national standards.

(5) High-performance structural concrete: Ultrafine Yellow River sand enabled high-strength UHPC with a refined pore structure even at high substitution levels [26]. Yuan et al. [139] applied it to ECC, achieving full quartz sand replacement. At 75% substitution, the material showed optimal ductility, crack control, and mechanical performance, supported by finite element modeling.

5.2. Fine-Grained Sediment as Binder Replacement

(1) Foam concrete for sound insulation and air purification: Foam concrete combines sound insulation, low thermal conductivity, and photocatalytic performance. However, sediment addition lowers pH, weakening the foaming effect. At 40% cement replacement, the mixture achieves optimal performance: best sound insulation (1767 m/s, 9% foaming agent), lowest thermal conductivity (0.2831 W/m·K, 6% foaming agent), and excellent photocatalytic efficiency (14.1%, $Bi_4Ti_3O_{12}$). Under

optimized sediment and foaming agent ratios, it shows strong multifunctionality, making it suitable for green building applications [5]. Heavy metals in the sediment are well encapsulated, with low leaching even in acidic conditions. Silica fume can also be added as a pore-refining agent [38]. Jiang et al. [27] used Yellow River silt in alkali-activated fly ash foam concrete and studied the effects of sediment and alkali content on fluidity, mechanical properties, pore structure, and thermal performance, confirming its feasibility as a supplementary material.

(2) Self-compacting and high-flow mortar: Mehdizadeh et al. [28] prepared self-compacting mortar by replacing 5–15% of cement with ultrafine Yangtze River sediment. The resulting mortar maintained good flowability and mechanical strength, meeting construction needs for complex structures.

(3) Alkali-activated cementitious materials (AAMs) concrete: Li et al. [45,106] used sediment from the lower Yangtze River to prepare AAMs concrete and found that a 25% replacement rate improved strength, microstructure, and shrinkage resistance, offering good durability for green infrastructure. Yu et al. [29] combined Yellow River silt with fly ash and cement to develop alkali-activated materials for coal mine backfilling. They studied the effects of Ca(OH)2, NaOH, and water glass, revealing that the formation of C–(A)–S–H gel enhanced hydration, pore structure, strength, and workability, achieving both resource utilization and environmental benefits.

(4) Application of Sediments in Ternary Cementitious Systems: Literature confirms sediments are a promising component in ternary systems. Some studies show sediments as key ternary blend components, enhancing mechanical properties and refining microstructure. First, explorations have focused on ternary systems with calcined sediment, limestone filler, and cement. Bellara, Zeraoui, Hadj Sadok, and others [13,14,140,141] prepared low-carbon binders by combining GGBS and cement with clay dam, flash-burned, or canal sediments. By optimizing the sediment/GGBS/cement ratio and moisture content, they enhanced fluidity and strength, developing an eco-friendly hydraulic road binder (HRB). The hydration mechanism was clarified: flash-burned sediment provides activity, GGBS adds strength, and cement supplies alkalinity synergy. Furlan et al. [142] studied fly ash reinforcement in lime–cement stabilized dredged sediment. They detailed the pozzolanic and micro-filling effects of fly ash on pore structure and products, linking them to improved strength and water resistance. Second, other ternary systems combined sediments with different mineral admixtures. Zhang et al. [143] showed that mixtures of sediment, slag, and fly ash achieved good compactness and mechanical performance. Yu [29] and Wang [75] focused on Yellow River sediment, formulating alkali-activated or cementitious ternary systems (sediment–fly ash–cement) for backfill and mortar. These studies achieved high strength and workability while controlling efflorescence by lowering alkaline ion concentrations. Collectively, these works confirm the strong potential and practicality of using sediments in ternary cementitious systems.

By replacing sand or cement, sediment-based concrete enables material recycling and functional enhancement. It meets structural safety requirements and offers energy-saving, environmental, and multifunctional advantages. Current applications include urban infrastructure, green buildings, functional materials, and ecological restoration. Future work should focus on standardizing classification, dosage control, and engineering adaptability to promote broader application.

6. Exploring the Classification and Application Scenarios of Sediment-Based Multifunctional

Urbanization has increased domestic and industrial wastewater discharge into rivers, leading to heavy metal accumulation in dredged sediments. For sediment concrete to be safely applied, the heavy metal content in leachate must not exceed that of control concrete or inert waste limits [39].

Environmental studies show that appropriate sediment incorporation can effectively immobilize heavy metals, ensuring environmental safety. Kai [25] used inductively coupled plasma mass spectrometry to test heavy metal levels in aerated concrete blocks. Except for Cr (average 4.23 μg/L), other metals were below detection limits. Leachate tests at 12 h and 18 h showed variation within 0.1%, confirming stable immobilization and environmental safety during use.

Mostafaei et al. [144] showed that replacing part of cement and sand with zeolite achieved 85 MPa compressive strength and reduced the carbon footprint to 659.72 kg CO_2/m^3, supporting the feasibility of sustainable materials such as sediment. Economic analysis showed that sediment-based C30 concrete costs 41% less than conventional concrete. If the quarry is over 30 km away from the sediment site, sediment concrete can reduce the carbon footprint equivalent to 5% added cement [39]. For high-performance cementitious materials, Jun Yan [26] showed that replacing quartz sand with Yellow River ultrafine sediment in UHPC reduced primary energy use by up to 7% while maintaining mechanical strength, as assessed by EN ISO 14040 [145]. Costs were cut to 55% under full substitution, highlighting the potential of sediments in green and high-value materials.

Based on a case study in Zhengzhou, China, where Yellow River sediment replaced 25% of cement in mortar production, a life-cycle cost and carbon emission analysis was carried out. The functional unit was defined as 1 m^3 of ready-mixed mortar, in line with industry standards, to ensure comparability of environmental and economic impacts [146]. The system boundary followed a cradle-to-gate approach, with analysis focusing on key cost and carbon emission factors [146–148]. Key assumptions were as follows: cement transportation distance was set at 30 km, with a cost of 0.6 RMB/kg; Yellow River sediment transportation distance was set at 20 km, classified as waste utilization with no raw material cost. The results indicated that using Yellow River sediment reduced cost by about 24.2% and carbon emissions by 24.8% per cubic meter of mortar, highlighting its considerable economic and environmental potential.

In summary, sediment used in cementitious materials can significantly reduce production costs while ensuring environmental safety. It also offers clear advantages in carbon emission reduction and ecological performance, supporting the green transformation of construction materials and high-value utilization of solid waste. Future work should focus on assessing long-term environmental stability under complex conditions to facilitate engineering applications and industrialization of sediment-based materials.

7. Conclusions and Outlook

7.1. Conclusions

Based on an extensive review of the literature and experimental results, this paper systematically evaluates the use of river sediments in concrete. Key findings and research directions are as follows:

(1) The resource properties and application potential of river sediments were evaluated. With wide particle size distribution, high SiO_2 content, and cementitious potential, sediments can replace natural sand, gravel, and partial cement as fine aggregates, lightweight aggregates, or pozzolanic materials after proper grading and decontamination.

(2) The activation mechanisms and property enhancement strategies were summarized. Synergistic activation with alkali (NaOH or $Ca(OH)_2$) and water glass promotes full consumption of $Ca(OH)_2$ and formation of dense C–S–H/C–A–S–H networks. Thermal treatment above 650 °C enhances the activity of clay minerals like kaolinite and chlorite, though activity declines beyond 900 °C. Mechanical milling and incorporation of additives such as biochar and fibers form a "micro-cement + filler" composite structure, improving 28-day compressive strength by 10–20%.

(3) Optimized mix design strategies were established. Combining minimum paste theory with packing density optimization reduces paste volume by 8–12% while maintaining a slump $\geq$ 180 mm. Optimal mechanical and durability performance is achieved when the sediment replacement rate is controlled at 25% $\pm$ 5%.

(4) The environmental and economic benefits of sediment reuse were confirmed. Life cycle assessment shows that replacing 30% of cement with sediment can reduce CO_2 emissions by approximately 180 kg/m^3 and material costs by 10–15%, offering substantial ecological and economic advantages.

7.2. Outlook

(1) A unified evaluation system for sediment grading, activation level, and application classification is urgently needed to support large-scale engineering deployment.

(2) Multi-scale coupling mechanisms should be explored using in situ neutron/X-ray techniques and molecular dynamics to uncover sediment–cement interface reactions and long-term degradation behavior.

(3) Future work should study the durability of mud–sand concrete under coupled degradation, focusing on synergistic effects between carbonation and other stresses such as chloride intrusion, dry–wet cycling, or mechanical loading.

(4) Low-energy activation processes such as microwave–alkali synergy should be developed to reduce energy use and secondary emissions.

(5) Future research should focus on intelligent functionalization, including sediment-based materials with temperature control, phase-change energy storage, and photocatalytic functions to achieve multifunctionality and high-value applications.

Author Contributions: Y.Z. (Yuanxun Zheng): Conceptualization, Methodology, Investigation, Formal analysis, Funding acquisition. Y.X.: Conceptualization, Investigation, Formal analysis, Writing—original draft. Y.Z. (Yu Zhang): Supervision, Investigation, Writing—original draft. C.W.: Supervision, Project administration, Writing—review and editing. L.M.: Investigation, Visualization. P.Z.: Formal analysis. All authors have read and agreed to the published version of the manuscript.

Funding: The authors would like to acknowledge the financial support received from the Science Foundation Project for Outstanding Youth of Henan Province (Grant No. 232300421014), the Key scientific research projects of colleges and universities in Henan Province (Grant No. 23ZX014), and the National Natural Science Foundation of China (Grant No .52279144/523791374).

Data Availability Statement: The authors confirm that the data supporting the findings of this study are available within the article.

Conflicts of Interest: The authors declare that they have no known competing financial interests or personal relationships that could have appeared to influence the work reported in this paper.

References

1. Chen, W.; Yang, S.; Zhang, X.; Jordan, N.D.; Huang, J. Embodied energy and carbon emissions of building materials in China. *Build. Environ.* **2022**, *207 Pt A*, 108434. [CrossRef]
2. Liu, T.; Zhao, R.; Xie, Z.; Xiao, L.; Chen, A.; Feng, W.; You, Z.; Feng, M.; Li, R. Carbon emissions from accumulated stock of building materials in China. *Build. Environ.* **2023**, *240*, 110451. [CrossRef]

3. Sousa, V.; Bogas, J.; Real, S.; Meireles, I.; Carriço, A. Recycled cement production energy consumption optimization. *Sustain. Chem. Pharm.* **2023**, *32* (Suppl. C), 101010. [CrossRef]
4. Ma, M.; Huang, Z.; Wang, J.; Niu, L.; Zhang, W.; Xu, X.; Xi, F.; Liu, Z. Carbon uptake by cement in China: Estimation and contribution to carbon neutrality goals. *Sci. China Earth Sci.* **2024**, *67*, 2056–2067. [CrossRef]
5. Kou, R.; Guo, M.Z.; Shi, Y.; Mei, M.; Jiang, L.; Chu, H.; Zhang, Y.; Shen, H.; Xue, L. Sound-insulation and photocatalytic foamed concrete prepared with dredged sediment. *J. Clean. Prod.* **2022**, *356*, 131902. [CrossRef]
6. Wang, J.; Yang, Y.; Zhang, M.; Zhu, L.; Li, S.; Wen, Y. Critical threshold of periodic point bar scour and sediment body transport path in tidal reaches: A case study of Fujiangsha reach, Yangtze River. *J. Geogr. Sci.* **2023**, *33*, 1334–1358. [CrossRef]
7. Tian, X.; Tian, P.; Zhao, G.; Gómez, J.; Guo, J.; Mu, X.; Gao, P.; Sun, W. Sediment source tracing during flood events in the Huangfu River basin in the northern Loess Plateau, China. *J. Hydrol.* **2023**, *620 Pt B*, 129540. [CrossRef]
8. Xue, C.; Yang, Y.; Xu, C.; Wang, M.; Gao, J.; Han, X.; Jia, J. Sedimentary records reveal two stages of evolution of the Abandoned Yellow River Delta from AD1128 to AD1855: Vertical accretion and land-forming. *Anthr. Coasts* **2023**, *6*, 1–14. [CrossRef]
9. Sun, Z.; Zhou, W.; Yuan, J.; Yang, Z.; Chen, L. Hydrological and sediment-transport characteristics of the middle and lower Yangtze River: Analysis from a magnitude-frequency perspective. *CATENA* **2023**, *231* (Suppl. C), 107293. [CrossRef]
10. Wang, Y.; Wang, Z.; Chen, Y.; Cao, T.; Yu, X.; Rui, P. Experimental study on bio-treatment effect of the dredged Yellow River silt based on soybean urease induced calcium carbonate precipitation. *J. Build. Eng.* **2023**, *75* (Suppl. C), 106943. [CrossRef]
11. Ni, Z.; Wang, S.; Zheng, X.; Qi, C. Application of geopolymer in synchronous grouting for reusing of the shield muck in silty clay layer. *Constr. Build. Mater.* **2024**, *419*, 135345. [CrossRef]
12. Duan, D.; Song, H.; Wei, F.; Feng, Z.; Cheng, H.; Cheng, F. Mechanical properties of solid waste-based composite cementitious system enhanced by CO_2 modification. *Constr. Build. Mater.* **2024**, *426*, 136187. [CrossRef]
13. Bellara, S.; Hidjeb, M.; Maherzi, W.; Mezazigh, S.; Senouci, A. Optimization of an Eco-Friendly Hydraulic Road Binders Comprising Clayey Dam Sediments and Ground Granulated Blast-Furnace Slag. *Buildings* **2021**, *11*, 443. [CrossRef]
14. Zeraoui, A.; Maherzi, W.; Benzerzour, M.; Abriak, N. Optimization of Ternary Binders Based on Flash-Calcined Sediments and Ground Granulated Blast Furnace slag Using a Mixture Design. *Preprints* **2021**. [CrossRef]
15. Wang, B.; Li, G.; Han, J.; Zheng, Y.; Liu, H.; Song, W. Study on the properties of artificial flood-prevention stone made by Yellow River silt. *Constr. Build. Mater.* **2017**, *144*, 484–492. [CrossRef]
16. Siham, K.; Fabrice, B.; Edine, A.; Patrick, D. Marine dredged sediments as new materials resource for road construction. *Waste Manag.* **2008**, *28*, 919–928. [CrossRef]
17. He, H.; Yue, Q.; Su, Y.; Gao, B.; Gao, Y.; Wang, J.; Yu, H. Preparation and mechanism of the sintered bricks produced from Yellow River silt and red mud. *J. Hazard. Mater.* **2012**, *203–204*, 53–61. [CrossRef]
18. Wang, H.; Guo, J.; Liu, W.; Song, H.; Yan, T.; Fu, D. Use of COVID-19 personal protective equipment pollutants to improve physical properties of silty sand in Yellow River flooded area. *Front. Environ. Sci.* **2022**, *10*, 1011685. [CrossRef]
19. Wu, Y.; Wan, Y.; He, X.; Cai, Y.; Xu, W.; Zhao, B.; Shen, Y. Improving the impermeability and mechanical properties of the Yellow River sediment with polymer gels. *Case Stud. Constr. Mater.* **2024**, *20*, e03246. [CrossRef]
20. Yang, J.; Xu, L.; Hao, H.; Yang, S. Effect of TiO_2 on the thermal conductivity of eco-friendly silica bricks fabricated by yellow river silt(Conference Paper). *Mater. Sci. Forum* **2009**, *610–613 Pt 1*, 206–210. [CrossRef]
21. Liu, J.; Hai, R.; Zhang, L.; Bolf, N. Modification of Yellow River Sediment Based Stabilized Earth Bricks. *Kem. u Ind.* **2016**, *65*, 613–618. [CrossRef]
22. Tang, C. Producing synthetic lightweight aggregates by treating waste TFT-LCD glass powder and reservoir sediments. *Comput. Concr.* **2014**, *13*, 325–342. [CrossRef]
23. Wang, S.; Yang, L.; Ma, X.; Mei, R.; Li, C.; Sun, Z. The formation of porous light ceramsite using Yellow River sediment and its application in concrete masonry production. *Case Stud. Constr. Mater.* **2022**, *17* (Suppl. C), e01340. [CrossRef]
24. Beddaa, H.; Tchiotsop, J.; Fraj, A.B.; Somé, C. Reuse of river sediments in pervious concrete: Towards an adaptation of concrete to the circular economy and climate change challenges. *Constr. Build. Mater.* **2023**, *368* (Suppl. C), 130443. [CrossRef]
25. Zhang, K.; Wei, Q.; Jiang, S.; Shen, Z.; Zhang, Y.; Tang, R.; Yang, A.; Chow, C. Utilization of Dredged River Sediment in Preparing Autoclaved Aerated Concrete Blocks. *J. Renew. Mater.* **2022**, *10*, 2989–3008. [CrossRef]
26. Yan, J.; Zhong, S.; Chen, S.; Lv, Y.; Yang, L.; Peng, G.; Deng, A. Study on the Application of Sediment-Based Embankment Building and Ultra-High-Performance Concrete (UHPC) Preparation in the Resource Utilization of Yellow River Sediment. *Materials* **2022**, *15*, 5668. [CrossRef]
27. Jiang, S.; Xu, J.; Song, Y.; Xu, Y. Alkali-activated fly ash foam concrete with Yellow River silt: Physico-mechanical and structural properties. *Constr. Build. Mater.* **2023**, *373* (Suppl. C), 130879. [CrossRef]
28. Mehdizadeh, H.; Guo, M.; Ling, T. Ultra-fine sediment of Changjiang estuary as binder replacement in self-compacting mortar: Rheological, hydration and hardened properties. *J. Build. Eng.* **2021**, *44* (Suppl. C), 103251. [CrossRef]

29. Yu, Z.; Wang, B.; Li, T.; Fan, C.; Yu, H. Effect and mechanism of activators on the properties of Yellow River sediment/fly ash/cement-based alkali-activated cementitious materials used for coal mine filling. *Constr. Build. Mater.* **2024**, *445*, 137955. [CrossRef]
30. Guo, Y.; Gong, H.; Shi, W.; Fang, N.; Tan, Y.; Zhou, W.; Huang, J.; Dai, L.; Dai, X.; Guo, Y. Insights into multisource sludge distributed in the Yangtze River basin, China: Characteristics, correlation, treatment and disposal. *J. Environ. Sci.* **2023**, *126*, 321–332. [CrossRef] [PubMed]
31. Huang, Z.; Liu, X.; Wen, J.; Fang, H.; Lin, S.; Li, W.; Wang, J.; Zeng, F.; Du, H.; Shi, L. Characteristics and fractionations of sediment oxygen demand in a complex tidal river network area. *J. Environ. Manag.* **2024**, *354*, 120352. [CrossRef]
32. Rahman, M.; Ali, M. Properties of dredged material and potential scope of its beneficial use: A case study of the Pussur River in Bangladesh. *Water Sci. Eng.* **2024**, *17*, 336–343. [CrossRef]
33. Marzouki, M.; Samet, B.; Tounsi, H. Application of Plackett–Burman and Box-Behnken designs for the optimization of Tunisian dam sediment-based geopolymers. *J. Build. Eng.* **2022**, *50* (Suppl. C), 104162. [CrossRef]
34. Slimanou, H.; Bouziane, A.; Bouzidi, N.; Bouzidi, M.; Quesada, D. Marine dredged sediment based cementitious matrix: Thermal treatment, physical properties and prediction using response surface methodology. *Environ. Sci. Pollut. Res. Int.* **2025**, *32*, 8284–8306. [CrossRef]
35. Zhang, J.; Kang, S.; Shen, Y.; Song, C.; Lei, H.; Xie, W.; Chen, X.; Wang, J.; Wu, W.; Wang, X. Effects of Sand Type and Alkali Equivalent on Drying Shrinkage and Microstructure of Seawater–Sea Sand Alkali-Activated Slag Concrete. *Materials* **2025**, *18*, 1005. [CrossRef]
36. Fernandes, I.; Lima, V.; Nascimento, C.; Carvalho, H.; Santos, C.; Neto, A. Valorization of textile sludge for use as supplementary cementitious material–Benefiting processes, pozzolanic activity, and application in no-slump concrete. *Constr. Build. Mater.* **2025**, *458*, 139619. [CrossRef]
37. Hazarika, A.; Huang, L.; Erlingsson, S.; Weerdt, K.; Löfgren, I.; Iftikhar, S.; Babaahmadi, A. Characterization, activation and reactivity—A case study of Nordic volcanic materials for application as Supplementary Cementitious Materials. *Case Stud. Constr. Mater.* **2025**, *22*, e04096. [CrossRef]
38. Yang, X.; Zhao, L.; Haque, M.; Chen, B.; Ren, Z.; Cao, X.; Shen, Z. Sustainable conversion of contaminated dredged river sediment into eco-friendly foamed concrete. *J. Clean. Prod.* **2020**, *252*, 119799. [CrossRef]
39. Beddaa, H.; Fraj, A.; Ducléroir, S. Experimental study on river sediment incorporation in concrete as a full aggregate replacement: Technical feasibility and economic viability. *Constr. Build. Mater.* **2021**, *313* (Suppl. C), 125425. [CrossRef]
40. Yang, L. Research on the Preparation of High-Performance Concrete Using Yellow River Sand. Master's Thesis, North China University of Water Resources and Electric Power, Zhengzhou, China, 2022. (In Chinese)
41. Zhao, M.; Dai, M.; Li, J.; Li, C. Case study on performance of pumping concrete with super-fine river-sand and manufactured-sand. *Case Stud. Constr. Mater.* **2023**, *18* (Suppl. C), e01850. [CrossRef]
42. Zajac, M.; Bremeier, R.; Deja, J.; Król, M.; Haha, M.B. Carbonation hardening of Portland cement with recycled supplementary cementitious materials. *Cem. Concr. Compos.* **2025**, *157*, 105904. [CrossRef]
43. Zhou, Y.; Yu, P.; Yang, H.; Xia, X.; He, S.; Huang, X. Utilization of municipal solid waste incinerator fly ash under high temperature sintering and alkali excitation for use in cementitious material. *J. Build. Eng.* **2024**, *94*, 110005. [CrossRef]
44. Rong, X.; Zhang, X.; Zhang, J.; Xu, W.; Zhang, Z. Study on mechanical and thermal properties of alkali-excited fly ash aerogel foam concrete. *Constr. Build. Mater.* **2023**, *408* (Suppl. C), 133770. [CrossRef]
45. Li, S.; Chen, X.; Zhang, W.; Ning, Y.; Casas, J. Utilization of ultra-fine dredged sand from the Yangtze River in alkali-activated slag/fly ash mortars: Mechanical properties, drying shrinkage and microstructure. *Case Stud. Constr. Mater.* **2023**, *107*, e02264. [CrossRef]
46. Ferone, C.; Liguori, B.; Capasso, I.; Colangelo, F.; Cioffi, R.; Cappelletto, E.; Di Maggio, R. Thermally treated clay sediments as geopolymer source material. *Appl. Clay Sci.* **2015**, *107*, 195–204. [CrossRef]
47. Huang, W.; Chen, X.; Luan, J.; Ning, Y.; Ji, T.; Shi, Z. Deep insight into mechanical behaviour and microstructure mechanism of dredged sand in the lower reaches of the Yangtze River and manufactured sand concrete. *J. Build. Eng.* **2023**, *68* (Suppl. C), 106105. [CrossRef]
48. Benkabouche, A.; Amar, M.; Benzerzour, M.; Abriak, N.; T'kint, M.; Mouli, M. The Influence of External Sulfate Attack on the Durability of Reinforced Mortars in the Presence of Calcined River Sediments. *Materials* **2023**, *16*, 6684. [CrossRef]
49. Shen, W.; Yang, Z.; Cao, L.; Cao, L.; Liu, Y.; Yang, H.; Lu, Z.; Bai, J. Corrigendum to: Characterization of manufactured sand: Particle shape, surface texture and behavior in concrete [Constr. Build. Mater. 114 (2016) 595–601]. *Constr. Build. Mater.* **2016**, *119*, 385. [CrossRef]
50. He, H.; Wang, Y.; Wang, J. Compactness and hardened properties of machine-made sand mortar with aggregate micro fines. *Constr. Build. Mater.* **2020**, *250*, 118828. [CrossRef]
51. Bayesteh, H.; Sharifi, M.; Haghshenas, A. Effect of stone powder on the rheological and mechanical performance of cement-stabilized marine clay/sand. *Constr. Build. Mater.* **2020**, *262 Pt 2*, 120792. [CrossRef]

52. Tomasz, Z.; Tomasz, T.; Marcin, A. Effect of the amount of river sediment on the basic properties of cement mortars. *MATEC Web Conf.* **2020**, *322*, 1032. [CrossRef]
53. Nakayenga, J.; Cikmit, A.; Tsuchida, T.; Hata, T. Influence of stone powder content and particle size on the strength of cement-treated clay. *Constr. Build. Mater.* **2021**, *305* (Suppl. C), 124710. [CrossRef]
54. Tian, E.; Ren, W.; Zhuang, Y.; Zeng, W. Effect of steel slag powder and stone powder by-product from manufactured sand on the mechanical properties and microstructure of cementitious materials. *J. Clean. Prod.* **2024**, *452*, 142128. [CrossRef]
55. Tittarelli, F.; Carsana, M.; Ruello, M. Effect of hydrophobic admixture and recycled aggregate on physical–mechanical properties and durability aspects of no-fines concrete. *Constr. Build. Mater.* **2014**, *66*, 30–37. [CrossRef]
56. Zaetang, Y.; Sata, V.; Wongsa, A.; Chindaprasirt, P. Properties of pervious concrete containing recycled concrete block aggregate and recycled concrete aggregate. *Constr. Build. Mater.* **2016**, *111*, 15–21. [CrossRef]
57. Hai, R.; Liu, J.; Zhang, L.; Yang, J. The Effect and Mechanism of $CaCl_2$ Composite Activation of Yellow River Sediment. *J. Build. Mater.* **2016**, *19*, 654–658. (In Chinese)
58. Zhao, Z.; Benzerzour, M.; Abriak, N.; Damidot, D.; Courard, L.; Wang, D. Use of uncontaminated marine sediments in mortar and concrete by partial substitution of cement. *Cem. Concr. Compos.* **2018**, *93*, 155–162. [CrossRef]
59. Jha, P.K.; Vaithiyanathan, P.; Subramanian, V. Mineralogical characteristics of the sediments of a Himalayan river: Yamuna River—A tributary of the Ganges. *Environ. Geol.* **1993**, *22*, 13. [CrossRef]
60. Elsayed, H.; Beusen, A.; Bouwman, A.F. Nutrient transport from the Ganga–Brahmaputra–Meghna River system to the Bay of Bengal: Past and future trends. *Environ. Res. Lett.* **2025**, *20*, 024054. [CrossRef]
61. Li, C.; Shi, X.; Gao, S.; Chen, M.; Liu, Y.; Fang, X.; Lv, H.; Zou, J.; Liu, S.; Qiao, S. Composition Characteristics and Material Sources of Clay Minerals in River Sediments in Taiwan. *Chin. Sci. Bull.* **2012**, *57*, 169–177.
62. Singh, P.; Rajamani, V. Geochemistry of the Floodplain Sediments of the Kaveri River, Southern India. *J. Sediment. Res.* **2001**, *71*, 50–60. [CrossRef]
63. Siddique, R.; Klaus, J. Influence of metakaolin on the properties of mortar and concrete: A review. *Appl. Clay Sci.* **2008**, *43*, 392–400. [CrossRef]
64. Snellings, R.; Suraneni, P.; Skibsted, J. Future and emerging supplementary cementitious materials. *Cem. Concr. Res.* **2023**, *171* (Suppl. C), 107199. [CrossRef]
65. Nofalah, M.; Ghadir, P.; Hasanzadehshooiili, H.; Aminpour, M.; Javadi, A.; Nazem, M. Effects of binder proportion and curing condition on the mechanical characteristics of volcanic ash- and slag-based geopolymer mortars; machine learning integrated experimental study. *Constr. Build. Mater.* **2023**, *395* (Suppl. C), 132330. [CrossRef]
66. Shi, C.; Jimenez, A.F.; Palomo, A. New cements for the 21st century: The pursuit of an alternative to Portland cement. *Cem. Concr. Res.* **2011**, *41*, 750–763. [CrossRef]
67. Scrivener, K.; Ouzia, A.; Juilland, P.; Mohamed, A. Advances in understanding cement hydration mechanisms. *Cem. Concr. Res.* **2019**, *124*, 105823. [CrossRef]
68. Tan, H.; Yuan, P.; Sun, D.; Fan, X.; Wang, C.; Liu, J. Ratio of water to cement and supplementary cementitious materials on mechanical and impact resistance properties of reactive powder concrete. *Sci. Rep.* **2025**, *15*, 7480. [CrossRef] [PubMed]
69. Li, C.; Zhang, T.; Wang, L. Mechanical properties and microstructure of alkali activated Pisha sandstone geopolymer composites. *Constr. Build. Mater.* **2014**, *68*, 233–239. [CrossRef]
70. Rabehi, B.; Ghernouti, Y.; Driss, M. Potential Use of Calcined Silt of Dam as a Pozzolan in Blended Portland Cement. *Int. J. Concr. Struct. Mater.* **2014**, *8*, 259–268. [CrossRef]
71. Zhang, B.; Peng, Z.; Fahimizadeh, M.; Yu, T.; Faheem, M.; Belaroui, L.; Hamada, B.; Yuan, P. Recycling of an ion-adsorption type rare earth tailing in a low-carbon construction material: Performance modulation and life cycle assessment. *Constr. Build. Mater.* **2025**, *475*, 141167. [CrossRef]
72. Jing, X.; Li, G.; Zhang, Y.; Han, J.; Wang, B. Experimental Research on the Modification of the Yellow River Sediment. *Iran. J. Sci. Technol. Trans. Civ. Eng.* **2021**, *45*, 1031–1037. [CrossRef]
73. Junakova, N.; Junak, J. Sustainable Use of Reservoir Sediment through Partial Application in Building Material. *Sustainability* **2017**, *9*, 852. [CrossRef]
74. Martinez-Ramirez, S.; Palomo, A. Microstructure studies on Portland cement pastes obtained in highly alkaline environments. *Cem. Concr. Res.* **2001**, *31*, 1581–1585. [CrossRef]
75. Wang, Z. Research on the Activation and Application of Multi-Grain-Size Yellow River Sediment. Master's Thesis, North China University of Water Resources and Electric Power, Zhengzhou, China, 2023. (In Chinese)
76. Buchwald, A.; Hohmann, M.; Posern, K.; Brendler, E. The suitability of thermally activated illite/smectite clay as raw material for geopolymer binders. *Appl. Clay Sci.* **2009**, *46*, 300–304. [CrossRef]
77. Li, C.; Dong, J.; Zhao, S.; Liu, H.; Yao, W.; Wang, L. Development of low cost supplementary cementitious materials utilizing thermally activated Pisha sandstone. *Constr. Build. Mater.* **2018**, *174*, 484–495. [CrossRef]

78. Snellings, R.; Horckmans, L.; Van Bunderen, C.; Vandewalle, L.; Cizer, Ö. Flash-calcined dredging sediment blended cements: Effect on cement hydration and properties. *Mater. Struct.* **2017**, *50*, 241. [CrossRef]
79. Chu, D.; Amar, M.; Kleib, J.; Benzerzour, M.; Betrancourt, D.; Abriak, N.; Nadah, J. The Pozzolanic Activity of Sediments Treated by the Flash Calcination Method. *Waste Biomass Valorization* **2022**, *13*, 4963–4982. [CrossRef]
80. Dang, T.; Kamali-Bernard, S.; Prince, W. Design of new blended cement based on marine dredged sediment. *Constr. Build. Mater.* **2013**, *41*, 602–611. [CrossRef]
81. He, C.; Makovicky, E.; Osbaeck, B. Thermal stability and pozzolanic activity of calcined kaolin. *Appl. Clay Sci.* **1994**, *9*, 165–187. [CrossRef]
82. Földvári, M. *Handbook of Thermogravimetric System of Minerals and Its Use in Geological Practice*; Geological Institute of Hungary Budapest: Budapest, Hungary, 2011; Volume 213.
83. García, R.; de la Villa, R.; Vegas, I.; Frías, M.; de Rojas, M.S. The pozzolanic properties of paper sludge waste. *Constr. Build. Mater.* **2008**, *22*, 1484–1490. [CrossRef]
84. Cook, D. Calcinated clay, shale and other soils. *Cem. Replace. Mater.* **1985**, 40–72.
85. He, C.; Makovicky, E.; Øsbæck, B. Thermal stability and pozzolanic activity of calcined illite. *Appl. Clay Sci.* **1995**, *9*, 337–354. [CrossRef]
86. Bonavetti, V.; Rahhal, V.; Irassar, E. Studies on the carboaluminate formation in limestone filler-blended cements. *Cem. Concr. Res.* **2001**, *31*, 853–859. [CrossRef]
87. Faure, A.; Smith, A.; Coudray, C.; Anger, B.; Colina, H.; Moulin, I.; Thery, F. Ability of Two Dam Fine-Grained Sediments to be Used in Cement Industry as Raw Material for Clinker Production and as Pozzolanic Additional Constituent of Portland-Composite Cement. *Waste Biomass Valorization* **2017**, *8*, 2141–2163. [CrossRef]
88. Benzerzour, M.; Maherzi, W.; Amar, M.; Abriak, N.; Damidot, D. Formulation of mortars based on thermally treated sediments. *J. Mater. Cycles Waste Manag.* **2018**, *20*, 592–603. [CrossRef]
89. Junakova, N.; Junak, J. Recycling of reservoir sediment material as a binder in concrete. *Procedia Eng.* **2017**, *180*, 1292–1297. [CrossRef]
90. Zhang, H.; Cao, M.; Xing, Z. Early-age properties of cement paste with mechanically ground Yellow River sediment. *Constr. Build. Mater.* **2024**, *411*, 134635. [CrossRef]
91. Lian, H.-Z.; Zhang, Z.-L.; Wang, Y.-H. Rapid evaluation on activity of pozzolanic materials. *J. Build. Mater.* **2001**, *4*, 299–304.
92. Deboucha, W.; Leklou, N.; Khelidj, A.; Oudjit, M. Hydration development of mineral additives blended cement using thermogravimetric analysis (TGA): Methodology of calculating the degree of hydration. *Constr. Build. Mater.* **2017**, *146*, 687–701. [CrossRef]
93. Taylor, M.; Lydon, F.; Barr, B. Mix proportions for high strength concrete. *Constr. Build. Mater.* **1996**, *10*, 445–450. [CrossRef]
94. Liu, G.; Cheng, W.; Chen, L. Investigating and optimizing the mix proportion of pumping wet-mix shotcrete with polypropylene fiber. *Constr. Build. Mater.* **2017**, *150*, 14–23. [CrossRef]
95. Arora, A.; Almujaddidi, A.; Kianmofrad, F.; Mobasher, B.; Neithalath, N. Material design of economical ultra-high performance concrete (UHPC) and evaluation of their properties. *Cem. Concr. Compos.* **2019**, *104*, 103346. [CrossRef]
96. Wang, J.; Yu, R.; Ji, D.; Tang, L.; Yang, S.; Fan, D.; Shui, Z.; Leng, Y.; Liu, K. Effect of distribution modulus (q) on the properties and microstructure development of a sustainable Ultra-High Performance Concrete (UHPC). *Cem. Concr. Compos.* **2022**, *125*, 104335. [CrossRef]
97. Zhang, W.; Zheng, M.; Zhu, L.; Lv, Y. Mix design and characteristics evaluation of high-performance concrete with full aeolian sand based on the packing density theory. *Constr. Build. Mater.* **2022**, *349* (Suppl. C), 128814. [CrossRef]
98. Xue, Z.; Qi, P.; Yan, Z.; Pei, Q.; Zhong, J.; Zhan, Q. Mechanical Properties and Crack Resistance of Basalt Fiber Self-Compacting High Strength Concrete: An Experimental Study. *Materials* **2023**, *16*, 4374. [CrossRef]
99. Akhtar, M.; Albatayneh, O.; Bani-Hani, K.; Malkawi, A. Performance of modified desert sand concrete: An experimental case study. *Case Stud. Constr. Mater.* **2024**, *21*, e03465. [CrossRef]
100. Murtaza, M.; Zhang, J.; Yang, C.; Cui, X.; Su, C.; Ramadan, A. Performance analysis of self compacting concrete by incorporating fly ash, coal gangue powder, cement kiln dust and recycled concrete powder by absolute volume method. *Constr. Build. Mater.* **2024**, *431*, 136601. [CrossRef]
101. Maherzi, W.; Ennahal, I.; Benzerzour, M.; Mammindy-Pajany, Y.; Abriak, N. Study of the polymer mortar based on dredged sediments and epoxy resin: Effect of the sediments on the behavior of the polymer mortar. *Powder Technol.* **2020**, *361*, 968–982. [CrossRef]
102. Ji, T.; Chen, C.; Zhuang, Y.; Chen, J. A mix proportion design method of manufactured sand concrete based on minimum paste theory. *Constr. Build. Mater.* **2013**, *44*, 422–426. [CrossRef]
103. Ennahal, I.; Maherzi, W.; Mamindy-Pajany, Y.; Benzerzour, M.; Abriak, N. Eco-friendly polymers mortar for floor covering based on dredged sediments of the north of France. *J. Mater. Cycles Waste Manag.* **2019**, *21*, 861–871. [CrossRef]

104. Mehdipour, I.; Khayat, K.H. Effect of particle-size distribution and specific surface area of different binder systems on packing density and flow characteristics of cement paste. *Cem. Concr. Compos.* **2017**, *78*, 120–131. [CrossRef]
105. Luan, J.; Chen, X.; Ning, Y.; Shi, Z. Beneficial utilization of ultra-fine dredged sand from Yangtze River channel as a concrete material based on the minimum paste theory. *Case Stud. Constr. Mater.* **2022**, *16* (Suppl. C), e01098. [CrossRef]
106. Li, S.; Chen, X.; Zhang, W.; Ning, Y.; Casas, J.R. Mechanical properties of alkali activated slag concrete with ultra fine dredged sand from Yangtze River. *Fuhe Cailiao Xuebao/Acta Mater. Compos. Sin.* **2022**, *39*, 335–343.
107. Van Bunderen, C.; Benboudjema, F.; Snellings, R.; Vandewalle, L.; Cizer, Ö. Experimental analysis and modelling of mechanical properties and shrinkage of concrete recycling flash calcined dredging sediments. *Cem. Concr. Compos.* **2021**, *115*, 103787. [CrossRef]
108. Altuki, R.; Ley, M.; Cook, D.; Gudimettla, M.; Praul, M. Increasing sustainable aggregate usage in concrete by quantifying the shape and gradation of manufactured sand. *Constr. Build. Mater.* **2022**, *321* (Suppl. C), 125593. [CrossRef]
109. Junakova, N.; Junak, J.; Balintova, M. Reservoir sediment as a secondary raw material in concrete production. *Clean Technol. Environ. Policy* **2015**, *17*, 1161–1169. [CrossRef]
110. Her-Yung, W. Durability Of Self-consolidating Lightweight Aggregate Concrete Using Dredged Silt. *Constr. Build. Mater.* **2009**, *23*, 2332–2337. [CrossRef]
111. Jin, W.; Chen, Y.; Lv, Y.; Jiang, L.; Bai, W.; Zhang, K.; Song, C.; Zhang, X. Mechanical Properties and Mechanism of Geopolymer Cementitious Materials Synergistically Prepared Using Red Mud and Yellow River Sand. *Materials* **2024**, *17*, 3810. [CrossRef]
112. Lv, Y.; Chen, Y.; Dai, W.; Yang, H.; Jiang, L.; Li, K.; Jin, W. Preparation and Properties of Porous Concrete Based on Geopolymer of Red Mud and Yellow River Sediment. *Materials* **2024**, *17*, 923. [CrossRef]
113. Zhang, Y.; Xu, H.; Fang, S.; Li, D.; Xue, W.; Chen, B.; Zhao, L. Biochar as additive for improved building performances and heavy metals solidification of sediment-based lightweight concrete. *Environ. Sci. Pollut. Res. Int.* **2022**, *30*, 4137–4150. [CrossRef] [PubMed]
114. Lang, L.; Li, J.; Chen, X.; Han, L.; Wang, P. Tensile strength behavior of cement-stabilized dredged sediment reinforced by polypropylene fiber. *Front. Struct. Civ. Eng.* **2024**, *18*, 380–392. [CrossRef]
115. Luo, D.; Lang, L.; Zhang, B. Splitting tensile strength behavior of dredged sediment with cement stabilization and straw fiber reinforcement. *J. Mater. Cycles Waste Manag.* **2025**, *27*, 1379–1393. [CrossRef]
116. Lang, L.; Chen, B. Strength Properties of Cement-Stabilized Dredged Sludge Incorporating Nano-SiO_2 and Straw Fiber. *Int. J. Geomech.* **2021**, *21*, 4021119. [CrossRef]
117. Lang, L.; Chen, B.; Li, D. Effect of nano-modification and fiber-reinforcement on mechanical behavior of cement-stabilized dredged sediment. *Mar. Georesources Geotechnol.* **2021**, *40*, 1–17. [CrossRef]
118. Leite, M.; Filho, J.; Lima, P. Workability study of concretes made with recycled mortar aggregate. *Mater. Struct./Mater. et Constr.* **2013**, *46*, 1765–1778. [CrossRef]
119. Luan, J.; Chen, X.; Ning, Y.; Zhang, W. Mechanical characteristics and energy dissipation characteristics of dredged sand concrete during triaxial loading. *J. Build. Eng.* **2022**, *55* (Suppl. C), 104700. [CrossRef]
120. Rozière, E.; Granger, S.; Turcry, P.; Loukili, A. Influence of paste volume on shrinkage cracking and fracture properties of self-compacting concrete. *Cem. Concr. Compos.* **2007**, *29*, 626–636. [CrossRef]
121. Mohammadi, M.; Wu, Y. Modified plastic-damage model for passively confined concrete based on triaxial tests. *Compos. Part B-Eng.* **2019**, *159*, 211–223. [CrossRef]
122. Zhang, T.; Xu, W.; Wang, R.; Yan, L.; He, M. Deformation characteristics of cement mortar under triaxial cyclic loading: An experimental investigation. *Int. J. Fatigue* **2021**, *150* (Suppl. C), 106305. [CrossRef]
123. Zhang, S.; Wang, J.; Lin, G.; Yu, T.; Fernando, D. Stress-strain models for ultra-high performance concrete (UHPC) and ultra-high performance fiber-reinforced concrete (UHPFRC) under triaxial compression. *Constr. Build. Mater.* **2023**, *370* (Suppl. C), 130658. [CrossRef]
124. Falade, F. An investigation of periwinkle shells as coarse aggregate in concrete. *Build. Environ.* **1995**, *30*, 573–577. [CrossRef]
125. Martínez-García, C.; González-Fonteboa, B.; Martínez-Abella, F.; Carro-López, D. Performance of mussel shell as aggregate in plain concrete. *Constr. Build. Mater.* **2017**, *139*, 570–583. [CrossRef]
126. Zivica, V.; Bajza, A. Acidic attack of cement-based materials—A review Part 2. Factors of rate of acidic attack and protective measures. *Constr. Build. Mater.* **2002**, *16*, 215. [CrossRef]
127. Ghrici, M.; Kenai, S.; Said-Mansour, M. Mechanical properties and durability of mortar and concrete containing natural pozzolana and limestone blended cements. *Cem. Concr. Compos.* **2007**, *29*, 542–549. [CrossRef]
128. Felekoğlu, B.; Selçuk, T.; Bülent, B. Effect of water/cement ratio on the fresh and hardened properties of self-compacting concrete. *Build. Environ.* **2007**, *42*, 1795–1802. [CrossRef]
129. Ibrahim, I.A.; ElSersy, H.H.; Abadir, M.F. The use of thermal analysis in the approximate determination of the cement content in concrete. *J. Therm. Anal. Calorim.* **2004**, *76*, 713–718. [CrossRef]
130. Singh, M.; Garg, M. Refereed paper Activation of gypsum anhydrite-slag mixtures. *Cem. Concr. Res.* **1995**, *25*, 332–338. [CrossRef]

131. Ma, X.; Zhang, C.; Li, R.; Zheng, L.; Xu, J. Effect of temperature and humidity environment on the microstructure and physicochemical properties of SBS modified asphalt. *Case Stud. Constr. Mater.* **2025**, *22*, e04192. [CrossRef]
132. Chang, J. A study on the setting characteristics of sodium silicate-activated slag pastes. *Cem. Concr. Res.* **2003**, *33*, 1005–1011. [CrossRef]
133. Lilkov, V.; Petrov, O.; Tzvetanova, Y.; Savov, P. Mossbauer, DTA and XRD study of Portland cement blended with fly ash and silica fume. *Constr. Build. Mater.* **2012**, *29*, 33–41. [CrossRef]
134. Safhi, A.; Rivard, P.; Yahia, A.; Benzerzour, M.; Khayat, K. Valorization of dredged sediments in self-consolidating concrete: Fresh, hardened, and microstructural properties. *J. Clean. Prod.* **2020**, *263*, 121472. [CrossRef]
135. Gong, J.; Zhang, W. The effects of pozzolanic powder on foam concrete pore structure and frost resistance. *Constr. Build. Mater.* **2019**, *208*, 135–143. [CrossRef]
136. Achour, R.; Zentar, R.; Abriak, N.; Rivard, P.; Gregoire, P. Durability study of concrete incorporating dredged sediments. *Case Stud. Constr. Mater.* **2019**, *11*, e00244. [CrossRef]
137. Silva, L.; Nehring, V.; de Paiva, F.; Tamashiro, J.; Galvin, A.; Lopez-Uceda, A.; Kinoshita, A. Use of blast furnace slag in cementitious materials for pavements-Systematic literature review and eco-efficiency. *Sustain. Chem. Pharm.* **2023**, *33* (Suppl. C), 101030. [CrossRef]
138. Sim, S.; Her, S.; Suh, H.; Cho, S.; Im, S.; Li, P.; Bae, S. Influences of alumina type and sulfate content on hydration and physicochemical changes in Portland–limestone cement. *Constr. Build. Mater.* **2024**, *426*, 135989. [CrossRef]
139. Yuan, C.; Raza, A.; Manan, A.; Ahmad, S.; Chao, W.; Umar, M. Numerical and experimental study of Yellow River sand in engineered cementitious composite. *Proc. Inst. Civ. Eng.-Eng. Sustain.* **2025**, *178*, 3–20.
140. Hadj Sadok, R.; Maherzi, W.; Benzerzour, M.; Lord, R.; Torrance, K.; Zambon, A.; Abriak, N. Mechanical Properties and Microstructure of Low Carbon Binders Manufactured from Calcined Canal Sediments and Ground Granulated Blast Furnace Slag (GGBS). *Sustainability* **2021**, *13*, 9057. [CrossRef]
141. Zeraoui, A.; Maherzi, W.; Benzerzour, M.; Abriak, N.; Aouad, G. Development of Flash-Calcined Sediment and Blast Furnace Slag Ternary Binders. *Buildings* **2023**, *13*, 333. [CrossRef]
142. Furlan, A.; Razakamanantsoa, A.; Ranaivomanana, H.; Amiri, O.; Levacher, D.; Deneele, D. Effect of fly ash on microstructural and resistance characteristics of dredged sediment stabilized with lime and cement. *Constr. Build. Mater.* **2021**, *272*, 121637. [CrossRef]
143. Zhang, G.; Li, K.; Shi, H.; Chen, C.; Yuan, C. Study on the Effects and Mechanisms of Fly Ash, Silica Fume, and Metakaolin on the Properties of Slag-Yellow River Sediment-Based Geopolymers. *Materials* **2025**, *18*, 1845. [CrossRef] [PubMed]
144. Mostafaei, H.; Bahmani, H. Sustainable High-Performance Concrete Using Zeolite Powder: Mechanical and Carbon Footprint Analyses. *Buildings* **2024**, *14*, 3660. [CrossRef]
145. *DIN EN ISO 14040:2006+A1:2020*; Environmental Management—Life Cycle Assessment—Principles and Framework. Deutsches Institut für Normung (DIN): Berlin, Germany, 2020.
146. *ISO 14075:2024*; Environmental Management—Principles and Framework for Social Life Cycle Assessment. International Organization for Standardization (ISO): Geneva, Switzerland, 2024.
147. Zhu, S.; Lu, Y.; Wang, S.; Liu, W.; Tang, K.; Li, N. Characteristics and reduction potential of carbon dioxide emission in China's cement industry from 2020 to 2050. *Huanjing Kexue Xuebao/Acta Sci. Circumstantiae* **2024**, *44*, 453–463.
148. Nian, T.; Li, Y.; Jin, X.; Wang, Z.; Wang, M.; Wang, Y.; Moacir, K. Toward Carbon Balance in Life Cycle: The Carbon Emission Assessment for the Recycled Coarse Aggregate Concrete. *Adv. Civ. Eng.* **2025**, *2025*, 9184976. [CrossRef]

MDPI AG
Grosspeteranlage 5
4052 Basel
Switzerland
Tel.: +41 61 683 77 34

Gels Editorial Office
E-mail: gels@mdpi.com
www.mdpi.com/journal/gels

www.ingramcontent.com/pod-product-compliance
Lightning Source LLC
Chambersburg PA
CBHW061830210926
51850CB00006B/851